THE RELEVANCE OF SOCIAL SCIENCE FOR MEDICINE

CULTURE, ILLNESS, AND HEALING

Studies in Comparative Cross-Cultural Research

VOLUME 1

THE RELEVANCE
OF SOCIAL SCIENCE
FOR MEDICINE

Edited by

LEON EISENBERG

Harvard Medical School, Boston

and

ARTHUR KLEINMAN

University of Washington, School of Medicine,
Seattle

D. REIDEL PUBLISHING COMPANY

DORDRECHT : HOLLAND / BOSTON : U.S.A.
LONDON : ENGLAND

Library of Congress Cataloging in Publication Data

Main entry under title:

The Relevance of social science for medicine.

    (Culture, illness, and healing)
    Includes bibliographies and index.
    1.   Social medicine.   I.   Eisenberg, Leon, 1922–
II.   Kleinman, Arthur.
III.   Series.   [DNLM: 1.   Sociology, Medical.   WA 31 R382]
RA418.R44   362.1   80–24965
ISBN 90–277–1176–3
ISBN 90–277–1185–2 (pbk.)

Published by D. Reidel Publishing Company,
P.O. Box 17, 3300 AA Dordrecht, Holland.

Sold and distributed in the U.S.A. and Canada
by Kluwer Boston Inc.
190 Old Derby Street, Hingham, MA 02043, U.S.A.

In all other countries, sold and distributed
by Kluwer Academic Publishers Group,
P.O. Box 322, 3300 AH Dordrecht, Holland.

D. Reidel Publishing Company is a member of the Kluwer Group.

TABLE OF CONTENTS

SECTION 5: SOCIAL LABELING AND OTHER PATTERNS OF SOCIAL COMMUNICATION

SECTION 6: SOCIOPOLITICAL AND SOCIOECONOMIC ANALYSES

To Carola and Joan

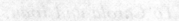

PREFACE

The central purpose of this book is to demonstrate the relevance of social science concepts, and the data derived from empirical research in those sciences, to problems in the clinical practice of medicine. As physicians, we believe that the biomedical sciences have made — and will continue to make — important contributions to better health. At the same time, we are no less firmly persuaded that a comprehensive understanding of health and illness, an understanding which is necessary for effective preventive and therapeutic measures, requires equal attention to the social and cultural determinants of the health status of human populations. The authors who agreed to collaborate with us in the writing of this book were chosen on the basis of their experience in designing and executing research on health and health services and in teaching social science concepts and methods which are applicable to medical practice.

We have not attempted to solicit contributions to cover the entire range of the social sciences as they apply to medicine. Rather, we have selected key approaches to illustrate the more salient areas. These include: social epidemiology, health services research, social network analysis, cultural studies of illness behavior, along with chapters on the social labeling of deviance, patterns of therapeutic communication, and economic and political analyses of macro-social factors which influence health outcomes as well as services. Particular emphasis is placed on patient-oriented teaching of social science in clinical training programs, teaching which attempts to translate knowledge and skills from anthropology and sociology in order to conceptualize sickness more adequately and to care for patients more successfully. We have chosen the chapters to reflect distinctive, clinically relevant examples of this new and potentially very important field of research.

We have in mind a primary audience of medical and other health science students, physicians and other health workers in practice, and clinical investigators and teachers who wish to learn what is relevant in social science. We have asked our contributors to write for such an audience and where possible to spell out the practical significance of their work. While the chapters vary in their accessibility to a clinical audience, we believe all of them can be read with profit and that many will have immediate value for the applied interests of clinicians. In addition, we believe that a number of the chapters in this book will be of use to social scientists whose field of interest includes health and the health professions.

The Editors share the view that social science has much to contribute to medicine, but that its practical implications need to be more precisely defined; strategies must be developed by which the new understanding can be more

ix

L. Eisenberg and A. Kleinman (eds.), The Relevance of Social Science for Medicine, ix—x.
Copyright © 1980 by D. Reidel Publishing Company.

effectively applied in medicine's distinctive domains. The chapters that follow disclose both successful examples and the difficulties in the process of transfer across disciplines. While some of the obstacles to this process arise within medicine, others emanate from social science. Although this volume does not pretend to have provided a recipe for the removal of these barriers, we believe that some of the major problems facing the integration of social science within medicine are identified and experiences in efforts to resolve them are shared.

Quite clearly, there is at present no rigorous and systematic means for deciding what is most relevant, how it can be applied and how its efficacy can be assessed. In the absence of a common agreement on strategy, the best that we can do is to share "state of the art" experiences and to compare outcomes critically. Many of the chapters in this book will advance this process and thereby indicate to readers significant directions for future collaboration. At the same time, others suggest (either explicitly or tacitly) where the limits of social science contributions may lie.

In preparing a book for a non-specialist audience, we have attempted to avoid lengthy expositions of highly technical questions of interest primarily to the separate social science disciplines themselves. At the same time, this is no mere primer. We take our readers seriously and ask them to join us in confronting issues at the critical juncture of sociology and anthropology with health problems. We hope that the chapters will be sufficiently exciting that readers will be impelled to use the extensive bibliographies appended to them in order to consult original sources as well as general reviews.

The Editors wish to acknowledge the outstanding secretarial assistance of Carla Millhauser and Marge Healy, and the editorial assistance of Leslie Morris.

We would also like to thank our students and colleagues at Harvard and at the University of Washington whose sometimes jaundiced responses to our own early efforts to relate social science to medicine prompted the concerns which resulted in the creation of this volume. The undergraduate and graduate students who attended our seminars and conferences most always took the position: "I'm from Missouri; prove it to me." While we did not always succeed, the demand to "prove it" resulted in sharpening our own awareness of the limits of our understanding and of the need for a clearer and more logical exposition of what we thought we understood. We hope they profited from our interchange; we know we did.

Boston and Seattle   LEON EISENBERG
April 1980   ARTHUR KLEINMAN

1. CLINICAL SOCIAL SCIENCE

IS MEDICAL PRACTICE IMPEDED BY "TOO MUCH SCIENCE"?

In the three and a half decades since the Second World War, there have been remarkable gains in the effectiveness of preventive and therapeutic measures in medicine. To mention but a few examples of the former: vaccines which can prevent poliomyelitis, rubella and measles; Rh_0 (D) immune human globulin administered to Rh negative mothers at the birth of an Rh positive infant to prevent sensitization of the mother and hemolytic disease in subsequent children; screening measures leading to appropriate management to minimize the consequences of inherited metabolic disorders; and prenatal diagnosis to assure a normal birth. As examples of the latter, consider only: antibiotic treatment of infectious diseases; diuretics and alpha blockers to control hypertension; open heart surgery to correct valvular defects; total hip replacement; chemotherapy for childhood leukemias; drugs capable of aborting acute psychotic episodes and of minimizing their recurrence. To a medical graduate of the mid-1940's who has seen these changes during his own professional lifetime, the new capabilities are a continuing source of wonder and gratification.

Despite the physician's daily observation of impressive results from modern treatments, it is a different matter to ask how far these treatments can be given credit for the improvements in the general health of the U.S. population over the same time period. Life expectancy for males, which was 64.4 years at birth in 1946 had increased to 69.3 years by 1977; the corresponding figures for females went from 69.4 to 77.1 (National Center for Health Statistics 1978, 1979). Some measures, no matter how effective for the particular patient, address disorders which are rare (dietary treatment for phenylketonuria, for example, improves the quality of life for one in eleven thousand live born infants); others, like total hip replacement, have little effect on mortality despite dramatic benefit for function; even those which are life-preserving may not add appreciably to longevity because the diseases they combat occur in the elderly who die not long after from other causes.

It is undoubtedly true, as McKeown (1976) has argued, that the incidence of many infectious diseases had begun to decline in the last century well before the introduction of contemporary treatments because of improved sanitation, nutrition and general living conditions, tuberculosis being a notable example. Nonetheless, the further decline of these once-dreaded ailments has been measurably hastened by chemotherapy (McDermott 1977). For example, over the past 20 years, the mortality rate for tuberculosis fell from about 60/100,000 in 1947, the year chemotherapy was introduced, to about 6 in 1967. If the rate

1

L. Eisenberg and A. Kleinman (eds.), The Relevance of Social Science for Medicine, 1–23.

of change in the curve had remained the same for that 20 year period as it had been for the earlier years of this century, the expected death rate would have been five times as large. Changes in the death rate from tuberculosis in New Zealand both among the Maori (from 300 to 15) and among Europeans (from 30 to 3) show similarly increased benefits, despite the very marked differences in living conditions between the indigenous and the Caucasion populations (McDermott 1977). Furthermore, it is the vaccines against polio, measles and rubella which alone account for the marked reduction in the incidence of these diseases in the United States. If medicine cannot claim sole credit for the tenfold reductions since 1900 in infant and child mortality and for the threefold reduction in adolescent and young adult mortality (Surgeon General 1979), the evidence is persuasive that it has made an important contribution to these gains.

Mortality statistics understate the contribution of modern therapeutics to patient welfare. Relief of pain and enhancement of function in individuals with chronic disease may yield few cures and little detectable effect on longevity but the gain in quality of life for the millions of individuals at risk has been sizable. Death is, after all, inevitable. The prolongation of life, by whatever means, inescapably brings with it a higher prevalence of the degenerative diseases of old age for which palliation rather than cure is the most likely outcome of the physician's efforts (Gruenberg 1978).

Yet, despite the impressive gains which have resulted from the application of biomedical science to the understanding and control of disease, the American public views itself, in John Knowles' (1977) pithy phrase, as "doing better and feeling worse." At least, this is what one would conclude from the chorus of articulate critics of medicine. It is not altogether clear that the dissatisfactions expressed in the journals of opinion are an accurate reflection of the attitudes of the general public who like their own doctors at the same time they have reservations about medicine as an institution. In a recent opinion poll conducted by the Center for Health Administration Studies at the University of Chicago, 88% of Americans reported general satisfaction with the care they receive, although 61% simultaneously believe that there is a "general crisis in health care" (Johnson Foundation 1978).

When complaints are registered, they include: escalating costs; maldistribution of physicians; disappearance of the house call and its replacement by the trip to the emergency room; fear of iatrogenic disease produced by new diagnostic and treatment methods; and resentment at treatment failures, a resentment which is all the greater because of the expectations aroused by publicity about each new "breakthrough." These complaints converge on the conviction that today's doctors are less responsive to the personal needs of their patients than the old-fashioned family doctor is thought to have been.

It has become the conventional wisdom that the increased dissatisfaction, in the face of the manifest improvement in medical effectiveness, stems from the very success of technological achievement. Doctors, it is alleged, have lost the human touch precisely because their preoccupation with laboratory tests and technical fixes obscures their awareness of the patient as a person. Is there evidence for the proposition that doctors are less sensitive to patient needs *because* they are more competent in curing disease? We do not argue that doctors are as responsive to personal and social needs as they should be; indeed, concern about that problem lies behind the writing of this book. The question we raise is this: were doctors ever the compassionate, humane and wise figures nostalgia would have us believe they once were? We are not persuaded that such was the case.

What Were the "Good Old Days" Like?

From classical antiquity (Edelstein 1967) to the present (Sigerist 1958), there have been outstanding medical practitioners who knew what was to be known, individualized the care they provided and were actuated by the highest ethical standards of the time. They have left us a legacy of eloquent treatises on medical practice; but these shining moments in the historical record do not represent the performance of the generality of their contemporaries. During the eighteenth and nineteenth centuries, medicine in England and America was practiced by doctors of every stripe and persuasion, rigid in their adherence to the tenets of a particular school of thought, varying in the degree of their acquaintance with the scientific knowledge of the day. King (1958) has provided an example of the rancor of the quarrels and the bitter competition between physicians by extracts from a pamphlet consisting of an exchange of defamatory letters between William Withering (the discoverer of the diuretic properties of foxglove in cardiac edema) and Robert Darwin (the father of Charles). Withering had infuriated the 22 year-old Darwin, one year out of medical school, by taking over the care of the latter's patient, arriving at a new diagnosis and changing the treatment radically. Wrote Dr. Darwin:

Every liberal person sees through the paltry motives which have always induced you to slander those of your own professions, among the other mean arts by which you attempt to support your business.

Replied Dr. Withering:

That I have slandered you ... is untrue ... As I could not protect you in any way in which I ever wished to cover the errors of a young physician, I could not, in justice to myself and my patients, act otherwise than I have done.

Rejoined Darwin:

You are one of those characters of whom the enmity is far less dangerous than the friendship.

Riposted Withering:

Possessed, therefore, as I am of self-satisfaction, of the good opinion of the world at large and of medical men in particular, your enmity or your friendship, your good or your bad opinion, are to me equally insignificant.

English novels of the nineteenth century make evident the ambivalence toward medical science by their emphasis on the demonic character of the physician-investigator (Millhauser 1973). Just how far the French physician of that period embodied empathy for the patient can be inferred from the passage in the last chapter of Balzac's *Pere Goriot* written in 1834; the medical student Bianchon, in reassuring his friend Rastignac that he cares for the dying Goriot, comments: "Doctors already in practice see only the [disease]; I can still see the sick man, my dear boy."

American medicine of the nineteenth century went from a cycle of bleeding and purging to what some condemned as therapeutic nihilism; advocates of each school roundly condemned the others (Rosenberg 1979). One American news-paper of the midcentury condemned "poisoning and surgical butchery;" another large daily declared that the whole medical guild was "a stupendous humbug" (Shryock 1947). There were, of course, amidst the polemics, compassionate physicians who responded in a very human way to the tragedies they faced. Rosenberg (1979:11) quotes from the diary of Dr. Samuel W. Butler in 1852 in which Butler recorded his response to the unexpected death of a child he had been treating:

Remedies altho' slow in their action, acted well but were powerless to avert the arm of death. The decrees of Providence . . . cannot be set aside. Man is mortal, and tho' remedies often seem to act promptly and effectually to the saving of life – they often fail in an unaccountable manner! 'So teach me to number my days that I may apply my heart unto wisdom.'

Nonetheless, what is noteworthy is how acerbic the quarrels continued to be even as the century reached its end. Abraham Jacobi, the first President of the American Pediatric Society, protested in 1908:

Expectant treatment is often a combination of indolence and ignorance . . . It is the sin of omission, which not infrequently rises to the dignity of a crime.

Yet Sir William Osler (1920), speaking at the Johns Hopkins Historical Club in 1901 asserted that the great accomplishment of the new school of medicine was:

. . . firm faith in a few good, well tried drugs, little or none in the great mass of medicine still in general use. Imperative drugging – the ordering of medicine in any and every malady – is no longer regarded as the chief function of the doctor.

These excerpts, it is important to recall, are from the writings of distinguished physicians. What can be said about the generality of practicing doctors? Abraham Flexner (1910), in his *Report on Medical Education in the United States and Canada*, commented:

The profession has been diluted by the presence of the great number of men who have come from weak schools with low ideals both of education and of professional honor (p. xiv) . . . We have indeed American practitioners not inferior to the best elsewhere; but there is probably no other country in the world in which there is so great a distance and so fatal a distance between the best, the average and the worst (1910:20).

The Flexner Report was to transform medical education by its recommendations for a four year curriculum, a full time faculty, clinical clerkships, the incorporation of medical schools within universities and the introduction of research into the teaching program. Within a decade of its publication, one-third of the existing medical schools closed their doors and the number of graduates in 1919 fell to half of what it had been at the turn of the century, a level it would not achieve again until after World War II (Richmond 1969). Nonetheless, struggles between the clinician and the laboratory scientist continued. Sir James MacKenzie (1919), an outstanding cardiologist, wrote:

Laboratory training *unfits* a man for his work as a physician, for the reason that, not only does the laboratory man fail to educate his senses, but he puts so much trust in his mechanical methods that he never recognizes their limitations and he fails to see that there are other methods which are essential to the interpretation of disease.

Alfred E. Cohn (1924), founding Editor of the Journal of Clinical Investigation, distinguished sharply between the bacteriology laboratory, remote from the bedside, and the contributions of the clinical investigator:

Dependence on the outside world (i.e. on the bacteriologist) for solution of its problems is in part a reproach to medicine . . . The task which academic medicine in the United States, now become self-conscious, has set itself . . . is the task of Clinical Investigation.

Cohn (1928) insisted that:

The history of medicine since the Renaissance has shown plentifully that whenever the approach to an understanding of disease is made by scholars trained primarily in the other pursuits of knowledge . . . the result, so far as understanding disease is concerned, is disappointing and sometimes grotesque.

Perhaps the most eloquent defense of the physician's clinical skills and their importance for patient care, is to be found in the writings of Francis W. Peabody (1930), Professor of Medicine at Harvard and Chief of the Fourth Medical Service of the Boston City Hospital, to whom we owe the moving words: "The secret of the care of the patient is in caring for the patient" (1930:57). In describing the attitudes of his medical contemporaries in 1927, he wrote:

The most common criticism made at present by older practitioners is that young graduates have been taught a great deal about the mechanism of disease, but very little about the practice of medicine — or to put it more bluntly, they are too 'scientific' and do not know how to take care of patients (1930:27).

Commenting on public attitudes, he noted:

The layman of the older generation, who has been disappointed in his medical experience and who feels that something has been lacking in the way of warmth, sympathy and understanding of his case as a whole, is very apt to hark back to earlier days. 'What we need,' he says, 'is a general practitioner!' (1930:7).

Thus, the tension between "science" and "care" was already present in the early stages of the thrust toward specialization, well before specialty boards were formally organized. Peabody argued forcefully for the role of the general practitioner:

The more a doctor knows of his patient's general background, the greater advantage he has in handling the case ... [The general practitioner] knows the patient from childhood up – his physical health, the nervous and mental strain to which he has been subjected, the conditions of his social, business and domestic life, and more even than this, he may have the same detailed knowledge of the patient's parents and of the circumstances of their lives ... The only person who can really gather together this fundamental knowledge of his patients is the general practitioner (1930:24–25).

Peabody's comments illuminate two issues. First, contentions that there is too little care *because* of too much science antedate today's era of high technology by 50 years; second, the virtues of the family doctor which Peabody spoke for so eloquently stemmed, when they were present, from continuing intimate acquaintance with patient, family and community, and not from medical theory or education. To a considerable extent, those virtues resided in the doctor's role in an America of family farms, small towns and multigenerational families. Generalist or specialist, the physician no longer has the opportunity to come to know the extended family for several generations, now that one in five American families moves each year; familiarity with "the conditions of the patient's social, business and domestic life" is no longer readily available to even the so-called neighborhood doctor now that our population has shifted to a predominantly urban locus, with its anonymity, fragmentation and weakening of identification with a neighborhood. Moreover, few doctors are likely to spend their medical lifetimes in one place.

Not quite ten years after Peabody's remarks, L. J. Henderson, Professor of Biological Chemistry at Harvard Medical School, issued a call for a theory to guide the physician in understanding doctor and patient as a social system. Henderson (1936) reminded the leaders of academic medicine that the Hippocratic tradition had emphasized a:

general view of the patient as a human being living in an environment that is social as well as physical. All this is particularly due to a clear appreciation of restrictions on mere technology in practice. It leads to the perception that in the practice of medicine there is much beyond mere technology (1936:8).

In his view, the grand accomplishments of laboratory science had "defeated the clinical party" and had brought about a condition:

in which the patient is ... often a mere *case* which (not who) passes through the doctor's office, his past, present and future unknown, except within the meager abstractions of etiology, diagnosis and prognosis; and his personality and relations with other persons not even thought of (1936:9–10).

Henderson emphasized the necessity for:

somebody to understand and treat real men and women, not mere medical, surgical or social cases (1936:10).

He contended that:

> when the ancient and empirical methods of acquiring a skill have lost their efficacy, there
> seems to be only one way of recovering what has been lost. This is through scientific for-
> mulation (p. 10) . . . There is scientific sociologic knowledge that can be applied by anyone
> who possesses a native capacity for the skilled management of his own relations with others
> and for understanding the role of human beings in the everyday world. Being scientific, such
> knowledge can be stated clearly and generally. It can therefore be taught and, within narrow
> limits, applied (1936:11).

Henderson (1935) believed that Pareto's sociology provided such a scientific
theory. Whether or not Pareto's formulations constitute an adequate basis for
conceptualizing "the role of human beings in the everyday world," what is
pertinent to this discussion is Henderson's injunction to physicians that:

> a physician and a patient taken together make up a social system . . . In any social system
> the interaction of the sentiments is likely to be at least as important as anything else (p. 14)
> . . . The doctor must not only appear to be but must really be interested in what the patient
> says . . . In an interview listen, first, for what the patient wants to tell, secondly, for im-
> plications of what he does not want to tell, thirdly, for implications of what he cannot tell
> (p. 17) . . . Beware, then, when talking to a patient, of your own arbitrary assumptions, of
> your own beliefs, of your own feelings (p. 18) . . . If physician and patient constitute a
> social system, it is almost a trivial one compared with the larger social system of which the
> patient is a permanent member and in which he lives. This system, indeed, makes up the
> greater part of the environment in which he *feels* that he lives. I suggest that it is impossible
> to understand any man as a person without knowledge of this environment and especially
> of what he thinks and feels it is; which may be a very different thing (1935:20).

TRADITIONAL HEALERS AND HOLISTIC MEDICINE: THE MYTH OF THE GARDEN OF EDEN

One further digression is necessary before we take up Henderson's avowal of
the importance of "scientific sociologic knowledge" for medical practice. As
anthropologic studies of cultures exotic to the West have become part of popular
lore, the romantic myth has arisen that traditional healers possess the very
understanding of patient care which is lacking in Western medical practice.
Precisely because we advocate the value of anthropologic methodology for a full
understanding of the doctor's role, it is necessary to clearify just how far this
belief is warranted. Irrelevant to our present concern is the extent to which
herbal remedies (Indian: rauwolfia; Peruvian: quinine; Chinese: ephedrine; Greek
and Arabic: morphine) have been shown (and others will be shown) to represent
the empirical discovery of active principles which, when further purified by
pharmaceutical chemistry, are incorporated into the modern pharmacopeia.
What matters to this argument is the set of therapeutic relationships and rituals
which characterize the forms of traditional medicine still to be found in developing countries and which are thought to represent major integrative forces within
the community.

If this thesis holds at all, it is true primarily for those small groups of hunter-gatherers and early agriculturalists, so remote geographically that they have been largely isolated from contact with other cultures and so continue to adhere to a central cosmology unchallenged by competing beliefs. Turner (1967) has explicated the Ndembu healer's view of illness as a manifestation of dissonance within the social order and therapeutic rituals as means to resolve conflict and reaffirm threatened cultural values. Many societies, like the Dobuans (Fortune 1932), are full of suspicion, ill will and treachery. Illness beliefs and healing rituals are central to the maintenance of cohesion. Since shamans and other sacred folk healers frequently can cause illness (via sorcery) as well as treat it, the threat of sorcery and the strongly negative feelings that attend it give healers unusual power over patients — power that may effectively silence patients' dissatisfaction and leave them without therapeutic recourse (Kleinman 1980:240). The belief in sorcery as a major cause of illness can wreak havoc when the epidemiology of disease is not at a steady state and therefore "control" by magic fails.

Lindenbaum (1979) has provided a graphic account of the crisis provoked by the spread of *kuru* among the Southern Fore in the Eastern Highlands of Papua New Guinea. *Kuru* is an invariably fatal, slowly progressive disease of the central nervous system, caused, in the Western meaning of cause, by an atypical neurotropic virus (Gajdusek and Gibbs 1975). In the medical classification scheme of the Fore, *kuru* is one of a group of diseases caused by the malicious actions of human sorcerers. Accordingly, the appropriate response to the onset of the disease is to summon a curer to identify the sorcerer and offset his malignant influences by appropriate magical remedies. As the pandemic intensified, accusation and suspicion mounted; curers themselves were denounced as frauds because their rituals failed to heal; villages turned against one another; warfare was imminent. Unable to control the disease at the local level, the Fore assembled in mass meetings known as *kibungs*. Sorcerers were publicly reproached for crimes against society and urged to confess their misdeeds; some public "confessions" were indeed elicited. Speakers called for brotherhood and unity:

Our ancestors were the same. We living men are the ones who split apart and gave separate names to our groups. At this *kibung* let us adopt the customs of our ancestors. We will stop making *kuru* on our own people. *Ibubuli* is our all-inclusive name (1979:104).

The *kibungs* served to minimize internecine warfare but they too fell into disuse as the disease persisted. It was only when modern virology had identified agent and mode of transmission and when modernization and civil regulation gradually transformed the social customs of the Fore that *kuru* was controlled; transmission was intercepted by ending the practice of ritual cannibalism as a rite of mourning and respect for dead kinsmen.

In most, if not all, developing countries, no single world view predominates. Rather, there are sets of competing ideologies which have resulted from commerce between cultures and different degrees of access to specialized knowledge.

The notion that healer and patient are united by a common cosmology is belied by the presence of many contradictory belief systems; most sick persons are pragmatists and are willing to consult, either simultaneously or in succession, a series of healers with divergent methods. For example, Crapanzano (1973) has studied the disease theory and therapeutic practices of the *Hamadsha* brotherhood (an order of Islamic Sufism). The cause of disease is *jinn* (spirit or devil); the task of the healer is to drive the *jinn* out or, failing that, to establish a working relationship with it. However, a contemporary Moroccan may also turn for help when ill, not merely to the Islamic brotherhoods (*Hamdushiyya, Gnawiyya, Isawiyya, Rahaliyya* and *Jilaliyya*) but also to *fuqaha* (Koranic teachers who write amulets and talismans), herbalists, specialists in traditional Arabic medicine; *aguza* (old women familiar with magical brews and midwifery); and exorcists. Along side these traditional healers are Western medical practitioners, each with stylistic and social class differences: European physicians; Western-trained Morrocans; pharmacists; male nurses; European missionaries; and local infirmaries and hospitals. Kunstadter (1975) working in Northern Thailand, Leslie (1976) in India, Janzen (1977) in the central Congo, Press (1969) in urban Colombia, and many other medical ethnographers offer detailed documentation of this marked pluralism of indigenous healing systems and of patients' pragmatic orientation to available therapeutic resources.

In an epidemiologic study of the village of Kota in India, Carstairs and Kapur (1976) identified three major types of traditional practitioners in addition to the Western-trained physicians who served the population. The *Vaids*, practitioners of Ayurveda, an indigenous system of empirical medicine with a vast pharmacopeia, ascribe illness to an imbalance between the natural elements leading to an excess of heat, cold, bile, wind or fluid secretions which can be caused by such things as eating wrong food or uninhibited sexual indulgence; at the same time, disease can be caused by *pishachis* or evil spirits; treatment is by herbs, roots and pills. *Mantarwadis* are masters of the zodiac and of potent secret verses termed mantras; cause is discovered through the zodiac and cure is carried out through the mantra. The *Patris* act as mediums for a *Bhuta* or spirit which uses the healer's body and voice as a means of communicating to the patient the ways of exorcising evil. A survey of the populace revealed that although Western practitioners were used as the sole source (40% of the time) more often than indigenous healers only (14% of the time), the most common pattern of patient care was to employ both Western and indigenous healers simultaneously (46%).

In a study in Taipei, Taiwan, Kleinman (1980) emphasizes the flourishing side by side of Western-trained physicians; practitioners of classical Chinese medicine; bone setters; pharmacists; fortune tellers; medicinal tea shops; physiognomists; geomancers; *ch'ien* interpreters; herbalists; Taoist priests and *tâng-kis* (shamans); experts in massage; midwives; and still other folk practitioners. Some are licensed; some are illegal; all seem to be in use. Each tradition conceptualizes the hidden causes underlying the manifest illness in a different but nonetheless narrow way. To illustrate the point, we need only compare the practices of modern Western-trained physicians with those of the classical Chinese physicians who still command a large clientele in Taiwan. Their medical behavior, no less than ours, is circumscribed by a set of theories which determine the questions they ask in taking a history and the way they go about a physical examination. In contrasting the patient encounters of Chinese-style with Western-style physicians, Kleinman found that the mean time for the office transactions was 7.5 minutes for the former as against 5 minutes for the latter, hardly an impressive difference; moreover, both types of physicians limited their curiosity to phenomena defined as relevant by their theories of disease; they afforded the patient precious little time for discussion of personal concerns. As Kleinman notes:

The popular medical ideology [in Taiwan] holds that the skills of the physician are demonstrated by his ability to ascertain what is wrong from the pulse and perhaps from a few short questions. The fewer the questions the better. A great doctor need ask nothing (1980:262).

The theories of the two types of practitioners could hardly be further apart; the former utilizes almost no technology whereas the latter is heavily dependent upon it. Yet the Chinese-style physician is no less remote than his Western counterpart from the social and interpersonal dimensions of illness and health. Recent outcome studies in Taiwan (A. Kleinman and J. L. Gale, unpublished data) demonstrate that even those shamans, who may be on occasion strikingly successful in responding to patients' personal troubles, do not systematically recognize or attempt to relieve the psychosocial burden of illness (nor do they practice without toxicity).

Thus, even the briefest epitome of traditional medicine in the developing world makes evident its diversity and complexity; the term "traditional healer" tells us almost nothing about a given practitioner without a detailed specification of the culture and the locus in that culture within which he practices. The celebration of the wisdom of *the* folk healer is part of the myth of a Golden Age, when life was simpler and men healthier, a myth embedded in Western as well as Eastern traditions. Edelstein (1967a, b) has contrasted the idea of progress and the belief in an idyllic past during classical Greek antiquity. Dubos (1959) quotes a Chinese scholar, Lieh-tzu of the fourth century B.C., who depicted the Taoist vision of the ancient paradise on earth:

The people were gentle, following Nature without wrangling and strife . . . Not till the age of 100 did they die, and disease and premature death were unknown. Thus they lived . . . having no decay and old age . . . (1959:9).

The readiness to believe in the fantasy of "primitive man" living in a Garden of Eden accounts for the widely prevalent view of peasant society as somehow more "organic" than our own, although Oscar Lewis (1951) long ago reported how profoundly suspicion and envy permeate that world. Romanticism about traditional healers obscures the far greater complexity of the reality of healing practices. Healing ceremonies can be efficacious, but hardly substitute for antibiotics or surgery. Healers can be shrewd and insightful; but some are rigid technicians who adhere (or are required to adhere) to a mechanical recitation of ritual; and others are primarily concerned with personal gain. Few of the systems of apprenticeship or formal training in traditional medicine include explicit attention to social and interpersonal considerations except in symbolic terms. Healers are indeed taught the *etiquette* of medical behavior but often emphasis is on impressing the client, rather than on understanding interpersonal interactions. In precisely such terms the Hippocratic physician was exhorted to wear proper garments, behave in a dignified fashion, refuse to treat hopeless cases lest he be blamed, consider the impression his manner made on others, and so on (Edelstein 1967a:87—110). In those instances when traditional healers modify standard practice by taking into account the idiosyncracies of a given family within a particular community, they rely on their tacit knowledge of village life rather than on the formal doctrines of their sects, much as did the vanishing general practitioners Peabody extolled.

Romanticism in anthropology and sociology leads to an overvaluation of the skills of traditional healers; in consequence, it results in a reverse ethnocentrism toward health care and the healing professions in our own society. In its most grotesque form, we are presented with a caricature of the patient as a victim and the physician as a jailer in Western medicine; whereas, the folk healer is portrayed as an infinitely wise guru with an intuitive knowledge of sociology and political science. This so distorts the real world as to turn clinicians away from the cross-cultural literature in social science. The fact of the matter is that, while traditional healing has many positive features, systematic understanding of the psychosocial aspects of illness is largely a modern accomplishment based on clinical and epidemiological studies of patients and healers in this and other societies by social scientists and psychiatrists.

To recapitulate our argument, then, the deficits in the doctor's understanding of the clinical encounter long antecede the contemporary era; narrow specialization and high technology have further accentuated the dichotomy between the patient's experience of illness and the doctor's concern with disease. The patient who seeks yesteryear's nostalgic image of a family doctor in place of today's biomedical expert would serve himself ill by foregoing remedies of proven value in the search for illusory compassion. Doctors may rationalize an exclusively biological focus by insisting on the priority of "facts" over "sentiments." Such physicians were no less common 50 years ago or 500 years ago; they differed only in what they consider to be "facts."

The key task for medicine is not to diminish the role of the biological sciences in the theory and practice of medicine but to supplement it with an equal application of the social sciences in order to provide both a more comprehensive understanding of disease and better care of the patient. The problem is not "too much science," but too narrow a view of the sciences relevant to medicine.

Why Social Science? Why Not More Biological Science?

The reader may object: Biomedical sciences have contributed greatly to more effective medical practice. By definition, science is unfinished business;

all answers are provisional. The one thing we can be certain of having is better answers tomorrow than we have today. Why doubt that the remaining problems of medicine will be solved by extending the very methods which have worked so well to now? Why insist that modern biology is intrinsically incapable of providing a comprehensive account of sickness and a complete recipe for cure?

We reply: The factors that determine who is and who is not a patient can only be understood by taking non-biological variables into account; *patienthood is a social state*, rather than simply a biological one. Psychosocial variables influence, not only the social and personal meanings of illness, but also the risk of becoming ill, the nature of the response to illness and its prognosis.

The assertion that patienthood is a social condition may seem absurd. To most physicians, patients are persons afflicted by disease ("real" patients) or those who erroneously believe themselves to be so afflicted (the "worried well"). From this standpoint, getting well is a matter of being treated properly if one is diseased or of being reassured accordingly if one is not. Since the central problem is the presence or absence of disease, the only issues of interest to the doctor are the agents, the mechanisms and the treatments of diseases.

Far from being self-evident, this disease-centered view completely overlooks the complexity of the processes leading to the decision to see the doctor; that is, the decision to become a patient. Community surveys regularly identify many more individuals with symptoms and many more with abnormal findings than are under medical care at any given time (White et al. 1961; Mechanic and Newton 1965), even in countries with comprehensive health care (Ingham and Miller 1976). Every clinician is familiar with the patient whose disease has been treated successfully but who obstinately persists in complaining of symptoms, as well as the patient who drops out of treatment despite active disease.

The study by Peterson et al. (1977) of the treatment of peptic ulcer provides a telling illustration. The investigators wished to study the effectiveness of high dose antacid therapy for peptic ulcer. In order to provide as objective a measure of outcome as possible, each patient was endoscoped at the beginning of the investigation and at the completion of the four week treatment period, after having received active drug or placebo on a double blind protocol. The endoscopic results were unequivocal: high dose antacid produced a much higher rate of ulcer healing than did placebo (78% versus 45%). Yet, simultaneous assessment of symptomatic change on antacid and placebo revealed no difference in clinical outcome at the end of four weeks; symptom scores had been reduced to 20% of the initial level in both groups. The discrepancy between ulcer healing rates and symptom improvement rates makes it clear that some patients with healed ulcers continued to have symptoms whereas others whose ulcer persisted had no complaints of pain. As the authors comment: "Loss of ulcer symptoms did not guarantee ulcer healing or even decrease in size." Other studies, which cannot be reviewed in detail here, document the influence of culture on the complaint pattern of patients with the same "objective" disease (Zola 1966), the significance of the circumstances under which injury occurs for the amount of pain the patient experiences (Beecher 1956) and the different criteria by which patients and physicians judge the outcome of surgery (Cay et al. 1975).

To highlight these clinical phenomena, we propose to make a semantic distinction between "disease" and "illness," terms synonymous in contemporary English usage. Physicians diagnose and treat diseases; that is, abnormalities in the structure and function of body organs and systems. Patients suffer illnesses; that is, experiences of disvalued changes in states of being and in social function (Eisenberg 1977). Disease and illness do not stand in a one-to-one relationship. Similar degrees of organ pathology can generate quite different reports of pain and distress; illness may occur in the absence of detectable disease; the course of the disease is distinct from the trajectory of the accompanying illness. A visit to the doctor is more likely when disease is present, but it is essential to understand that contracting a disease, feeling ill and being a patient are overlapping but not co-extensive states.

En route to becoming a patient, the individual must make, almost always with the advice of others, a self-diagnosis of being ill, a judgement made against implicit standards of what it means to be well. Just as there is no completely satisfactory medical definition of health, wellness means different things to different people: feeling good, not having symptoms, being able to get the job done, not believing oneself to be at risk or being told by the doctor that one is well. Against this background of values which vary with social class and culture, the process of decision-making is initiated by an experience of unexpected discomfort, decrease in previous functional capacities and/or change in physicial appearance.

A first decision must be made: is the change an important deviation or is it a normal part of living? Can it be dismissed as transient? Is it to be attributed to a recent event: something eaten, a muscle strain, the time of the month? Threshholds for ascribed significance vary with life expectations; for the poor, pain and fatigue may be part of life. Familiar symptoms are rarely frightening.

When ready or easily fabricated ways of explaining symptoms away are not at hand, they suggest that there is something wrong. Among individuals under stress, symptoms are not only more likely to occur but they are more likely to lead to a search for help (Mechanic and Volkart 1961; Tessler et al. 1976). Family members and friends are almost always consulted at this stage of evaluation; they may be decisive in determining the actions taken (Twaddle 1977). Once it has been decided that something must be done, the individual has to identify the appropriate type of help: a family remedy, a folk healer, the local druggist, a chiropracter, a physician, etc. The selection will reflect a judgement about what is wrong and what type of treatment is needed, an expectation which can lead to an impasse if the treatment prescribed by the practitioner differs from the anticipated one.

Up to this point, a whole series of health care transactions has occurred outside the official medical network. Community studies indicate the some 75–90% of episodes self-identified as illness are managed entirely without recourse to the health system (Hulka et al. 1972; Zola 1972). Yet, medicine has barely begun to pay attention to the cumulative evidence that what doctors see in offices and hospitals is a grossly unrepresentative sample of the illnesses and diseases which occur in the community. Failure to appreciate the dimensions of the sampling problem has consequences for disease diagnosis as well as for illness treatment.

The stubborn fact, the one that won't go away and that doesn't fit the medical lexicon, is that what doctors choose to call "delay" is the rule in patient behavior rather than an aberration. Severe trauma and overwhelming infection aside, most patients appear in the office with symptoms which have been present for weeks and months. Most people don't come in for most of their complaints most of the time; that's normal illness behavior. Thus, it is a useless putdown to ask a patient: "Why didn't you come in earlier?" when the meaningful question is "Why did you come now?" The better we understand the triggers for deciding to see the doctor, the better will we be able to respond to the patient's needs. For example, Roghmann and Haggerty (1973), in a study of 512 young families, asked each mother to keep a diary in which she recorded each day any upsetting events which had occurred in the family. Analysis of the stressful events in relation both to illness episodes and to the use of medical care revealed different effects on care patterns for the mother herself and for her children. The presence of stress in the family *and* illness in the child *increased the likelihood* that medical care would be utilized for the child (from 1% to 15%). On the other hand, if the mother was ill, family stress *decreased* the likelihood she would seek medical care whereas it *increased* the likelihood she would see the doctor at times when she was *not* ill. In a prepaid group practice, Tessler et al. (1976) found that physician utilization increased in direct ratio to the amount of stress the patient experienced; at the same level of health impairment, the individual under greater stress was more likely to consult a physician. In the view of David Mechanic (1978), the leading investigator in this area, the available evidence indicates that distress has as powerful an effect on utilization behavior as does health status itself.

HOW DOES THE MEDICAL CONSUMER VIEW SOCIAL SCIENCE?

However persuasive to us and to our readers the evidence that nonbiological variables influence illness and care-seeking behavior and that social science research therefore has high relevance to medical practice, the question remains: what do doctors in practice think about applied social science? It is they who will be the ultimate consumers of applied social science. The evidence is scanty. Surveys of pediatricians in practice (Shonkoff et al. 1979) do indicate an awareness of the inadequacy of conventional medical training for the behavioral aspects of practice and a wish for more systematic instruction. Although research reports and survey articles on social science are clearly under-represented in medical journals, they have been considerably more frequent in the past decade than they were earlier. The new programs in primary care and family practice, and the journals devoted to these fields, both in England and in this country, reflect growing sophistication in social science.

What is the attitude of medical educators, those who make the decisions on whether the information the social scientist purveys will be included in formal instruction to their students? That is what Professors Petersdorf and Feinstein have endeavored to ascertain by a survey whose results are reported in the next chapter of this book. They asked the Chairpersons of Departments of Medicine, Pediatrics and Family Medicine their opinions of the current status of "medical sociology," otherwise undefined. On the basis of an unusually high response rate to a mailed questionnaire, they provide a fascinating if disquieting snapshot of current attitudes among the Professoriate.

They found, as expected, a "gradient of enthusiasm" with family medicine most receptive, pediatrics less so and internal medicine the least. The gradient from positive to negative parallels (a) the extent to which social scientists are represented on departmental faculties in each area and (b) the amount of time devoted to social science instruction during student clerkships and house officer education. Whether familiarity leads to enthusiasm or enthusiasm to familiarity cannot be said. What is evident from their responses is that even where the attitude is the most favorable the time commitment remains quite limited and the coverage spotty and unsystematic. Teaching and research in social science continue to have relatively low priority in the allocation of departmental resources.

If the utility of social science for clinical practice is to be judged from the response to the Petersdorf—Feinstein questionnaire, the most optimistic conclusion would be the Scot's verdict: not proven. The data also suggest another conclusion: that medical educators, particularly those oriented to specialty practice rather than primary care, reflect their prejudices rather than considered judgements when they dismiss social science without much evidence of a serious effort to familiarize themselves with its methods and findings. The topics included by the respondents under the rubric of "medical sociology" reflect a confusion of humanism, psychodynamics and medical ethics with social science; the latter may have much to contribute to the clarification of each of these areas (just as it does to the identification of host factors in resistance to disease) but it should not be equated with any of them any more than with biology. Helping to make young doctors humane is more likely to be achieved by providing role models of humane internists and pediatricians than by courses in literature or philosophy. Humanism is a criterion by which all of us must be measured; we are not convinced it is more often found among Professors of Romance Languages or American History than among Professors of Physics or Molecular Biology.

Nonetheless, it would be a grievous error, in our estimation, to dismiss the negative appraisal of those who collectively do much to determine the content of medical education. The extent of their negative bias, at the least, serves to define the size of the barrier to be overcome; more than that, it is likely to reflect unsatisfactory experiences at the interface between medicine and social science. When they object to "jargon," it simply will not do to point out that the medical literature is hardly a model of clarity, unambiguous language and sparkling logic. Social science *is* afflicted by neologisms, unwieldy abstractions and large conclusions based upon limited data.

When doctors complain of anti-physician bias among social scientists, they may be guilty of faulting an entire discipline for the strong positions taken by a few, but they are hardly being paranoid. As an example, sociologic critics complain that alcoholism has been captured by medicine (Conrad 1975; Zola 1977); in support of this contention, they stress the fact that official medical groups from the American Medical Association to the World Health Organization have pronounced that alcoholism is a "disease." However, they conviently omit to mention an equally consisting finding; namely, that very few physicians regard alcoholism as a disease about which *they themselves* could or should do very much (Hanna 1978; Strong 1978). Most physicians, psychiatrists included, refer alcoholic patients elsewhere when at all possible. Thus, despite official pronouncements, which are grist for the sociologic mill, actual practice is a far different matter.

Doctors do, as sociologists have been forthright enough to tell us, overrate the importance of their work (a stance hardly unique among the professions); we are organized to maintain the prestige and income which it brings our way. Yet as Strong (1979) has pointed out so cogently, the "thesis of medical imperialism is part of a more general sociologic analysis of professional ambition — an analysis which can, in its turn, also be applied to sociology."

In considering the self-interest of sociology in competing with medicine for a share in the health care largesse, Strong cites Susser (1974) to the effect that:

The history of social science in general is perhaps exemplified in the parochial history of (its) evolution . . . in relation to health policy in Britain . . . In a first phase, social science srruggled for a place, any kind of place, in the health field. In a second phase, social science gained a place . . . and was perceived as useful in health policy by those who had the power to frame policy. At this stage of its evolution, social science proved threatening to many individual clinicians, but was no longer seen as threatening by the administration at the center of political power. Administrators perceived the utility of social science in its capacity to function within the *status quo* while illuminating special problems. In a third phase, social science can be said to have been co-opted by those at the administrative center of power in forming health policy . . .

The incursion of sociology into health has by now become a permanent occupation of territory. The moment seems appropriate for a review of the conduct of the occupying troops . . . (Susser 1974:407–408).

The sociological critique of the medicalization of everyday life has been a major contribution to the identification of an important problem area but it overstates the case by attributing the phenomenon to a conspiracy by doctors. Contrast the doctrine of deliberate medical imperialism with the views expressed by a prominent leader of what has been termed the biomedical establishment,

Lewis Thomas (1977), President of the Memorial Sloan-Kettering Cancer Center, who states that the biggest source of waste in burgeoning health care costs:

results from the general public conviction that contemporary medicine is able to accomplish a great deal more than is in fact possible. This attitude is in part the outcome of overstated claims on the part of medicine itself in recent decades, plus medicine's passive acquiesence while even more exaggerated claims were made by the media ... The system is being overused, swamped by expectant overdemands for services that are frequently trivial or unproductive. The public is not sufficiently informed in the facts about the things that medicine can and cannot accomplish. Medicine is surely not in possession of special wisdom about how to live a life ... If our society wishes to be rid of the diseases, fatal and nonfatal, that plague us the most, there is really little prospect of doing so by mounting a still larger health care system at still greater cost for delivering essentially today's kind of technology on a larger scale (1977:35–36).

Thomas contends that it is only investment in fundamental science which will yield the new knowledge to enable the medicine of the future to make more of a difference to health outcomes. Whether one shares his view or not, it is hardly medical imperalism to call doctors back to the laboratory bench and to acknowledge the limits of their skills.

The forces in contemporary society which thrust doctors into areas which many, like Thomas, would prefer to abjure, are embedded in our culture (Fox 1977). If sociologists have done the public and the profession a service by criticizing the unwarranted extention of the biomedical model beyond its domain of applicability, they themselves, by arguing for a "social model," advocate a position which implies the involvement of health experts (albeit nonmedical ones; sociologists, in fact) in the management of an even wider range of everyday activities (Strong 1979).

The absurd lengths to which a social structural analysis of the role of medicine and society can be carried is evident in a recent paper by Taussig (1980) which argues that the signs and symptoms of a disease "signify critically sensitive and contradictory components of our culture and social relations" and that medical practice conceals this meaning "within the realm of biological signs ... In this way disease is recruited into serving the ideological needs of the social order, to the detriment of healing and our understanding of the social causes of misfortune" (1980:3). Taussig argues that the social role of the Western doctor is much like that of the Ndembu healer (Turner 1967:32) in which the doctor has the task of domesticating "the raw energies of conflict ... in the service of the traditional social order." Taussig maintains that the social interaction between doctor and patient serves to reinforce the culture's basic premises and that "the moral and metaphysical components of disease and healing are concealed by the use of the natural science model" (1980:5).

In specific, Taussig criticizes a paper (Kleinman et al. 1978) in which we have put forth the view that clinical social science can lead to measurable improvement in management and compliance, patient satisfaction and treatment outcomes. He complains that our proposal to incorporate knowledge of anthropology into medical practice contains "the danger that the experts will avail themselves of that knowledge only to make the science of human management all the more powerful and coercive." He derides the possibility of a constructive alliance between doctor and patient because "one party avails itself of the other's private understandings in order to manipulate them all the more successfully" (1980:12).

In this self-proclaimed Marxist analysis, it is manipulation rather than education for the doctor to take the patient's view of the illness into account in order to persuade the patient of the scientific logic for the treatment prescribed. We find it a remarkable brand of egalitarianism which accords equal value to lay and professional models of illness without regard for evidence of efficacy. In its obsession with power relationships, it entirely ignores the central fact that the patient comes to the doctor in search of relief from distress, a relief which can only be obtained *if* effective medical measures are available and *if* the patient agrees to apply them. The social and metaphorical view of disease is so dominant in this analysis that Taussig implies that sickness contains the seeds of revolution by challenging:

the complacent and everyday acceptance of conventional structures of meaning . . . The doctor and the patient are curing the threat posed to convention and society, tranquilizing the disturbance that sickness unleashes against normal thought which is not a static system but a system waxing, consolidating and dissolving on the reefs of its contradictions (1980:13).

It is difficult for practicing clinicians to recognize any correspondence between this abstraction and clinical reality. It is indeed true, as a number of the chapters in this book will make clear, that socioeconomic forces are major determinants of health. Correction of the differentials in morbidity and mortality between the advantaged and disadvantaged castes and classes in society demand social reform and not simply *post facto* medical rescue (Kitagawa and Hauser 1973; Holtzman 1977). Nonetheless, the patient who seeks help from the doctor is today's victim, not salvageable by tomorrow's hoped-for reform. His or her distress will not be put aright by injunctions for political action, to say nothing of the doctor's dubious credentials for making such recommendations. We find the implication bizarre that withholding from the physician such knowledge of anthropology as can increase clinical effectiveness in patient care will serve the patient — or lead to social change. Indeed, about the only thing Taussig and we agree upon is that the application of anthropological knowledge to clinical practice can enhance medical care, though we are rather more modest in our expectations of it.

It is precisely that conviction which we believe to be borne out by the chapters in this book. Berkman demonstrates persuasively the impact of the social environment on physical health status and McKinlay the ways in which the patient's social network influences episodes of illness and the pathways the patient chooses in seeking help. Twaddle develops the concept of the sickness career and traces out its implications for the understanding of sick behavior and the search for care. Bergner and Gilson provide a methodology for measuring the impact of sickness by means of a profile which enables the clinician to pinpoint the dysfunctions which require correction. The essay by Lewis illustrates the ways in which culture shapes illness behavior.

The Goods stress the metaphorical meaning of symptoms and the importance of understanding that meaning in the practice of primary care. Zola sets out for the reader the dynamic factors which underlie what doctors label as "noncompliance." Katon and Kleinman provide a *vademecum* of practical strategies to improve clinical care.

Waxler states the case forcefully for the impact of the social label applied to deviant behavior on the subsequent evolution of the trajectory of illness and Alexander analyzes the relationship between dialysis patients and the health professionals who care for them in terms of a double bind of conflicting messages. In the final chapters, Brenner provides the statistical evidence for the thesis that socioeconomic indices correlate with health status; Waitzkin argues the case that the structure of capitalism is reflected in health care institutions and in illness patterns.

We acknowledge that the viewpoints presented in this book lack an overarching integrated theoretical viewpoint; indeed, some of the positions taken are at variance with others; the units of analysis extend from doctor and patient as a dyad – to populations – to institutions – to cultures – and to broad economic forces. Indeed, the positions taken are not always those with which the Editors would be in agreement. But each chapter, in our opinion, makes an explicit and forthright statement of an important area of scholarship in social science and will provide the reader with an exciting view of the ferment in the field, its implications for current practice and its potential for contributing toward a more effective medicine in this future.

The fulfillment of that promise is by no means inevitable. It depends, as all scientific progress does, on the effort and the resources expended on it, the openness of the intellectual environment to it, and leadership. The sad fact is that social science is barely present in medical institutions and the thoughtful dialogue we hope this book will provoke is as yet only an occasional and often bitter conversation. Just as physicians need an appreciation of what social science can conribute to the understanding of patienthood and healing (Eisenberg 1980), social scientists must immerse themselves in the clinic in order to relate theory to practice with a better appreciation of the urgencies and immediacies of patient care (Kleinman 1980:375–389). The field awaits theoreticians with the breadth and depth to integrate the disparate and often contradictory concepts which are the best today's social science is able to offer. But we are convinced that the time has come for clinical departments in teaching institutions to encourage young physicians to undertake graduate study in the social sciences just as they have done in the fields of microbiology and molecular biology, to the enormous enrichment of the clinic. It is our prediction that similar gains will result when individuals who have mastered the two cultures (of the consulting room and the social sciences) are full members of the medical faculty. Those individuals will not supplant the social scientist per se (any more than clinician-investigators do the biochemist) but they will be uniquely able to take advantage of "experiments of culture," analogous to inherited metabolic disorders as experiments of nature (Garrod 1923), in contributing both to medicine and to social science.

REFERENCES

Bain, S. T. and W. B. Spaulding
　1967　The Importance of Coding Presenting Symptoms. Canad. Med. Assoc. J. 97:953–959.
Beecher, H. K.
　1956　Relationship of Significance of Wound to the Pain Experienced. J. Amer. Med. Assoc. 161:1609–1613.
Carstairs, G. M. and R. L. Kapur
　1976　The Great Universe of Kota: Stress, Change and Mental Disorder in an Indian Village. Berkeley: University of California Press.
Cay, E. L., A. E. Phillips, W. P. Small, et al.
　1975　Patients' Assessment of the Result of Surgery for Peptic Ulcer. Lancet 1:29–31.
Cohn, A. E.
　1924　Purposes in Medical Research: an Introduction to the Journal of Clinical Investigation. J. Clin. Invest. 1:1–11.
Cohn, A. E.
　1928　Medicine and Science. J. Philos. 25:403–416. Cited in Geison, G. L. op cit.
Conrad, P.
　1975　The Discovery of Hyperkinesis: Notes on the Medicalization of Deviant Behavior. Soc. Problems 23:12–21.
Crapanzano, V.
　1973　The Hamadsha: A Study in Moroccan Ethnopsychiatry. Berkeley: University of California Press.
Dubos, R.
　1959　Mirage of Health: Utopias, Progress and Biological Change. New York: Harper Brothers.
Duffy, J.
　1979　The Healers: A History of American Medicine. Urbana: University of Illinois Press, pp. 180–188.
Edelstein, L.
　1967a Ancient Medicine. Baltimore: The Johns Hopkins Press, pp. 87–110; 319–366.
Edelstein, L.
　1967b The Idea of Progress in Classical Antiquity. Baltimore: The Johns Hopkins Press.
Eisenberg, L.
　1977　Disease and Illness: Distinctions between Professional and Popular Ideas of Sickness. Culture, Medicine and Psychiatry 1:9–23.
Eisenberg, L.
　1980　What Makes Persons "Patients" and Patients "Well?" Amer. J. Med. 169:277–286.
Flexner, A.
　1910　Medical Education in the United States and Canada. Carnegie Foundation for the Advancement of Teaching, Boston: D. B. Updike, The Merrymount Press.

Fortune, R. F.
  1932 Sorcers of Dobu. New York: Dutton.
Fox, R.
  1977 The Medicalization and Demedicalization of American Society. Daedalus 106: 9–22.
Gajdusek, D. C. and C. J. Gibbs
  1975 Slow Virus Infections of the Nervous System. In The Nervous System Vol. 2: The Clinical Neurosciences. Chase (ed.) New York: Raven Press, pp. 113–135.
Garrod, A.
  1923 Inborn Errors of Metabolism. London: Oxford University Press.
Gruenberg, E. M.
  1978 The Failures of Success. Milbank Mem. Fund. Quart. 55:3–24.
Hanna, E.
  1978 Attitudes Toward Problem Drinkers: a Critical Factor in Treatment Recommendations. Quart. J. Stud. Alcohol 39:98–109.
Helman, C. G.
  1978 'Feed a Cold, Starve a Fever' — Folk Models of Infection in an English Suburban Community and Their Relation to Medical Treatment. Culture, Medicine and Psychiatry 2:107–138.
Henderson, L. J.
  1935 Pareto's General Sociology: A Physician's Interpretation. Cambridge: Harvard University Press.
Henderson, L. J.
  1936 The Practice of Medicine as Applied Sociology. Trans. Assoc. Amer. Physicians 51:8–22.
Holtzman, N. A.
  1977 The Goal of Preventing Early Death. In Conditions for Change in the Health Care System, Washington: DHEW Publ. No. (HRA) 78–642, pp. 107–132.
Horton, R.
  1967 African Traditional Thought and Western Science. Africa 37:50–71; 155–187.
Hulka, B., L. L. Kupper, and J. C. Cassell
  1972 Determinants of Physician Utilization. Med. Care 10:300–309.
Ingham, J. G. and P. McC. Miller
  1976 The Concept of Prevalence Applied to Psychiatric Disorders and Symptoms. Psychol. Med. 6:217–226.
Jacobi, A.
  1908 Nihilism and Drugs. N.Y. State J. Med. 8:57–65. Cited in Rosenberg, C. E. op cit.
Janzen, J.
  1978 The Comparative Study of Medical Systems as Changing Social Systems. Soc. Sci. Med. 12(2B):121–130.
Robert Wood Johnson Foundation
  1978 Special Report — Access. Princeton, N.J. 08540, P.O. Box 2316.
King, L. S.
  1958 The Medical World of the Eighteenth Century. Chicago: University of Chicago Press, pp. 237–239.
Kitagawa, E. M. and P. Hauser
  1973 Differential Mortality in the United States: A Study in Socioeconomic Epidemiology. Cambridge: Harvard University Press.
Kleinman, A. M.
  1973 Medicine's Symbolic Reality. Inquiry 16:203–216.
Kleinman, A.
  1980 Patients and Healers in the Context of Culture. Berkeley: University of California Press.

Kleinman, A., L. Eisenberg, and B. Good
    1978 Culture, Illness and Care. Ann. Int. Med. 88:251–258.
Knowles, J.
    1977 Doing Better and Feeling Worse: Health in the United States. New York: Norton.
Kunstadter, P.
    1975 Do Cultural Differences Make Any Difference? Choice Points in Medical Systems
          Available in Northwestern Thailand. *In* Medicine in Chinese Cultures. Kleinman,
          A. et al. (eds.) Washington: DHEW Publication No. (NIH) 75–653, pp. 351–
          383.
Leslie, C. (ed.)
    1976 Asian Medical Systems. Berkeley: University of California Press.
Lewis, O.
    1951 Life in a Mexican Village: Tepoztlan Restudied. Urbana: University of Illinois
          Press.
Lindenbaum, S.
    1979 Kuru Sorcery: Disease and Danger in the New Guinea Highland. Palo Alto:
          Mayfield Publishing Company.
Mackenzie, J.
    1919 The Future of Medicine. Cited by Geison, G. L.: Divided We Stand: Physiologists
          and Clinicians in the American Context. *In* M. J. Vogel and C. E. Rosenberg op
          cit., pp. 67–90.
McDermott, W.
    1977 Medicine: the Public Good and One's Own. Persp. in Biol. and Med. 21:167–187.
McKeown, T.
    1976 The Role of Medicine: Dream, Mirage or Nemesis? London: Nuffield Provincial
          Hospitals Trust.
Mechanic, D.
    1978 Effects of Psychological Distress on Perceptions of Physical Health and Use of
          Medical and Psychiatric Facilities. J. Human Stress 4:26–32.
Mechanic, D. and M. Newton
    1965 Some Problems in the Analysis of Morbidity Data. J. Chronic Dis. 18:569–580.
Mechanic, D. and E. H. Volkart
    1961 Stress, Illness Behavior and the Sick Role. Amer. Sociol. Rev. 26:51–58.
Millhauser, M.
    1973 Dr. Newton and Mr. Hyde: Scientists in Fiction from Swift to Stevenson. Nine-
          teenth Century Fiction 28:287–304.
National Center for Health Statistics
    1978 Health: United States. Washington: DHEW Publ. No. (PHS) 78–1232, pp. 174–
          175.
Osler, W.
    1920 Aequanimitas. 3rd edition. New York: McGraw-Hill, p. 254.
Peterson, W. L., R. A. L. Sturdevant, H. D. Frankl, et al.
    1977 Healing of Duodenal Ulcer with an Antacid Regimen. N. Eng. J. Med. 297:341–
          345.
Peabody, F. W.
    1930 Doctor and Patient. New York: The Macmillan Company.
Press, I.
    1969 Urban Illness: Physicians, Curers and Dual Use in Bogota. J. Health and Illness
          Behav. 10:209–218.
Richmond, J. B.
    1969 Currents in American Medicine: A Developmental View of Medical Care and
          Education. Cambridge: Harvard University Press, pp. 3–6.

CLINICAL SOCIAL SCIENCE 23

Roghmann, K. J. and R. J. Haggerty
  1973 Daily Stress, Illness and Use of Health Services in Young Families. Pediat. Res.
       7:520–526.
Rosenberg, C. E.
  1979 The Therapeutic Revolution: Medicine, Meaning and Social Change in Nineteenth
       Century America. *In* The Therapeutic Revolution: Essays in the Social History of
       American Medicine. M. J. Vogel and C. E. Rosenberg, eds. pp. 3–26. Philadelphia:
       University of Pennsylvania Press.
Shonkoff, J. P., P. H. Dworkin, A. Leviton, et al.
  1979 Primary Care Approaches to Developmental Disabilities. Pediatrics 64:506–514.
Shryock, R. H.
  1947 The American Physician in 1846 and 1946. J. Amer. Med. Assoc. 134:417–424.
Sigerist, H. E.
  1958 The Great Doctors. New York: Doubleday Anchor Books.
Stoeckle, J., I. K. Zola, and G. Davidson
  1964 The Quantity and Significance of Psychological Distress in Medical Practice.
       J. Chronic Dis. 17:959–970.
Strong, P.
  1978 The Alcoholic, the Sick Role and Bourgeois Medicine. Mimeographed.
Strong, P.
  1979 Sociological Imperialism and the Profession of Medicine: A Critical Examination
       of the Thesis of Medical Imperialism. Soc. Sci. Med. 13A:199–215.
Surgeon General
  1979 Healthy People. Washington: DHEW (PHS) Publ. No. 79–55071.
Susser, M.
  1974 Introduction to the Theme: a Critical Review of Sociology in Health. Int. J.
       Health Serv. 4:407–409.
Taussig, M. T.
  1980 Reification and the Consciousness of the Patient. Soc. Sci. Med. 14B:3–13.
Tessler, R., D. Mechanic, and M. Dimond
  1976 The Effect of Psychological Distress on Physician Utilization: a Prospective Study.
       J. Health Soc. Behav. 17:353–364.
Thomas, L.
  1977 On the Science and Technology of Medicine. Daedalus 106:35–46.
Turner, V.
  1967 The Forest of Symbols. Ithaca: Cornell University Press.
Twaddle, A.
  1977 Sickness Behavior and the Sick Role. Boston: Schenkman-Hall.
Unschuld, P. A.
  1979 Medical Ethics in Imperial China: A Study in Historical Anthropology. Berkeley:
       University of California Press.
Vogel, M. J. and C. E. Rosenberg, eds.
  1979 The Therapeutic Revolution: Essays in the Social History of American Medicine.
       Philadelphia: University of Pennsylvania Press.
White, K. L., T. F. Williams, and B. G. Greenberg
  1961 The Ecology of Medical Care. N. Eng. J. Med. 265:885–892.
Zola, I. K.
  1966 Culture and Symptoms: an Analysis of Patient's Presenting Complaints. Amer.
       Sociol. Rev. 31:615–630.
Zola, I. K.
  1972 Studying the Decision to See the Doctor. Advan. Psychosom. Med. 8:216–236.
Zola, I. K.
  1977 Healthism and Disabling Medicalisation. *In* Disabling Profesisons. I. Illich (ed.)
       London: Marion Boyars.

SECTION 1

HOW ACADEMIC PHYSICIANS VIEW THE SOCIAL SCIENCES

2. AN INFORMAL APPRAISAL OF THE CURRENT STATUS OF
'MEDICAL SOCIOLOGY'

Medical sociology has become a distinctive entity among the different disciplines associated with medicine. During the past decade alone, at least sixteen text-books[1] and two new journals[2] have appeared with titles that contain some combination or congeners of *sociology* and *medicine*; and appropriate articles on this topic have begun to occur with increasing frequency in traditional medical journals.[3]

Like many disciplines that were initially created as hybrids, medical sociology is not easy to describe; and its definition, content, and scope have varied greatly with each author who attempts a description. The diverse rubrics and topics that seem to be included in *medical sociology* can be summarized with the following array of nouns and prepositions:

(1) *Sociology in Medicine*. This rubric contains perhaps the most common of the different ideas about medical sociology. It refers to the way that social phenomena can either predispose people to the development of disease or affect their medical and other behavior after disease has occurred. Examples of such topics are the prevalence and incidence of disease in different socioeconomic classes, and the way that social factors may influence both the itinerary that leads to medical care when illness occurs and the patient's compliance with therapeutic recommendations. Classically these topics have been regarded as part of traditional medical education, but they are often neglected in an age of technology and hence tend to receive special emphasis as a part of medical sociology.

(2) *Sociology of Medicine*. This rubric refers to the various medical personnel, administrative arrangements, community resources, or other social structures that are involved in the delivery of health care. The rubric includes topics often previously cited under such titles as health care systems, health care delivery, medical manpower, training of paramedical personnel, etc.

(3) *Sociology for Medicine*. This rubric refers to clinical or investigative contributions that employ the methodologic strategies of sociology. It includes the techniques (described with such eponyms as Thurstone, Likert, and Guttman) that are used to create attitudinal scales and ratings for previously unmeasured entities, such as patient satisfaction with medical care. The rubric also includes certain multivariate mathematical procedures, such as factor analysis and path analysis, that are often used in the statistical appraisals of sociologic data.

(4) *Sociology from Medicine*: In this rubric, medical people become the social groups whose education, behavior, and professional life-styles are described as a subject of sociologic investigation. Examples of such research are Fox's well-known studies of physicians and patients at a clinical investigative unit (1959) and of the "socialization" that occurs during the education of medical students

27

L. Eisenberg and A. Kleinman (eds.), The Relevance of Social Science for Medicine, 27–48.
Copyright © 1980 by D. Reidel Publishing Company.

(1957). Certain other studies, such as Duff and Hollingshead's (1968) appraisal of in-patient care and Freidson's commentaries on issues of "dominance" (1970) and "control" (1975), provide critical (and often controversial) evaluations of professional activities.

(5) *Sociology at Medicine*: This rubric contains issues in political orientation and ideology. Such issues were being discussed more than a century ago by Rudolf Virchow (Miller 1973) who said, "Medicine is a social science and politics nothing else but medicine on a large scale". Authors of modern treatises in this field appraise (and usually condemn) the current structure of medical care within Western society, with recommendations for drastic changes in medicine, society, or both. Perhaps the best known of these treatises is Ivan Illich's *Medical Nemesis* (1976). Other authors have commented on the medicosociologic virtues of Marxism (Navarro 1977, Waitzkin and Waterman 1974), and the importance of social medicine as a substitute for the alleged failures of clinical medicine (Carlson 1975, McKeown 1976).

(6) *Sociology around Medicine*: This rubric refers to interactions, analogous to the five types just cited, that occur between medicine and several other social sciences, such as economics, anthropology, and ethnology. The rubric might also contain room for the medical activities and relationships of workers in such fields as ethics, philosophy, law, and linguistics.

These different rubrics and contributions from medical sociology have evoked, as might be expected, a variety of reactions from members of the academic and practicing community. Our general impression of these reactions, before undertaking any specific research, was as follows:

Sociology in Medicine has usually been welcomed and applauded for its obvious importance, although some medical educators believe that the material – being neither substantially new nor different from what was known and taught in the past – sometimes receives a distorted emphasis that suggests that its existence was first revealed by sociologists. *Sociology of Medicine* is generally regarded as a rearrangement of topics traditionally taught as part of what was formerly called public health. The methodologic contributions of *Sociology for Medicine* are readily accepted when useful, although the value of the methods has seldom been carefully tested against alternative techniques. *Sociology from Medicine*, a reasonable research activity for sociologists, has usually evoked satisfactory cooperation from the medical people under study although they do not always agree with the sociologic interpretation of the results. *Sociology at Medicine* has been a troublesome domain for many clinicians, who believe their distinctive concerns for individual people are lost in collectivist beliefs about society, and whose generally conservative political views have clashed with the strongly liberal, often radical positions of many sociologists. A few physicians have even contended that certain sociologists "love mankind but hate people". Since the last rubric, *Sociology around Medicine*, includes a series of non-sociologic disciplines, opinions about the roles of each of these disciplines in medicine are as varied as those just cited for the roles of sociology.

Among medical suggestions for improving the function of medical sociologists has been the proposal that they become more oriented toward social interventions in a manner analogous to clinicians' therapeutic activities. Such interventions might include "large-scale behaviour modification" with respect to "the dangers of smoking, over-eating, not wearing seat-belts and so on" (Lancet 1976). From sociologists have come two sets of warnings. One of these is that certain sociologic critiques of "medical expansion" have been "misleading or exaggerated", and that sociologists need to beware of their own "sociological imperialism" (Strong 1979). The other warning refers to "the dilution or alteration of sociological perspectives" that may occur during collaboration "with members of powerful disciplines and professions" (Gold 1977).

Because of the growing attention and importance given to medical sociology, the editors of this book asked us to appraise the current and potential contributions of this new discipline. Rather than trying to review a vast literature and arriving at what would be merely a composite of two personal opinions, we decided to solicit comments from leaders who observe the scope of what is happening in medical education and practice today. This report contains the results of what was learned in that survey.

METHODS

To determine perceptions and attitudes about the current state of medical sociology, we sent a questionnaire to the chairpersons of Departments of Medicine, Pediatrics and Family Medicine at each medical school in the United States. To avoid any constraints on the scope of the inquiry, we deliberately did not define medical sociology, hoping that its contents would emerge from the responses received to the questions. The questionnaire, which is shown in the Appendix, was intended to be short enough to evoke a reply, but open-ended enough to allow diverse responses that were not restricted to a "check list". (The design of the questionnaire was discussed with Professor Renée Fox, to whom we are grateful for many useful suggestions, although she is not responsible for the final format.) In an appended covering letter, which is also shown in the Appendix, the purpose of the questionnaire was explained.

Except for a difference in the title of the department and a different color of paper for each department, the wording of the questionnaire was identical for all recipients, whose names were obtained from rosters of three American academic societies of "chairpersons": The Association of Professors of Medicine, the Association of Pediatric Chairmen and the Association of Chairmen of Family Medicine. Although the questionnaires could have been returned anonymously, most respondents identified themselves, so that recipients who failed to answer the initial request could be solicited a second time.

The results were tabulated from the total responses available after the second mailing. The response rates for the chairpersons were 111/129 (86%) among internists, 106/125 (85%) among pediatricians, and 70/101 (70%) among family medicine physicians. The relatively high rates of response were gratifying and encouraged further analysis of the data.

RESULTS

The results are presented in sections relating to each of the questions that was asked. For each question, the responses are divided according to departmental sources. In several instances, the results are cited entirely within the text, but most of the data is presented in separate tables.

Question #1: In your institution do the medical students receive formal instruction in medical sociology during the pre-clinical years? Table 1 shows that about 50% of medicine, 40% of pediatrics and 40% of family medicine chairpersons said medical sociology was formally taught to medical students. The departments mainly responsible for the teaching, when done, were psychiatry and behavioral

TABLE 1

Is medical sociology formally taught to medical students?

	Number of responses by chairpersons of		
Responses	Medicine	Pediatrics	Family medicine
Yes:	56	47	28
No:	46	39	20
Don't know:	9	20	11
Did not answer:	0	0	11
Departments responsible for instruction*			
Psychiatry and Behavioral science	20	20	13
Community medicine	19	13	14
Preventive medicine	12	3	5
Family medicine	9	5	14
Medicine	7**	4**	2
Pediatrics	1	8	1
Public health/epidemiology	4	1	6
Sociology/social medicine	5	5	0
Others (anthropology; obstetrics and gynecology; rehabilitation medicine; history of medicine; primary care)	3	10	5

* Number of involved departments add up to more than the *yes* answers because of teaching by multiple departments in many institutions.
** As part of introduction to clinical medicine.

sciences, community medicine, and preventive medicine. Other involved departments included family medicine, medicine (primarily as a part of the Introduction to Clinical Medicine), pediatrics, public health and community medicine, sociology and social medicine. In many instances, teaching was a multidisciplinary effort, involving participation by two, three or even more departments.

Departments answering the questionnaire invariably seemed to be more aware of their own participation than that of other primary care departments. In pediatrics, for example, eight pediatric chairmen cited the department of pediatrics as a participant in the teaching of medical sociology, but only one chairperson each in family medicine and medicine was aware of participation by the department of pediatrics.

Results of the next three questions are summarized in Table 2.

TABLE 2

Is formal instruction in medical sociology given by your department during . . .

	Number of chairpersons responding		
	Medicine	Pediatrics	Family medicine
. . . *Clerkships for medical students?*			
Yes	13 (12%)	27 (26%)	24 (34%)
No	98	78	46
Not answered	0	1	0
. . . *Programs for house officers?*			
Yes	15 (14%)	31 (30%)	32 (47%)
No	96	74	36
Not answered	0	1	2
. . . *Grand rounds or conferences*			
Yes	49 (44%)	74 (64%)	46 (68%)
No	62	42	22
Not answered	9	0	2

Question #2: During a major clerkship in your clinical discipline do students receive any formal instruction in medical sociology? The top segment of Table 2 shows that formal instruction in medical sociology occurred in only 13 of 111 departments of medicine, 27 of 106 departments of pediatrics, and 24 of 70 departments of family medicine. These data show a clear gradient of "instruction", from 12% in medicine to 26% in pediatrics and 34% in family medicine.

Question #3: Do residents in your program receive any formal instruction in medical sociology? The middle section of Table 2 shows that formal instruction in medical sociology was part of the house officers' curriculum in only 14% of departments of medicine, but in 30% of departments of pediatrics and in nearly half the departments of family medicine.

Question #4: Do your Grand Rounds or teaching rounds contain topics in medical sociology? As shown in the bottom section of Table 2, medical sociology was "discussed" more often than it was "taught". Subjects defined as being within the purview of medical sociology were presented at Grand Rounds or conferences in almost half the departments of medicine and in about two-thirds of the departments of pediatrics and family medicine.

Each of the foregoing questions also asked about the time committed to instruction in medical sociology for clinical clerks and house officers, and in conferences. Table 3 shows the responses. *Substantial teaching* to clinical clerks and house officers was defined as at least one conference a week, and *substantial involvement* in conferences and Grand Rounds was defined as more than four conferences a year. The results show that even when the curriculum for medical students and house officers included medical sociology, the time allotted was sporadic in departments of medicine, considerably greater in departments of pediatrics, and substantial in departments of family medicine. The ascending gradient of involvement from medicine to pediatrics to family medicine was again evident.

TABLE 3

Time commitment to instruction in medical sociology

Time committed	Number of chairpersons responding*		
	Medicine	Pediatrics	Family medicine
For medical students			
Substantial	3	9	18
Sporadic	10	18	2
For house officers			
Substantial	3	16	18
Sporadic	12	15	6
In grand rounds and conferences			
Substantial	5	15	16
Sporadic	41	47	17

* Numbers do not equal those in Table 2 because not all respondents answered question concerning time commitment.

Another section in questions 2—4 asked about the topics covered during the instruction. Table 4 summarizes the multiplicity of topics indicated as being in the realm of medical sociology. These topics were arbitrarily classified into five major categories. The first two, personal behavior (subdivided into activities of daily living, causes of illness, and response to illness) and interpersonal behavior are part of *Sociology in Medicine*. The next three categories — physician behavior, the community and the environment, and organization of health care — constitute part of *Sociology of Medicine*.

TABLE 4

Topics cited as covered in courses and conferences defined as medical sociology

I.   *Personal behavior*
     A. *Daily living*: nutrition; growth and development; health status; sexuality; contraception; abortion; delinquency; guidance and counseling; mystical beliefs.
     B. *Causes of illness*: perinatal problems; mental retardation; poisoning; accidents; alcoholism; drug abuse; lifestyle; venereal disease; suicide.
     C. *Response to illness*: detection of genetic diseases; ethnic or cultural values; perception of health care system; compliance with health behavior; chronic illness and disability; depression; attitude toward specific diseases — cancer, chronic renal failure, diabetes (diabetic recidivism).

II. *Interpersonal behavior*
     Family structure and function; birthing; parenting; child abuse; multiply deformed child; failure to thrive; sudden infant death; adoption; school problems; teenage pregnancy; aging.

III. *Physician behavior*
     Communication with parents; behavior of medical students; informed consent; malpractice; stress on physicians; ethical dilemmas; aging; death and dying.

IV. *The community and the environment*
     Socio-cultural influences on decision making; community resources; child advocacy; child care centers; health care in the third world; care and housing of the aged; cats and dogs as a menace.

V.   *Organization of care*
     Patterns of health care delivery; primary care; health planning; physician distribution; role of nurse practitioners; the health care team; cost/benefit analysis; technology assessment; cost of illness; other economic issues.

Within these broad classifications, the topics varied widely. For example, the subjects included among activities of daily living ranged from nutrition and growth and development to mystical beliefs. Among causes of illness were mental retardation, poisoning, accidents, alcoholism, drug abuse, and suicide. The topics included in "response to illness" were detection of genetic diseases, the role of ethnicity, and response to chronic disease.

Although this inventory was noted among responses from all three primary care specialities, the topics of child abuse, poisoning, teenage pregnancy, and child advocacy were mentioned most frequently in responses from chairpersons of departments of pediatrics. Responses from internal medicine dealt largely with aging, chronic illness and disability, and attitudes toward cancer, chronic renal failure, and diabetes as well as with death and dying. Responses from family medicine emphasized the role of the health care team, the structure and function of the family, and sociocultural influences on decision making. Other issues included such global problems as technology assessment and physician distribution as well as home-spun topics, such as "cats and dogs as a menace."

Question #5: Does anyone teach medical sociology in your department? As shown in Table 5, 20% of departments of medicine contained faculty who taught medical sociology. The corresponding percentages were 33% for departments of pediatrics and 57% for departments of family medicine. The proportions of faculty members with primary academic appointments in the clinical department were 73% for medicine, 80% for pediatrics, and 90% for family practice, but many of these faculty had joint appointments, usually in psychiatry, community medicine, or preventive medicine. In departments of pediatrics and family medicine, many faculty teachers of medical sociology were medical social workers, but the faculty in departments of medicine contained few medical social workers. The department of medicine teachers were usually generalists who were active in ambulatory care programs or in student health services.

TABLE 5

Location of faculty who teach medical sociology

Faculty in department	Number of chairpersons responding		
	Medicine	Pediatrics	Family medicine
No answer	0	1	1
No	89 (80%)	70 (67%)	30 (43%)
Yes	22 (20%)	35 (33%)	39 (57%)
Primary appointment in department	16 (73%)	28 (80%)	35 (90%)
Primary appointment elsewhere	6 (27%)	7 (20%)	4 (10%)

Table 6 shows the answers to Question 6, which was concerned with research in medical sociology. The occurrence rates of research activity showed the same gradients noted previously: 21% in departments of medicine, 34% in departments of pediatrics, and 41% in departments of family medicine. The research topics that were cited contained 20 issues in *Sociology in Medicine* and 11 issues in *Sociology of Medicine*. Topics pursued by investigators in all three clinical

TABLE 6

Research in medical sociology

Presence of research	Number of chairpersons responding		
	Medicine	Pediatrics	Family medicine
Yes	23 (21%)	35 (34%)	28 (41%)
No	87	68	41
Not answered	1	3	1

Topics covered

Sociology in medicine

Health status	+	+	
Growth and development		+	
Preventive care	+		
Health and illness behavior	+		+
Parental behavior		+	
Communication skills of children		+	
Self-opinion of children		+	
Family interaction			+
Failure to thrive		+	
Child abuse		+	
Problems of adolescence		+	+
Delinquency		+	
Mental retardation		+	
MD/Pt relationship	+		
Patient compliance	+	+	+
Patient's perception of care	+		
Sociocultural influences on decision making	+	+	+
Adaptation to chronic illness	+	+	
Geriatric issues	+		+
Rural health			+
Guidance and counseling		+	
Community resources		+	
Organization of care	+	+	
Ethical problems		+	
Screening		+	
Cost of technology	+		
Nurse practitioners	+	+	+
Cost containment	+		
Medical costs	+		
Patterns of health delivery	+		
Career choices of family physicians			+

departments included patient compliance, sociocultural influences on patient and physician decision making, and the role of nurse practitioners. Other topics seemed to be determined by the differences in the clinical practices. Thus, geriatric problems were studied in departments of medicine and family medicine but not in pediatrics; whereas problems of adolescence were investigated in departments of pediatrics and family medicine, but not in internal medicine. Topics pursued in only a single department included child abuse (pediatrics) and family interaction, the career choices of family physicians and issues in rural health (family medicine). Although these topics were arbitrarily tabulated in one of the parent clinical departments, the research often involved collaboration with departments of community medicine, preventive medicine, behavioral science and psychiatry and with Schools of Public Health.

Question #7: What do you view as the main contribution that medical sociology makes to your teaching program? If it is not part of your teaching programs, please state the reasons. Answers to these two questions could not be easily quantified and are simply listed in Tables 7 and 8. The contributions of medical sociology seemed regarded more highly by respondents from departments of pediatrics and family medicine than from departments of medicine. All three

TABLE 7

Contributions of medical sociology

| | Positive responses noted from | | |
	Medicine	Pediatrics	Family medicine
Enhanced perspective of medicine	+		+
Better understanding of illness behavior	+	+	+
Awareness of community and society	+	+	+
Improved curriculum	+		+
Research design	+		+
Better patient care	+	+	+
More attention to outcome	+		
More humanistic care	+		
New data base	+		
Better records	+		
Awareness of community resources	+	+	+
Better family interaction	+		+
Appreciation of other cultures	+	+	+
Better understanding of emotional problems		+	
Death and dying		+	
Medical-legal issues		+	
Better physician			+
Better understanding of health care system			+
Better understanding of students			+
Holistic medicine			+
Management skills			+

TABLE 8

Reasons for absence of medical sociology from curriculum

Reason	Departments citing this reason		
	Medicine	Pediatrics	Family medicine
Low priority	+	+	+
Lack of faculty	+	+	+
Lack of interest by Dept.	+	+	
Lack of time in curriculum	+	+	+
Lack of relevance	+		
Lack of financial resources	+	+	+
Adequately covered by other departments	+		+
Lack of knowledge by chairperson	+		
No need for subject	+	+	+
Inertia	+		
School (department) too young to develop	+		+
Subject matter poorly defined		+	+
Peripheral to clinical core		+	
Inability to form meaningful relationships with social scientists		+	

types of respondents listed contributions that fell into four realms: a better understanding of illness behavior both by the patient and the physician; an enhanced awareness of the community and society and the associated effect on illness; better knowledge of community resources; and improved appreciation of social groups. In many instances, the contributions of medical sociology to improved care of minority groups, that have specific social needs, were cited. Other contributions listed by individual department respondents were an enhanced perspective of medicine, improved curriculum, an aid in research design, more attention to outcomes, better medical records, more humanistic care, better family interaction, better understanding of the issues surrounding death and dying, an emphasis on medical/legal issues, better understanding of health care systems, more empathy with students, and improved management skills. Several respondents indicated that medical sociology was prototypical of holistic medicine.

The reasons for the absence of medical sociology from the curriculum, as noted in Table 8, were remarkably uniform among the three departments. The most frequently cited problems were lack of faculty, lack of curricular time, and lack of financial resources. Several respondents from all three departments felt that this subject had relatively low priority, particularly in some new and developing schools that needed to put their resources into teaching the more classical subjects of the medical curriculum. Although quantitative data are not displayed in Table 8, lack of relevance or interest were cited less frequently by Departments of Pediatrics and Family Medicine than by Departments of Internal Medicine.

Question #8: What have you found most appealing about what medical sociology offers to clinicians? As shown in Table 9, about half of the responding internists and pediatricians did not answer this question, and a few explicitly said that medical sociology offered nothing. In contrast, only 26% of family physician respondents failed to answer this question. The distinction probably reflects the generally more positive attitude toward medical sociology held by family physicians in comparison to the "negativism" of many internists and some pediatricians.

TABLE 9

Appealing features of medical sociology

Question not answered	Medicine 56/111 (50%)	Pediatrics 57/106 (54%)	Family medicine 18/70 (26%)
Features cited in answers			
Effect of society on practice	+	+	+
Relationship of pt to health care system	+	+	
Md sensitivity to non-medical issues	+	+	+
Sociology of family	+	+	+
Problems of elderly	+		
Urban medicine	+		
Focuses on patient compliance	+	+	
Ecological aspects of pt care	+	+	
Improves MD's logic	+		
Codifies the art of medicine	+		
Alcoholism and drug addiction	+		
Focuses on pt role	+	+	+
Emphasis on ethical issues	+		
Appreciation of cost of medical care	+	+	
Health care facilities and community resources	+	+	
Matrial counseling	+		
Awareness of community		+	+
More comprehensive care		+	+
Demographic issues		+	+
Technology assessment		+	
Use of social workers		+	
Helpful in health care research		+	+
Emphasis on chronic illness		+	
Attention to environment		+	
Humanization of medicine			+

The appealing features mentioned most commonly were that medical sociology provided knowledge about the effect of society on practice, an enhanced sensitivity to non-medical issues, greater appreciation of the patient's role in his illness, and an emphasis on the role of the family on illness. Other appealing features were: the focusing of medical sociology on the health care system as opposed to individual care; the problems of urban health; the issues of compliance; the role of the environment; the emphasis on societal ills, such as alcoholism and drug addiction; and the issues of cost containment and technology assessment.

Question #9: What have you found least appealing about what medical sociology offers clinicians? As shown in Table 10, this question was not answered by about

TABLE 10

Unappealing features of medical sociology

	Medicine	Pediatrics	Family medicine
Question not answered	67/111 (60%)	65/106 (61%)	31/70 (44%)
Features cited in answers			
Data soft and unquantitative	+	+	+
Data base inaccurate	+	+	+
No value to clinicians	+		+
Deals in generalities	+		
Deals with large populations, not individuals pts	+	+	+
Anti-MD stance	+	+	
Tendency to oversimplify	+	+	
Emphasis on psychosocial factors	+		+
Anti-intellectual	+		
Naive	+		
Impractical		+	
Jargon; verbose		+	+
Lack of objectivity		+	+
Fuzzy-thinking		+	
Maternal-infant bonding		+	
Too many expensive and non-productive programs		+	
Defensive		+	
Use of questionnaire methodology		+	
9–5 work ethic		+	
Elitist		+	
Inappropriate		+	
Problems too great for solution		+	
Biased against family role			+
Dull			+
Doctrinaire			+
Excessive detail			+
No evidence for improved patient care			+

60% of internists and pediatricians and by almost half of the family physicians. The features cited in the answers are not quantified, but were relatively uniform. Many respondents complained that medical sociology deals with "soft data that is not quantifiable," and with large populations rather than individual patients. Other negative comments included references to an inaccurate data base; to the anti-physician stance of medical sociology; and to the tendency of medical sociologists to over-simplify, to be unobjective, and to express themselves in a peculiar jargon that was difficult for clinicians to grasp. The question evoked strong responses particularly from the internists, some of whom used extraordinary amounts of space or eloquence to express their negative feelings. Some of the comments are quoted here:

(Sociologists) offer hypotheses that are not testable, conclusions that are poorly supported by experimental observations and a flavor of historicism better suited to metaphysics than medicine.

Medical sociology is a cult – a 'sophist'-oriented activity which attempts to legitimize itself as a scientific discipline (logical positivism) which has been abandoned long ago. Unfortunately, it has been popularized by pandering to public and professional anxieties and has had an increasingly negative effect on the formulation of both medical curriculum and decision making.

It is dangerous to let sociologists into medical schools. They cause divisiveness by emphasizing differences in care rather than commonalities.

Sociologists think they have the answer to the human condition.

(sociologists) "can't present succinctly. They tend to 'bull-shit.' They talk in 'generalities' when clinicians need specifics.

poor preparation of hypotheses and broad conclusions based on inadequate thinking.

they teach student material that is inhibitory. We have to de-program students and re-program them.

Lack of competent scholars who can relate to internists in a relevant manner.

Little knowledge of area in which they take a role.

In all fairness, we would like to quote from enthusiastic supporters of medical sociology, and there were a number of these. However, they were not nearly as eloquent in expounding their positive views, as the detractors were in relieving themselves of their negative biases. Rather, their comments were more muted and their descriptions listed in Table 9 and the commentary on this table are accurate.

DISCUSSION

These results clearly demonstrate that activities in medical sociology have become a distinct part of the total spectrum of events in the "primary care" departments of medical schools. The proportion of medical sociology occupied in that spectrum is greater in family medicine than in pediatrics, and least in internal medicine. The enthusiasm for this new discipline has a similar gradient of distribution; and the amount of apathy or overt hostility has a reversed gradient, being greatest among internists and least among academic family medicine physicians.

The scope of topics noted as "medical sociology" suggests that much of this new discipline is not new. Many of the topics contained as part of *sociology in medicine* have been studied and taught by clinicians for many years, although the activities have generally been regarded as part of ambulatory care, "general medicine or pediatrics", or clinical "art". Some of the negative reactions expressed, particularly by internists, may reflect a resentment either of the sociologic intrusion on their "turf" or of the increased attention now being given, by medical sociologists and others, to problems that occur beyond the traditional scientific, in-patient setting of academic clinical medicine. Topics such as costs, organization of care, and patterns of delivery that are noted as *sociology of medicine* have also been studied and taught for many years, but these subjects have usually been addressed in departments having such names as public health, social medicine, or community medicine. The titular reassignment of these topics to medical sociology probably indicates their greater educational access to clinicians and their increasing prominence as issues requiring clinical attention.

Very few of the topics contained in the rubrics of sociology *for, from,* or *at medicine* were cited as receiving active attention in either clinical education or clinical research, even though these features of medical sociology could be regarded as having distinctively sociologic origins. The predominance noted for clinical and public health topics in "medical sociology" can therefore help explain some of the negative reactions by clinicians, who may view sociologists as lacking a unique or distinctive contribution to the medical arena and as being inadequately trained for the medical subjects they pursue. Without adequate clinical and public health exposure beyond the contents of the "basic science," a sociologist whose education has emphasized the data, methodology, and theoretical paradigms of sociology may be as unprepared for medical phenomena as a physician whose education was concentrated solely on molecular biology, biochemistry, and membrane physiology. Some suitable analogy of a clinical clerkship, internship, or residency may therefore be highly desirable for sociologists who plan to work in medical sociology, particularly in association with clinical departments.

Some of the people whose responses are included here complained about the questionnaire and the research itself. The most common complaint was that we had not defined *Medical Sociology*. The reasons for this decision were noted earlier. We also thought that a specific definition might inhibit the responders and that a thorough definition might take a great deal of space that we wanted to save for asking questions.

Several of the respondents, all in departments of family medicine, accused us of bias in designing the research. Because we thought (and still think) we prepared a straightforward, balanced set of questions, we were puzzled about the reason for this accusation until we recalled that the phrase "no-holds-barred" had been used by one of us during a burst of rhetorical exuberance while dictating the letter that accompanied the questionnaire. Although the idea might have been expressed more felicitously, it correctly describes what we wanted to do: to discover supporters with evangelistic fervor, detractors with troglodyte nihilism, and whatever is present between those two extremes. We wanted our work to provide a "no-holds-barred" appraisal, because we thought it would be important for everyone to learn the actual views that were held on both sides. Regardless of the opinions of any particular physician or sociologist, we think it is valuable to find out what is going on, to rate the positive contributions attributed to medical sociology, to learn the negative features that might be improved, and to recognize the kind of opposition that must be overcome before this new discipline is fully accepted.

We should like, however, to cite a different reason for suggesting that our survey is biased: it is concerned only with medical sociology. If a similar survey were done to appraise the value of other components of medical education, such as molecular biology, community medicine, psychiatry, or surgery, the results might show similar polarities of opinion. We would also be curious to learn the results of an analogous questionnaire — concerned with the merits of internal medicine, pediatrics, and family medicine — sent to the chairpersons of departments of biochemistry, microbiology, and physiology. We shall leave that project for other investigators.

Finally, several respondents to the questionnaire wondered why we had not cited the authorization for the research and the agency supporting it. In an era of grantsmanship and massive team performances, these respondents may not have believed in the archaic, rugged nostalgia that allowed a research survey to be performed by two individuals, who planned their study mostly by long-distance telephone and who performed the work without a specific grant or project site visits, neglected the anointment of multiple institutional review committees, operated without a large consortium of technical advisers and assistants, and who tabulated the data by a manual process. Besides ourselves, our secretaries, and the single consultant we cited earlier, the entire research "team" consisted of one person who helped compile the bibliography. The result may not contain the reliability, validity, or profundity of a more formal professional project, but we met the deadline imposed for completing the manuscript, we had fun working on it, and we think the results are worthwhile.

NOTES

1. *The cited textbooks are*:
   Coe, R. M.
      1970 Sociology of Medicine. New York: McGraw-Hill.
   Cox, C. and A. Mead, eds.
      1975 A Sociology of Medical Practice. London: Collier-Macmillan.

Denton, J. A.
    1978 Medical Sociology. Boston: Houghton-Mifflin.
Fabrega, H., Jr.
    1974 Disease and Social Behavior: An Interdisciplinary Perspective. Cambridge,
          Massachusetts: MIT Press.
Freeman, H. E., S. Levine and L. G. Reeder, eds.
    1979 Handbook of Medical Sociology, III. Englewood Cliffs, New Jersey: Prentice-
          Hall.
Jones, R. K. and P. A. Jones
    1975 Sociology in Medicine. London: English Universities Press.
Litman, T. J.
    1976 The Sociology of Medicine and Health Care: A Research Bibliography. San
          Francisco: Boyd and Fraser.
Mechanic, D.
    1978 Medical Sociology. New York: Free Press.
Robertson, L. S. and M. C. Heagarty
    1975 Medical Sociology. A General Systems Approach. Chicago: Nelson-Hall.
Robinson, D.
    1978 Patients, Practitioners, and Medical Care: Aspects of Medical Sociology, II.
          London: Heinemann Medical Books.
Schwartz, H. D. and C. S. Kart, eds.
    1978 Dominant Issues in Medical Sociology. Reading, Massachusetts: Addison-
          Wesley.
Susser, M. W. and W. Watson
    1971 Sociology in Medicine. London: Oxford University Press.
Tuckett, D., ed.
    1976 An Introduction to Medical Sociology. London: Tavistock Publications.
Tuckett, D. and J. M. Kaufert, eds.
    1978 Basic Readings in Medical Sociology. London: Tavistock Publications.
Twaddle, A. C. and R. M. Hessler
    1977 A Sociology of Health. St. Louis: C. V. Mosby.
Wilson, R. N.
    1970 The Sociology of Health. New York: Random House.

2. *The cited journals are*:
Journal of Health and Social Behavior. Social Science and Medicine.

3. *The cited journal articles are*:
Chaska, N. L.
    1977 Medical Sociology for Whom? Mayo Clinic Proceedings 52:813–818.
Eisenberg, J. M.
    1979 Sociological Influences on Decision-making by Clinicians. Annals of Internal
          Medicine 90:957–964.
Hull, F. M.
    1972 Social Class and the General Practitioner. Practitioner 209:698–699.
Kleinman, A., L. Eisenberg and B. Good
    1978 Culture, Illness, and Care. Clinical Lessons from Anthropologic and Cross-
          cultural Research. Annals of Internal Medicine 88:251–258.
Najman, J. M., G. Isaacs and M. Siskind
    1978 Teaching Sociology to Medical Students. Medical Education 12:406–412.
Skyler, J. S., ed.
    1971 Symposium on Social Issues and Medicine. Archives of Internal Medicine
          127:49–110.

REFERENCES

Carlson, R. J.
  1975 The End of Medicine. New York: John Wiley.
Duff, R. S. and A. B. Hollingshead
  1968 Sickness and Society. New York: Harper and Row.
Fox, R. C.
  1957 Training for Uncertainty. In The Student-Physician: Introductory Studies in the
        Sociology of Medical Education. Merton, R., G. C. Reader and P. Kendall, eds.
        Cambridge, Massachusetts: Harvard University Press.
Fox, R. C.
  1959 Experiment Perilous. Physicians and Patients Facing the Unknown. New York:
        Free Press.
Freidson, E.
  1970 Professional Dominance: The Structure of Medical Care. New York: Atherton
        Press.
Freidson, E.
  1975 Doctoring Together: A Study of Professional Social Control. New York: Elsevier.
Gold, M.
  1977 A Crisis of Identity: The Case of Medical Sociology. Journal of Health and Social
        Behavior 18:160–168.
Illich, I.
  1976 Medical Nemesis: The Expropriation of Health. New York: Pantheon.
Lancet (editorial)
  1976 How Many Fingers in the Pie? Lancet 2:615.
McKeown, T.
  1976 The Role of Medicine: Dream, Mirage or Nemesis? London: Nuffield Provincial
        Hospitals Trust.
Miller, H.
  1973 Medicine and Society. London: Oxford University Press.
Navarro, V.
  1977 Social Security and Medicine in the U.S.S.R.: A Marxist Critique. Lexington,
        Massachusetts: Lexington Books.
Strong, P. M.
  1979 Sociological Imperialism and the Profession of Medicine. A Critical Examination
        of the Thesis of Medical Imperialism. Social Science and Medicine 13A:199–
        215.
Waitzkin, H. and B. Waterman
  1974 The Exploitation of Illness in Capitalist Society. Indianapolis: Bobbs-Merrill.

In addition to specifically cited references, the following publications are of interest:

Aakster, C. W.
  1972 Socio-cultural Variables in the Etiology of Health Disturbances: A Sociological
        Approach. Thesis. Groningen.
Berlant, J. L.
  1975 Profession and Monopoly: A Study of Medicine in the United States and Great
        Britain. Berkeley: University of California Press.
Bloom, S. W.
  1965 The Doctor and his Patient: A Sociological Interpretation. New York: Free
        Press.
Bosk, C. L.
  1979 Forgive and Remember: Managing Medical Failure. Chicago: University of Chicago
        Press.

Brenner, M. H.
  1973 Mental Illness and the Economy. Cambridge, Massachusetts: Harvard University
        Press.
Dreitzel, H. P.
  1971 The Social Organization of Health. New York: Macmillan.
Elling, R. H. and M. Sokolowska, eds.
  1978 Medical Sociologists at Work. Edison, New Jersey: Transaction Books.
Fox, R. C. and J. P. Swazey
  1978 The Courage to Fail: A Social View of Organ Transplants and Dialysis, II. Chicago:
        University of Chicago Press.
Freidson, E.
  1970 Profession of Medicine: A Study of the Sociology of Applied Knowledge. New
        York: Dodd, Mead.
Freidson, E. and J. Lorber, eds.
  1972 Medical Men and their Work. Chicago: Aldine-Atherton.
Henry, J. P. and P. M. Stevens
  1977 Stress, Health, and the Social Environment: A Sociobiologic Approach to Medi-
        cine. New York: Springer-Verlag.
Hollingshead, A. B. and F. C. Redlich
  1958 Social Class and Mental Illness. New York: John Wiley.
Kosa, J., A. Antomovsky and I. K. Zola, eds.
  1969 Poverty and Health: A Sociological Analysis. Cambridge, Massachusetts: Harvard
        University Press.
Merton, R. K., G. C. Reader and P. Kendall, eds.
  1957 The Student-Physician: Introductory Studies in the Sociology of Medical Educa-
        tion. Cambridge, Massachusetts: Harvard University Press.
Millman, M.
  1977 The Unkindest Cut: Life in the Backrooms of Medicine. New York: William
        Morrow.
Straus, R.
  1957 The Nature and Status of Medical Sociology. American Sociological Review
        22:200–204.
Vernon, G. M.
  1970 Sociology of Death: An Analysis of Death-Related Behavior. New York: Ronald
        Press.

UNIVERSITY OF WASHINGTON
SEATTLE, WASHINGTON 98195

Department of Medicine, RG–20 September 11, 1978
Office of the Chairman

Dear

Dr. Alvan Feinstein, Professor of Medicine and Epidemiology, and I have been invited to write a no-holds-barred evaluation of the contributions that medical sociology makes to education, research, and practice in primary care.

We decided that the best evaluation we might offer was to perform an objective survey of what was actually happening in medical education and to obtain the opinions of the academic clinicians who were most directly concerned.

Accordingly, the enclosed questionnaire is being sent to you and to all other Chairpersons of Departments of Family Practice in American medical schools. Because we know how busy you are, we have deliberately kept the questionnaire simple, short, and easy to answer. In order for the survey results to be meaningful, we need a high rate of response. I hope you will take a few minutes of your time now to answer the nine questions and to return it to me in the enclosed envelope.

Since the responses are anonymous, we have no way of letting you know the results. If you want to know them, please note your name and address on your response (or send your identity data in a separate letter) and we shall send you a summary of the findings. The detailed results will be published as a chapter in a forthcoming book, but we may also prepare a separate paper for the medical literature.

We shall be most grateful for the information you supply and we thank you for your cooperation.

Very sincerely yours,

Robert G. Petersdorf, M.D.
Professor and Chairman

RGP:cr

enclosure

Telephone: (206) 543-3293

QUESTIONNAIRE ON MEDICAL SOCIOLOGY

During the past few decades, Medical Sociology has been developed as a new discipline in which the concerns, methods, data, and principles of Sociology are applied to problems in medical care and health services. The purpose of this questionnaire is to obtain information about the way in which medical sociology has become (or has failed to become) a part of programs in clinical education and research. Because we have been asked to write an evaluation of the contributions of medical sociology to primary care specialties, our goal here is simply to find out what has been happening and what clinicians think about this subject. We shall be grateful for your candid responses to the questions that follow.

1. At your institution, do the medical students receive formal instruction in medical sociology during the pre-clinical years?   YES ☐   NO ☐ DON'T KNOW ☐   If YES, please indicate what department is responsible for the instruction.

2. During a major clerkship in your clinical discipline, do students receive any formal instruction in medical sociology?   YES ☐   NO ☐ If answer is YES, how much time is devoted and what topics are covered?

3. Do residents in your program receive any formal instruction in medical sociology?   YES ☐   NO ☐   If answer is YES, how much time is devoted and what topics are covered?

4. Do your grand rounds or teaching rounds contain topics in medical sociology? YES ☐   NO ☐   If answer is YES, how often and what topics are covered?

(over)

5. Does anyone teach medical sociology in your department? YES ☐   NO ☐
   If answer is YES, please indicate the faculty title and primary faculty appointment of the teacher(s).

6. Is anyone in your department doing research in medical sociology?   YES ☐
   NO ☐   If YES, what are the main topics under study?

7. What do you view as the main contribution that medical sociology makes to your teaching program? If medical sociology is not a part of your teaching program, please cite the reasons.

8. What have you found most appealing about what medical sociology offers clinicians? (Please include any published work that you think is particularly valuable.)

9. What have you found least appealing about what medical sociology offers clinicians? (Please include any published work that you think is particularly objectionable.)

Please use the rest of this page (or separate pages) for any additional comments you would like to offer.

PLEASE RETURN QUESTIONNAIRE TO: Dr. Robert G. Petersdorf
                                  Professor and Chairman
                                  Department of Medicine, RG 20
                                  University of Washington
                                  School of Medicine
                                  Seattle, Washington 98195

SECTION 2

SOCIAL SUPPORTS: INFLUENCES ON HEALTH AND ILLNESS

LISA F. BERKMAN

3. PHYSICAL HEALTH AND THE SOCIAL ENVIRONMENT: A SOCIAL EPIDEMIOLOGICAL PERSPECTIVE

Social variations in the distribution of health and disease have been observed for centuries; however, the reasons for these differences in physical health status are not well understood. For many years, it was assumed that these differences could be explained by variations in ethnicity or genetic stock, exposures to noxious stimuli in the physical environment, or access to medical care resources. While these factors undoubtedly account for some of the differences in disease rates among members of different social groups, evidence is now beginning to accumulate which indicates that certain conditions and circumstances within the social environment or socio-cultural milieu *per se* have disease consequences. It is these factors which are in the purview of the social epidemiologist.

In general, we might say that epidemiologists study the distribution of a disease or physical condition in human populations and factors that influence the distribution (Lilienfeld 1976). Social epidemiologists focus further on social conditions and disease processes (Syme 1974). Even though the boundaries of social epidemiology are somewhat vague and overlap with those of medical sociology and psychology and psychosomatic medicine, within this segment of social science and medicine collaboration, there is a primary concern with psychosocial determinants of the following: (a) illness or disease onset (incidence of new events), (b) course of illness or disease (exacerbations, repeat events), and (c) outcome of disease process and/or degree of recovery (Kasl 1977; Kasl and Berkman 1979).

In the first part of this paper, several examples of the ways in which the social environment may have an impact on health status are presented. These are meant more as illustrative cases rather than comprehensive reviews of socio-environmental variables and their relations to physical health status. For several more comprehensive reviews on this subject, the reader is referred to works by Cassel (1976), Antonovsky (1967), Syme (1967), Fox (1978) and Jenkins (1976). A serious concern in regard to the relationship between socio-environmental variables and health status is the mechanism(s) by which such environmental variables are linked to actual pathological/disease processes. Although there is not much evidence currently about such causal pathways, it is important to be assured that such potential pathways do exist. This issue is addressed briefly in the second section of the paper.

Finally, it is obvious the knowledge concerning disease etiology is useless unless there is also a way to intervene in the disease process through either prevention or cure. The perspective of epidemiology, as a branch of public health, has been to focus on ways to prevent unnecessary disease occurrence, for the most part, through either environmental intervention (e.g. water purification,

51

L. Eisenberg and A. Kleinman (eds.), The Relevance of Social Science for Medicine, 51–75.
Copyright © 1980 by D. Reidel Publishing Company.

pasteurization of milk) or alteration of host susceptibility to disease (e.g. immunization, dietary change). Though at first glance, it may seem difficult to imagine how factors in the social environment might fit into this traditional prevention approach, in fact there are several models of social intervention which may lend themselves quite easily to preventive efforts. The conclusion of this paper is a discussion of such social interventions.

1. THE IMPACT OF THE SOCIAL ENVIRONMENT ON MORBIDITY AND MORTALITY

A. *Social Class*

To start with one of the most consistently observed relationships, a vast body of evidence has shown that those in the lower social classes have higher mortality, morbidity, and disability rates than those in the middle and upper classes. In a nationwide study of mortality by Kitagawa and Hauser (1973), mortality rates among men and women 25–64 years of age, varied dramatically by level of income, education, and occupation considered together or separately. Since education was the variable least likely to be influenced by deterioration in health status, most of their analyses were confined to this variable. In Table 1, it can be seen that white males in the lowest education groups have higher age-adjusted mortality rates for every cause of death for which data are available. For white females, those in the lowest education group have an excess mortality rate for all causes except cancer of the breast and motor vehicle accidents. These social class gradients have been observed by other investigators examining both mortality (Nagi and Stockwell 1973; Ellis 1958; Yeracaris 1955; Graham 1957; Cohart 1954) and morbidity from many conditions (Hart 1972; Wan 1972; Hochstim et al. 1968; Elder and Acheson 1970; Cobb 1971; Graham 1963) including various mental illnesses (Srole et al. 1962; Hollingshead and Redlich 1958; and Gurin et al. 1960).

It should be clear from even this cursory review that social class is associated with a very wide range of disease consequences. While particular hypotheses may be offered to explain the gradient for one or another of these specific diseases, the fact that so many diseases exhibit the same gradient leads to speculation that a more general explanation may be more appropriate than a series of disease-specific explanations.

One of the more obvious explanatons might be that people in lower social classes have higher levels of risk factors traditionally associated with major diseases. Although, at least in most western countries, those in lower classes do tend to smoke cigarettes more, and are more likely to be obese and have higher blood pressure levels (Khosla and Lowe 1972; Ostfeld and D'Atri 1977; US.H.E.W. 1973; Oakes and Syme 1973), these differences seem to explain only a part of the social class gradient in disease risk. In one study of British civil servants, Marmot and his colleagues (1978) report a strong inverse gradient

TABLE 1

Percentage difference in mortality ratio between highest and lowest education level,
by cause of death, for whites, 25–63 years, United States, 1960*

Cause of death	Percentage difference in mortality ratio			
	White males		White females	
Tuberculosis	776		†	
Malignant neoplasms	31		23	
Stomach		123		†
Intestine, rectum		21		66
Lung, bronchus, trachea		93		37
Breast		†		−22
Uterus		†		109
Other neoplasms		5		12
Diabetes	45		332	
Cardiovascular-renal diseases	33		109	
Vascular lesions of the CNS		27		103
Rheumatic fever		24		26
Arteriosclerotic		25		139
Hypertensive		79		158
Other cardiovascular		71		72
Influenza, pneumonia	159		†	
Cirrhosis of the liver	2		16	
All accidents	127		24	
Motor vehicle accidents		84		−4
Other accidents		163		
Suicide	74			
Other causes of death	100		48	

* Adapted from Kitagawa and Hauser (1973) pp. 76–77. Mortality ratios for non-whites
are not shown due to insufficient data. In this table, the percentage differential in mortality
ratio is computed by dividing the *difference* in ratios by the ratio at the lowest education
level. Any given percentage figure in the table may be read as the percentage by which the
ratio at the lowest education level is *higher* than the ratio at the highest education level.
† Insufficient data to calculate ratios.
This table is reprinted from Syme and Berkman (1976).

between different employment grades and coronary heart disease (CHD) mortality which is independent of serum cholesterol, systolic blood pressure, smoking,
body mass, blood glucose levels, physical activity and height. Figure 1 reveals
that approximately 60 percent of the grade differences in CHD could not be
accounted for by differences in the above risk factors. Studies such as this one
are rare however, and should be replicated on different populations and in relation to different diseases so that we may increase our understanding of the role
of standard risk factors in the class/disease association.

Hypotheses focusing on the role of medical care and exposure to a toxic and
hazardous physical environment also seem capable of explaining a part of the

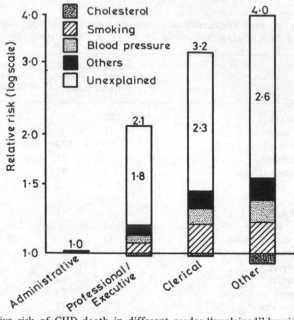

Fig. 1.   Relative risk of CHD death in different grades "explained" by risk factors (age-standardized) among British civil servants. (This figure is reprinted from Marmot et al. (1978).)

class gradient in disease but do not seem able to entirely explain class differences (Lipworth 1970; Fink et al. 1972; Syme and Berkman 1976). Thus, the identification of new factors is critical to our understanding of disease processes among people in different social classes. We are hampered in this search by a lack of understanding concerning specifically what it is about life in a particular social class which could predispose an individual towards illness. This lack of understanding stems from at least two difficulties: (1) it has been extremely difficult, methodologically, to establish a consistent, and valid measure of class which embodies the essence of the concept, (2) investigators have rarely focused on specific components of lifestyle associated with social class.

The methodological concern is quite serious and is centered on the definition of social class. When class is conceived of as unidimensional, measured generally by a system of occupational rankings, it has suffered because (1) occupation is often measured and ranked in arbitrary and unreliable ways (Duncan 1961; Robinson 1979); and (2) occupation is an incomplete measure of social class (Robinson and Kelly 1979; House 1979; Haug and Sussman 1971; Horan and Gray 1974). Rankings developed decades ago on small or medium sized communities have been used in large urban areas where the rankings are not equally valid. There is also some evidence that the rankings are not stable and may have changed over time. When class has been more accurately conceived of as multidimensional, including several components such as education, income, occupation, or residence, there is the additional possibility that the individual components of these multi-dimensional indices are not highly correlated with each other and will interact with each other in unforseen ways. It is also possible that they are not all similarly associated with the outcome variable of interest (House 1979). A final possibility is that variables which traditionally go unmeasured such as relationships to authority, work, etc., (Robinson and Kelly 1979) not only have more to do with class *per se*, but also with disease outcomes than more commonly used variables. The inclusion of such dimensions in future studies would be of help in obtaining a better grasp of the measurement of social class.

An equally important point concerns the elaboration of specific facets of lifestyle in different social classes. In examining these variables we might be wise to focus at first on factors which have also been reported to be associated with poor physical health status. Lower class persons report more high-impact life events of an undesirable nature (out of work, death of loved one, problems in school or job, foreclosure of mortgage) than middle and upper class people do (Myers, Lindenthal and Pepper 1974). They also seem to lack strong social networks especially in terms of formal affiliations and very intimate contacts (Berkman 1977). There is some evidence, particularly with regard to psychiatric disturbance that either life events and/or social networks may explain a great deal of the relationship between social class and psychiatric disturbance (Brown, Bhrolchain, and Harris 1975; Myers, Lindenthal,and Pepper 1974). Additional evidence indicates that those in the lower social classes, especially middle-aged men and women, are more likely to engage in poor health practices (cigarette smoking, lack of physical activity, alcohol consumption, obesity) than middle and upper class men and women. The increased prevalence of undesirable life events, social disconnection, and poor health practices gives us some indication of the kinds of socio-environment conditions which may be found among people in the lower social classes.

To explain the differential in morbidity and mortality rates among the social classes, it is important to identify socio-environmental factors that affect susceptibility and have diverse disease consequences; it is also important to determine which of these factors are more prevalent in the lower social classes. Thus, our understanding would be enhanced if it could be shown not only that those in the lower classes live in a more toxic physical environment with inadequate medical care, but also that they live in a social and psychological environment that increases their vulnerability to a whole series of diseases and conditions.

B. *Socio-cultural change*

Another part of the social environment which is associated with many disease consequences is social and cultural change. Much of the social epidemiological literature has been devoted to this topic, especially with regard to the impact of industrialization, urbanization, migration, and occupational and geographical mobility on coronary heart disease (CHD). The basis for much of this work has

evolved from the observation that CHD is, by and large, a disease of industrialized, urbanized countries.

Cardiovascular disease also seems to increase as people in predominantly non-
industrialized countries adopt an urban or "modern" way of life. Populations
isolated from western culture and industrialization have been located which
appear to have blood pressures which are uniformly low and do not rise with
age (Prior 1977). Zulus in South Africa (Scotch 1963), Polynesians in the Cook
Islands (Prior 1974) and in Palau (Labarthe et al. 1973) and people living in
different villages in Tonga (W.H.O. 1975) have all been observed to have increased blood pressure levels as they live in more "modern" social settings. In
several of these studies the higher blood pressure levels found among the group
living in modern settings was found to be independent of level of obesity or
dietary fat intake; however, in none of the studies could the direct effect of
psychosocial factors be established apart from other changes in weight, diet, or
smoking habits.

These observations have led investigators to pose three hypotheses which have
in turn led to many new studies on social, cultural and life changes: [1]

(1)   that modern industrialized countries produce stressful situations that
         may lead to coronary heart disease,
(2)   that the process of cultural and social *change* may in itself be stress-
         ful and predispose to coronary heart disease,
(3)   that there is some kind of selective bias occuring in which people
         prone to coronary heart disease migrate to certain social environ-
         ments.

The first two of these hypotheses center on the notion that if an individual
finds himself in a situation with which he is unprepared to cope (because of
some social discontinuity or disruption), the situation is stressful and will increase that person's vulnerability to illness (Cassel et al. 1960; Henry and Cassel
1969). Cassel and Tyroler (1961, 1964) in a series of investigations showed that
people who recently became factory workers had higher illness rates than second
generation factory workers, and that individuals who themselves remained stable
but whose community had urbanized had higher CHD mortality rates. This latter
study was carried out to refute the third hypothesis mentioned concerning
selection bias.

People who have experienced occupational and geographical mobility also
appear to have higher rates of disease than people who are more stable. In
studies of both urban and rural communities, Syme (1964, 1965, 1966) has
shown that men who had experienced occupational and geographical mobility
are at increased risk of acquiring coronary heart disease. However, recently new
studies have offered both supporting (Lehr et al. 1973; Kaplan et al. 1971) and
detracting evidence regarding the mobility hypotheses (Wardwell, Bahnson 1973;
Bengtsson et al. 1973). Without reviewing all this evidence, a statement by
Jenkins (1976) seems appropriate that "we are less optimistic than in former

years regarding these variables as simply understood pointers to be found." In addition, many of the studies of status mobility are plagued with the same methodological problems mentioned concerning social class.

Studies of immigrants provide us with information on another type of mobility and social change. Migrants to the United States have been uniformly found to have higher rates of coronary heart disease than those in their home country, regardless of country of origin (Marmot 1975). When compared to native-born U.S. residents, migrants generally have CHD rates intermediate between those of the country of origin and those of native born (Stamler et al. 1960; Krueger and Moriyama 1967). A study of Norwegian and British migrants to the United States confirms this trend for rates of chronic respiratory disease (Reid 1966). Cancer mortality rates among migrants from other countries to the U.S. reveals a general trend showing migrants having higher rates than native-born Americans. Migrants also generally have higher cancer mortality rates than their counterparts who remained in the home country (Lilienfeld et al. 1972).

In Israel, an interesting situation has emerged. Medalie (1973) found that persons born in Europe, where CHD rates are generally high, had high CHD rates when they migrated to Israel. Groups from Middle East and North Africa, where CHD are comparatively low, showed low rates of myocardial infarction when migrating to Israel. Perhaps most interesting were the intergenerational differences which were observed. For both men whose fathers migrated from Europe and those whose fathers had migrated from Asia or Africa, the rates among the first Israeli-born generation were higher than the rates for the migrant groups. Oddly, the lowest rates were found among the second-generation Israelis (those whose fathers were born in Israel). Incidentally, Medalie (1973a) found no relationship between their measures of fat intake and CHD incidence. While factors associated with European culture may be partially responsible for the European versus Asian CHD differences, it appears that something about change *per se* may be involved in the intergenerational differences. Marmot (1975) has speculated that:

Migrants only undergo a limited degree of culture change since to a large extent, they bring their own culture with them and live in their own cultural milieu; their children, who learn a new language and a new culture from the world around them are caught in conflict between the old ways and the new. This line of reasoning would then explain the drop in CHD rates among the second generation native born by arguing that members of this generation are no longer in cultural conflict as they now represent the dominant culture.

A longitudinal study of migrants from the Tokelau Islands (a group of small atolls near Western Samoa) to New Zealand provides additional evidence on the impact of social and cultural change. In this study, Tokelauans who migrated to New Zealand had higher blood pressures than they did before they migrated. Additionally, those Tokelauans who migrated and interacted with New Zealand institutions and Europeans during work and leisure times had higher pressures than immigrants who primarily worked and lived with other Tokelauans, attending Pacific Island churches and clubs. This association was found to be independent of body mass or length of stay in New Zealand (Prior 1977). These data are intriguing because they are contrary to Scotch's findings among the Zulus, that migrants to urban areas who retained their traditional cultural behaviors had higher pressures than those migrants who adopted more urban ways of life (Scotch 1963).

In any case, these data would indicate that something about western culture and change itself may have disease consequences, but what precisely is this phenomenon? Let us turn to studies of Japanese migrants.

Japan is an industrialized, urban, modern country with a very low rate of CHD. It is the exception to the pattern. Several investigators have reported a gradient in CHD mortality as Japanese migrate West (Gordon 1957; Worth and Kagan 1970). In order to better understand what it was about life in Japan, or being Japanese which seemed to infer some protective effect against CHD, a detailed study was undertaken to examine a wide range of risk factors in Japanese in Japan and Japanese-Americans in Hawaii and California. The results have been reported in several papers; however, the one that most directly addresses the issue concerning cultural effects examines the role of acculturation among Japanese-American men in California (Marmot and Syme 1976). In this study it was found that the most traditional group of Japanese-Americans (i.e. those with Japanese group relationships) had a CHD prevalence as low as that observed in Japan. The most acculturated group had a three-to-five-fold excess in CHD prevalence (see Figure 2). The differences between these two groups could not be accounted for by differences in the major coronary risk factors, i.e., blood

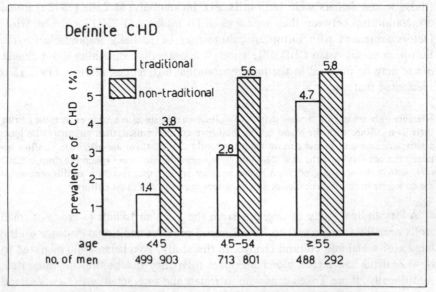

Fig. 2.   Prevalence of CHD by culture of upbringing among Japanese-American men in California. (This figure is reprinted from Marmot and Syme (1976).)

pressure, serum cholesterol, smoking, or diet. In this study it is interesting to note that it was the indicators of acculturation rather than the actual social and cultural attitudes which best predicted CHD prevalence.

At this time no one knows what the precise features of Japanese, or for that matter Tokelauan culture might be that are protective against CHD. However, there is general agreement that the social environment in Japan is significantly different from our own. Matsumoto (1970) has written clearly about some important differences:

(1)   "In the West the increasing importance of individualism focused on the relative autonomy of the person, has been emphasized as an outstanding correlative to modern industrial-urban growth. In spite of rapid social change in Japan, observers agree that Japan has not moved from group values toward individualism, but rather retains strong emphasis on collectivity orientations within the in-group." (Matsumoto 1970).

(2)   In a book called *The Anatomy of Dependence*, Doi, (1973) a Japanese psychiatrist has suggested the term "amaeru", the wish to be loved or dependency needs, is a key to the understanding of Japanese culture and a word missing in most other languages. Matsumoto writes that Western observers note a greater sense of dependence or interdependence in Japan.

(3)   "A third point is that it is not unusual for the individual in the West to spend the major portion of his working hours among persons in whom he cannot usually confide or from whom he can expect little guidance. The Japanese individual, however, is sheltered within his personal in-group community with built-in social techniques and maneuvers for diminishing tension" (Matsumoto 1970).

In addition to these differences in the social environment there is some evidence that Type A behavior, a behavior characterized by "intense striving for achievement; easily provoked impatience; competitiveness; time urgency; abruptness of gesture and speech; overcommitment to vocation or profession and excess of drive and hostility," (Jenkins 1976) is less common among Hawaiian Japanese than among white Americans (Cohen 1974). This behavior pattern has been shown to be significantly associated with increased risk of coronary heart disease among American men and women (Rosenman et al. 1976; Haynes et al. 1978) but not, as traditionally measured, among Hawaiian Japanese (Cohen 1974).

C. *Social networks*

It is evident that people who are occupationally and geographically mobile, those who become acculturated to a westernized lifestyle, as well as those who are poor, have higher than expected morbidity and mortality rates from many diseases; however, the reasons for these associations are not so readily apparent.

In exploring the social environment hypothesis, one is directed towards the search for some characteristic or set of characteristics which these groups have in common and which in itself has been thought to have deleterious health consequences. One potential set of factors, strongly implicated from the work just cited, is the kind of social links an individual has to other people. Individuals who are in some way isolated or disconnected from other people, who lack ties to others in either intimate or instrumental ways, have been shown to suffer from a wide variety of mental and physical disturbances (Cobb 1976; Kaplan et al. 1977). In addition, groups of people in certain structural positions in society, such as migrants, the poor, and the mobile, have also been shown to lack certain connections to others. Such phenomena as poverty, migration, mobility, and industrialization exert powerful influences on an individual's ability to maintain enduring and effective social ties.

A useful framework for viewing and conceptualizing the kinds of social relationships a person has with others is provided by social network analysis. Mitchell (1969) notes that this approach focuses not on the attributes of people in the network, but rather on the characteristics of the linkages in their relationship to one another. In order to measure relationships or linkages, network analysts look at two major categories of networks: the structure or morphology of networks and the types of quality of interaction occuring among linked people (Mitchell 1969). The first category includes such characteristics as size, range, and symmetry of links. Also included are the degree to which people connected to the individual are known to one another, "density," (Barnes 1969), and the number of steps it takes to contact a specified person from a given starting point, "reachability." In the second category, qualities such as intensity, durability over time, frequency of contact and content of interaction are measured. Since all these measures could be applied to one's family, friends, co-workers, neighbors and casual associates, it is clear that a myriad of types of relationships are possible for every individual. Health data, however, are available for very few of the measures. Several comprehensive reviews have been written on this topic (Cobb 1976; Kaplan et al. 1977; Kasl and Berkman 1979); in the following discussion we will highlight several of the more major of the network studies.

One of the first studies of the health effects of different support systems was conducted by Nuckolls, Cassel, and Kaplan (1972) on 170 white primaparous army wives who were followed through delivery of their babies. In this study, it was found that when women had undergone many changes in their lives, women with many psycho-social resources had one-third the pregnancy complication rate of women who scored low on the psychosocial asset scale. In the absence of many life changes, there was no significant relationship between psychosocial resources and complication rates.

In another study (Berkman and Syme 1979) the degree to which individuals maintained social and community ties was assessed in relation to their nine-year mortality risk. In 1965, 6928 adults were surveyed in The Human Population Laboratory Survey of Alameda County, California. Mortality data on respondents were collected for a nine year period from 1965 to 1974. From items asked on the 1965 survey, a Social Network Index was developed tapping four sources of contact: (1) marital status; (2) contacts with close friends and relatives; (3) church membership; and (4) informal and formal group associations. Figure 3 shows the age- and sex-specific mortality rates from all causes by the Social Network Index. The figure reveals a generally consistent pattern of increased mortality rates associated with each decrease in social connection. The age-adjusted relative risks are 2.3 for men and 2.8 for women ($p \leqslant 0.001$). In subsequent analysis, the Network Index was found to be associated with mortality risk independently of baseline physical health status, socioeconomic status, health practices such as cigarette smoking, physical activity, alcohol consumption, obesity, and sleeping and eating patterns, and a range of other psychosocial variables including general measure of preventive utilization of health services. However, it should be noted that while the Social Network Index/mortality relationship was independent of these variables, the relative risk was reduced somewhat when controlling for these factors, especially the health practices.

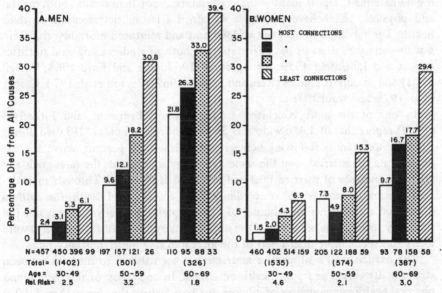

Fig. 3. Age and sex-specific mortality rates from all causes per 100 for Social Network Index, Human Population Laboratory study of Alameda County, 1965–1974. (This figure is reprinted from Berkman and Syme (1979).)

For the most part, other studies have not addressed the impact of a wide variety of network measures, or sources of contact on disease risk; although several of them have elucidated the role of one or another type of social ties.

Studies on marital status and health consistently reveal that those who are married have lower mortality rates than those who are single, widowed, or divorced (Ortmeyer 1974; Durkheim 1951; Price et al. 1971). This mortality risk does not seem to be as great for women as for men and seems to decline with age. Some evidence also suggests that the relationship between marital status and health is independent of many "traditional" physiologic risk factors. In a random sample 6,672 men and women between the ages of 18 and 79, Weiss (1975) examined the relationship between marital status, coronary heart disease and serum cholesterol, systolic and diastolic blood pressure, and a ponderal index. Although Weiss found increased CHD mortality rates present among the non-married to some extent at all ages above 25, his results revealed that no differences in any risk factor explained the married/non-married CHD mortality differential. In fact, there were no consistent differences in any of the risk factor levels between married and non-married men and women at any age levels. The excess risk in CHD found among the non-married is, thus, not due to any increases in any of the more obvious CHD physiologic risk factors.

The association between widowhood and increased morbidity and mortality is particularly striking. Maddison and Viola (1968), Marris (1958), and early studies by Parkes (1964) indicate that widows, especially in the first year following bereavement, report many more complaints about their health, both mental and physical, and believe they have sustained a lasting deterioration to their health. The relationship between widowhood and increased mortality risk from a wide variety of diseases has been reported both in studies using vital statistics (Kraus and Lillienfeld 1959; Young et al. 1963; Cox and Ford 1964; McNeil 1973) and in cohort studies (Rees and Lutkin 1967; Clayton et al. 1974; Gerber et al. 1975; and Ward 1976).

In one of the more conclusive studies, Parkes, Benjamin, and Fitzgerald (1969) report that of 4,486 widowers 55 years of age and older, 213 died during the first six months following bereavement. This is 40 percent above the expected rate for married men the same age. After six months, the rates gradually fell back to those of married men and remained at that level. Through an analysis of husbands' and wives' concordance rates for cause of death, the authors concluded that neither the sharing of similar pathogenic environment nor the tendency towards the selection of the unfit to marry the unfit (homogamy) were likely to explain more than a part of the increased six-month mortality rate.

The existence of a supportive marriage has been shown to mediate between stressful life events and poor health outcomes. In one study of the mental and physical health consequences of job loss due to a factory shutdown, Gore (1973) reports that those men who had "the emotional support of their wives while unemployed for several weeks had few illness symptoms, low cholesterol levels, and did not blame themselves for loss of job." In general, men who were both unemployed for a longer time and unsupported tended to have the worse health outcomes (Cobb and Kasl 1977). In another study of psychiatric disturbance among women, Brown, Bhrolchain, and Harris (1975) found that having a husband or boyfriend who was a confidant served as a powerful mediator between a severe event or major difficulty and onset of psychiatric disorder. In this sample of women 18—65 years old, 38 percent of those who had a stressful event and no husband or boyfriend as confidant had onset of disturbance. For those without such a confidant or without severe event, the percentage of psychiatric disturbance was under 4 percent. When the confidant named was a sister, mother or friend seen weekly, the relationship was not observed to mediate between life events and psychiatric disturbance.

These data suggest that there is something protective about a supportive spouse or partner which is capable of shielding an individual against the otherwise deleterious effects of some objective life circumstances. The morbidity and mortality findings also indicate that the loss of a spouse, a major enduring tie to another person, may be at least a precipitating factor in the increased death rates found among widowers. The relationship appears to be at least to some extent independent of the traditional CHD physiologic risk factors, homogamy, and equal exposure to pathogenic environments.

The studies reviewed give the reader some indication of the potential role social connections play in disease etiology. Clearly, there is much work left to be done in this area. Much more evidence linking social networks to disease processes is available in the fields of mental health, rehabilitation, and compliance with medical regimens (Haynes and Sackett 1974; Kasl and Berkman 1979; Doehrman 1977); however, the aim of this presentation has been to provide the reader with some evidence on the association between social connections and mortality and physical morbidity.

2. PATHWAYS LEADING FROM THE SOCIAL ENVIRONMENT TO PHYSICAL ILLNESS

The mechanisms by which conditions in the social environment might influence health status in human populations is a relatively unexplored area. In a search for such mechanisms, it is important to keep in mind that social conditions seem to be associated with a wide range of outcomes rather than any single disease entity. This observation would suggest that there are several pathways leading from social circumstances to illness and/or that such circumstances lead to a compromised resistance to disease in general. As Cassel (1976), a proponent of the latter hypothesis, suggests, it may also be that there are several clusters of diseases associated with different psychosocial situations. An elucidation of these issues is critical since by understanding the process by which social factors lead to poor health we can learn where to intervene most effectively and prevent unnecessary illness and death.

If we take the approach that there are likely to be multiple biological pathways, several potential processes can be outlined: (1) behavioral processes whereby people living in certain social and cultural cirucmstances maintain health practices which are either beneficial (e.g. physical activity) or harmful (e.g. cigarette smoking) to their health; (2) psychological processes whereby people respond to circumstances by becoming depressed or changing their coping and appraisal processes; (3) direct physiological changes in both known biological risk factors (e.g. blood pressure, serum cholesterol) and unidentified processes which are directly altered by exposure to certain environmental circumstances. In the exploration of this chain leading from environmental conditions to health outcomes, we must also recognize that factors which in this chain are considered mediators may also directly influence socio-environmental factors, reversing the causal chain. Thus, it is possible, for instance, that psychological states such as depression could influence social conditions. Studies in which these variables are being investigated will be most useful when the temporal chain of events will be able to be identified. It is also likely that characteristics of the person and the environment, combined, will ultimately be the best predictors of disease risk.

Behavioral factors including health practices, preventive utilization of health services, and compliance with treatment regimens are obvious and likely candidates for linking socio-environmental conditions to disease consequences; however, the evidence available thus far indicates that health practices are capable of explaining only a part of the environment/disease association. Studies in which this hypothesis was directly addressed, (Marmot et al. 1978; Berkman and Syme 1979; Marmot and Syme; Prior 1977) suggest that other pathways must also be involved, although in most cases a cross-sectional association between the social condition and health behavior was noted.

Psychological factors such as depression or coping processes also seem likely candidates as mediators between environmental conditions and illness responses; and there is some literature to support this view. Of particular interest is the recent work by Seligman (1974) and earlier work by Rotter (1966) and others interested in feelings of internal and external control and learned helplessness and a review on such coping mechanisms and social circumstances by Satariano and Syme (1979). These investigators have hypothesized that when individuals are habitually confronted with situations in which their responses either are or appear to be ineffective, they ultimately come to conclude that events in general are uncontrollable and that they are powerless to effect a particular outcome. Seligman (1974) indicates that such feelings are related to depression and perhaps to other health problems. Psychological responses may also predispose an individual to suicide or risk-taking behavior which could result in accidents. Engel and Schmale (1972) and Antonovsky (1979) also refer to the importance of "giving up" or maintaining a sense of control or "coherence" to health maintenance. There is, as yet, little strong evidence in support of these positions in terms of prospectively predicting physical health status or of linking socio-environmental processes to health outcomes in human populations. However, it is interesting to note the similarity of these positions with Cassel's (1976) characterization of stressful social situations as ones in which "the actor is not receiving adequate evidence (feedback) that his actions are leading to anticipated consequences."

While the previous hypothetical pathway suggests that the critical role social factors play in disease causation is not due to objective circumstances themselves, but to the way in which such circumstances are more subjectively perceived and mediated, it is also possible that there may be a pathway leading directly from social circumstances to physiologic changes in the body which increase either general or specific disease susceptibility. The finding in the Human Population Laboratory study that no psychological factors developed from items on the 1965 survey mediated between social isolation and mortality risk supports this view, although none of the factors were created to tap the psychological dimensions just described (Berkman 1977).

Neural, hormonal, and immunologic control systems have frequently been invoked as potential pathways by which stressful social circumstances might cause disease. In animal experiments, stressful social circumstances have been found to alter such control systems and to lead to disease consequences (Calhoun 1962; Ader et al. 1963; Ratcliffe 1958; Gross 1972). In human populations this series of links has not been established, but in cancer patients both cell mediated and humoral immunity are frequently depressed. Furthermore different hormonal patterns have been shown in cancers of the breast and prostate (Henderson, Gerkins, and Pike 1975) and the possibility exists that some estrogens and androgens are responsive to stress (Lemon 1969). Sympatho-adrenomedullary activity may link socio-environmental conditions to cardiovascular disease. Physiological concomitants of increased sympatho-adrenomedullary activity are: (1) increased blood pressure and heart rate; (2) increased myocardial oxygen utilization; (3) increased circulating levels of epinephrine and norepinephrine; (4) increased concentrations of plasma free fatty acids; and (5) increased plasma renin activity (Herd 1979).

In this discussion it is important to keep in perspective that socio-environmental conditions may serve as predisposing factors (Cassel 1976) which affect a person's general resistance to disease and that other factors (e.g. genetic susceptibility, exposure to noxious stimuli) may determine specific disease vulnerabilities.

3. SOCIAL INTERVENTION IN THE PREVENTION OF DISEASE

As stated in the beginning of this chapter, public health efforts have traditionally focused on primary prevention. With the increased prevalence of chronic diseases such as cancer and coronary heart disease, for which there are currently many unidentifiable causes, primary preventive efforts obviously must be limited. Clearly, the identification of causal factors in these diseases is of the utmost importance. If, as growing evidence suggests, there is a relationship between diseases and the social environment, primary preventive efforts aimed at modifying the disease promoting aspects of the social environment should be considered. Though such interventions are relatively new with regard to improving health status, there is a long history in the United States of using social intervention to improve mental health as well as social and economic well-being (Zurchen and Bonjean 1970; Caplan 1974). In the following discussion, intervention in the area of social networks will be taken as an example of potential interventions.

At least three routes may be taken in modifying an individual's social network depending upon the factors influencing the network: (1) socio-structural interventions: promoting opportunities for social contact; (2) social interventions: improving opportunities and skills for social contact; (3) psychosocial interventions: providing psychological treatment and opportunities for social contact.

A. *Socio-structural interventions*

Interventions directed at the socio-structural level assume that network configurations are at least in part determined by structural aspects of the social environment. Networks and the extent of social connections maintained by an individual are not seen as being primarily determined by personal variables, but by the very real lack of opportunities providing for such contact by social situations. According to this view such social circumstances as poverty, urbanization, migration, housing situations, and deviancy may be the major barriers to making social connections. If these factors are found to be determinants of networks, several interventions might be useful in promoting adequate contacts:

(1)   *Poverty*: Poor people appear to have economic barriers which prevent them from maintaining many kinds of social connections. Lack of adequate transportation and communication channels across distances, lack of economic ability to provide for families, as well as to join organizations, may encourage isolation and social disconnectedness. Interventions in this area may be mostly economic, providing income supplements, job opportunities, and access to good transportation and communication resources.

(2)   *Community disintegration*: Frequently because of changes in industrial sites, urban planning or renewal efforts, or population shifts, older communities begin to disintegrate, disrupting both family and community organizations. Ethnic working class communities, communities of older people and often even neighborhoods filled with transients have developed ways of functioning and surviving which are complex. When these communities are disbanded or relocated, new social connections are difficult to form. An example of such social disruption resulting from an urban renewal program in which predominantly Italian working-class residents of Boston's West End were relocated is poignantly documented by Gans and Fried (Gans 1963, Fried 1966). Appropriate community intervention may, in some cases, be a form of non-intervention. Leaving intact communities alone, and helping other communities to remain intact may be, literally, the healthiest kind of action. Of course, urban planning has the potential both to alleviate unhealthy housing conditions and to promote adequate social support systems. Planning which takes into consideration the importance of both the physical and social environment might be a powerful form of intervention.

(3)   *Deviancy*: Though this word often carries a negative connotation to it, many people are deviants in the sense that they are placed in a position different from many of their peers, a situation which often makes it difficult or awkward for them to maintain many social ties. People who are widowed early in life, single parents, migrants who come to a country and live isolated from other people with similar backgrounds, anyone who is surrounded by people in a different social position, frequently find themselves segregated from people around them. Blau (1973), in her work on structural constraints on friendships in old age, has described this phenomenon in some depth. Two sorts of interventions are possible to increase these people's social connections: (1) integration into the larger community through interventions aimed at increasing contact among these people and their work associates, neighbors, extended family; (2) development of what has been called "an intentional community," based on some common interest. Co-ops, child-care centers, retirement communities, drug and alcohol abuse centers, (e.g. Alcoholics Anonymous), Reach for Recovery, Parents without Partners, organizations for people who are physically disabled, such as the Center for Independent Living, and communes are just some examples of groups organized for some common purpose by people who were otherwise having a difficult time maintaining enough social contacts to fulfill emotional and/or pragmatic needs.

B. *Social Intervention*

While the only barrier against adequate social contact for some people is a simple matter of opportunity, others lack the social skills necessary to maintain and create opportunities for social contact. In fact, our culture, by encouraging independence and self-sufficiency, may in many ways be discouraging the development of such skills necessary to the development of strong and supportive social networks. For example, some men are socialized so that it is difficult for them to maintain intimate relationships. Other people are temporarily caught by a crisis, move, or job change with neither social contacts nor a vision of how to create opportunities for such contacts. Older lower class women and women from certain ethnic groups have been described as not ever being socialized to make friends outside their family. All these people are similar in that they probably have a variety of potential sources of social support of which they are either unaware or feel unable to utilize.

A form of intervention, appropriately called Social Network Intervention, has evolved which was created to deal with situations of just this nature. In this intervention, a team of intervenors assembles all members of a kinship system, all friends and neighbors and anyone else who is of significance to the individual. The process which then ensues is complex and has been described in greater detail than is possible here by Speck and Attneave (1971).

This form of network intervention provides both opportunities and skills for utilizing the potential links in an individual's network structure. In this way, it is possible to structure networks in homes for the aging, residence clubs for younger people, work groups in which many members are highly mobile, as well as in traditional family structures.

C. *Psychosocial Intervention*

Although many people are isolated because of few opportunities for contact or because they lack certain social skills, some people are isolated either by choice or because serious psychological difficulties prevent them from maintaining relationships with other people. The issue of appropriate intervention for the individual who actively refuses social contact is a difficult one. Certainly, if a person does so by choice and is satisfied with his or her circumstances, no intervention ought to be attempted. After all, many people who are isolated enjoy good health, are very satisfied with their lives (Berkman 1977), profit by it, and would be far more unhappy being forced into social situations.

For the group of isolates who would prefer having more social contacts but appear to be psychologically unable to do so, several different forms of intervention might be examined. Social Network Intervention might be appropriate under certain circumstances; other forms of family, crisis and group therapy might also be attempted. Encouraging those individuals to engage in non-threatening social encounters or providing protected living conditions such as half-way houses could be suggested.

These ideas are only examples of potential forms of intervention and are not presented as definitive answers to the problems of isolation and social disconnection. Rather, they are offered with the aim that people in the fields of public health, and medicine, will perceive that intervention in the social environment is not an impossible or utopian task. The issues raised here are complex and will not be resolved by a single formula or in a short time. However, if future research supports the importance of the social environment to the maintenance of health, hopefully this work will contribute to the development of sound and constructive social and health policies.

NOTE

1. I am indebted to Michael Marmot for his conceptualization of these hypotheses.

REFERENCES

Ader, R., A. Kreutner, and H. L. Jacobs
    1963 Social Environment, Emotionality and Alloxan Diabetes in the Rat. Psychosomatic Medicine 25:60–68.
Antonovsky, A.
    1967 Social Class, Life Expectancy, and Overall Mortality. Milbank Memorial Fund Quarterly 45(2):31–73.
    1979 Health, Stress and Coping. San Francisco: Jossey-Bass Publishing Co.
Barnes, J. A.
    1969 Networks and Political Process. *In* Social Networks in Urban Situations. J. C. Mitchell, ed. pp. 51–76. Manchester, University Press.

Bengtsson, C., T. Hallstrom, and G. Tibblin
1973 Social Factors, Stress Experience and Personality Traits in Women with Ischaemic Heart Disease, Compared to a Population Sample of Women. Acta Medica Scandanavica (Suppl) 549:82–92.
Berkman, L. F.
1977 Social Networks, Host Resistance, and Mortality: A Follow-up Study of Alameda County Residents. Ph.D. dissertation in Epidemiology. University of California, Berkeley.
Berkman, L. F. and S. L. Syme
1979 Social Networks, Host Resistance, and Mortality: A Nine-Year Follow-up Study of Alameda County Residents. American Journal of Epidemiology 109(2):186–204.
Blau, Z.
1973 Old Age in a Changing Society. New York: Franklin Watts.
Brown, G. W., M. N. Bhrolchain, and T. Harris
1975 Social Class and Psychiatric Disturbance Among Women in an Urban Population. Sociology 9:225–254.
Calhoun, J. B.
1962 Population Density and Social Pathology. Scientific American 206(2):139–148.
Caplan, G.
1974 Support Systems and Community Mental Health. New York: Behavioral Publications.
Cassel, J.
1976 The Contribution of the Social Environment to Host Resistance. American Journal of Epidemiology 104(2):107–123.
Cassel, J., R. Patrick, and D. Jenkins
1960 Epidemiological Analysis of Culture Change: A Conceptual Model. Annals of the New York Academy of Sciences 84:938–949.
Cassel, J. and H. Tyroler
1961 Epidemiological Studies of Culture Change. I. Health Status and Recency of Industrialization. Archives of Environmental Health 3:31–39.
Clayton, P. J.
1974 Mortality and Morbidity in the First Year of Widowhood. Archives of General Psychiatry 30:747–750.
Cobb, S.
1971 The Frequency of the Rheumatic Diseases. Cambridge: Harvard University Press, pp. 42–62.
1976 Social Support as a Moderator of Life Stress. Journal of Psychosomatic Medicine 38:300–314.
Cobb, S., and S. V. Kasl
1977 Termination: The Consequences of Job Loss. Cincinnati: DHEW (NIOSH) Publication No. 77–224.
Cohart, E. M.
1954 Socioeconomic Distribution of Stomach Cancer in New Haven. Cancer 7:455–461.
Cohen, J.
1974 Sociocultural Change and Behavior Patterns in Disease Etiology: An Epidemiologic Study of Coronary Heart Disease Among Japanese Americans. Ph.D. dissertation in Epidemiology, School of Public Health, University of California at Berkeley.
Cox, P. R. and J. R. Ford
1964 The Mortality of Widows Shortly After Widowhood. The Lancet 1:163–164.

Doehrman, S. R.
   1977 Psycho-Social Aspects of Recovery from Coronary Heart Disease: A Review. Social Science and Medicine 11:199–218.
Doi, T.
   1973 The Anatomy of Dependence. Tokyo: Kodansha International.
Duncan, D.
   1961 Occupational Components of Educational Differences in Income. Journal of American Statistical Association 56:783–792.
Durkheim, E.
   1951 Suicide. New York: The Free Press.
Elder, R. and R. M. Acheson
   1970 New Haven Survey of Joint Diseases XIV Social Class and Behavior in Response to Symptoms of Osteoarthrosis. Milbank Memorial Fund Quarterly 48(4):449–502.
Ellis, J. M.
   1958 Socio-economic Differentials in Mortality from Chronic Diseases. In Patients, Physicians, and Illness. E. G. Jaco, ed. pp. 30–37. Glencoe, Ill.: The Free Press.
Engel, G. L., and A. H. Schmale
   1972 Conservation-Withdrawal: A Primary Regulatory Process for Organismic Homeostasis. In Ciba Foundation, Symposium 8, Physiology, Emotion and Psychosomatic Illness, pp. 57–85. Amsterdam: Elsevier.
Fink, R., S. Shapiro, M. Human, C. Rosenberg, and M. Liebowitz
   1972 Health Status of Poverty and Non-Poverty Groups in Multiphasic Health Testing. Presented at the 100th Annual Meeting of the American Public Health Association, Medical Care Section, November 14, 1972, Atlantic City, New Jersey.
Fox, B. H.
   1978 Premorbid Psychological Factors as Related to Cancer Incidence. Journal of Behavioral Medicine 1(1):45–134.
Fried, M.
   1966 Grieving for a Lost Home: Psychological Costs of Relocation. In Urban Renewal. The Record and the Controversy. J. Q. Wilson, ed. pp. 359–379. Cambridge: M.I.T. Press.
Gans, H.
   1963 The Urban Villagers. Glencoe, Ill.: The Free Press.
Gerber, I., R. Rusualem, N. Hannon, D. Battin, and A. Arkin
   1975 Anticipatory Grief and Widowhood. British Journal of Psychiatry 122:47–51.
Gordon, T.
   1957 Mortality Experience Among the Japanese in the United States, Hawaii, Japan. Public Health Reports 72:543–553.
Gore, S.
   1978 The Effect of Social Support in Moderating the Health Consequences of Unemployment. Journal of Health and Social Behavior 19:157–165.
Graham, S.
   1957 Socio-economic Status, Illness, and the Use of Medical Services. Milbank Memorial Fund Quarterly 35:58–66.
   1963 Social Factors in Relation to Chronic Illness. In Handbook of Medical Sociology. H. E. Freeman, S. Levine, and L. G. Reeder, eds. pp. 65–98. Englewood Cliffs, New Jersey: Prentice-Hall.
Gross, W. B.
   1972 Effect of Social Stress on Occurrence of Marek's Disease in Chickens. American Journal of Veterinary Research 33(11):2275–2279.
Gurin, G., J. Veroff, and S. Feld
   1960 Americans View Their Mental Health. New York: Basic Books.

Hart, J. T.
    1972 Data on Occupational Mortality 1959–63, Too Little and Too Late. The Lancet
          1:192–193.
Haug, M. and M. Sussman.
    1971 The Indiscriminant State of Social Class Measurement. Social Forces 49:549–
          563.
Haynes, R. B., and D. L. Sackett
    1974 A Workshop Symposium: Compliance with Therapeutic Regimes – Annotated
          Bibliography. Department of Clinical Epidemiology and Biostatistics, McMaster
          University Medical Centre, Hamilton, Ontario.
Haynes, S., M. Feinleib, and S. Levine, N. Scotch, and W. B. Kannel
    1978 The Relationship of Psychosocial Factors to Coronary Heart Disease in the
          Framingham Study. II. Prevalence of Coronary Heart Disease. American Journal
          of Epidemiology 107(5):384–402.
Henderson, B. E., V. R. Gerkins, and M. C. Pike
    1975 Sexual Factors in Pregnancy. In Persons at High Risk of Cancer. J. F. Fraumeni,
          ed. pp. 267–284. New York: Academic Press.
Henry, J., and J. Cassel
    1969 Psychosocial Factors in Essential Hypertension. American Journal of Epidemiology
          40:171–200.
Herd, A.
    1979 Behavioral Factors in the Physiological Mechanisms of Cardiovascular Disease.
          Paper presented at the 1st Annual Meeting of Behavioral Medicine Research,
          June 4.
Hochstim, J., D. A. Athanasopoulos, and J. H. Larkins
    1968 Poverty Area Under the Microscope. American Journal of Public Health 58(10):
          1815–1827.
Hollingshead, A. B., and F. C. Redlich
    1958 Social Class and Mental Illness. New York: John Wiley and Sons.
Horan, P., and B. Gray
    1974 Status Inconsistency, Mobility and Coronary Heart Disease. Journal of Health
          and Social Behavior 15:300–310.
House, J.
    1979 Facets and Flaws of Hope's Diamond Model. American Sociological Review
          40(2):439–442.
Jenkins, D.
    1976 Recent Evidence Supporting Psychologic and Social Risk Factors for Coronary
          Disease. I. New England Journal of Medicine 294(18):987–994. and II. New
          England Journal of Medicine 294(19):1033–1038.
Kaplan, B. H., J. Cassel, H. Tyroler, et al.
    1971 Occupational Mobility and Coronary Heart Disease. Archives of International
          Medicine 128:938–942.
Kaplan, B. H., J. Cassel, and S. Gore
    1977 Social Support and Health. Medical Care (Supplement) 15(5):47–58.
Kasl, S. V.
    1977 Contributions of Social Epidemiology to Studies in Psychosomatic Medicine. In
          Advances in Psychosomatic Medicine: Epidemiologic Studies in Psychosomatic
          Medicine. S. V. Kasl and F. Reichsman, eds. pp. 160–223. Basel: S. Karger.
Kasl, S. V., and L. F. Berkman
    1979 Some Psycho-social Influences on the Health Status of the Elderly: The Per-
          spective of Social Epidemiology. Paper presented to the Conference on Biology
          and Behavior of the Elderly, National Academy of Sciences, Wood's Hole, June
          22–24.

Khosla, T., and C. R. Lowe
    1972 Obesity and Smoking Habits by Social Class. British Journal of Preventive and
          Social Medicine 26:249–256.
Kitagawa, E. M., and P. M. Hauser
    1973 Differential Mortality in the United States. Cambridge: Harvard University
          Press.
Kraus, A. S., and A. M. Lilienfeld
    1959 Some Epidemiologic Aspects of the High Mortality Rates in the Young Widowed
          Group. Journal of Chronic Diseases 10:207–217.
Krueger, D. and I. Moriyama
    1967 Mortality of the Foreign Born. American Journal of Public Health 57:496–503.
Labarthe, D., D. Reed, J. Brody, and R. Stallones
    1973 Health Effects of Modernization in Palau. American Journal of Epidemiology
          98:161–174.
Lehr, I., H. B. Messinger, and R. Rosenmann
    1973 A Sociobiological Approach to the Study of Coronary Heart Disease. Journal
          of Chronic Diseases 26:13–30.
Lemon, H. M.
    1969 Endocrine Influences on Human Mammary Cancer Information. Cancer 23:781–
          790.
Lilienfeld, A. M.
    1976 Foundations of Epidemiology. New York: Oxford University Press.
Lilienfeld, A. M., M. L. Levin, and I. Kessler
    1972 Cancer in the United States. Cambridge: Harvard University Press.
Lipworth, L., T. Abelin, and R. R. Connelly
    1970 Socio-economic Factors in the Prognosis of Cancer Patients. Journal of Chronic
          Diseases 23:105–116.
Maddison, D., and A. Viola
    1968 The Health of Widows in the Year Following Bereavement. Journal of Psychoso-
          matic Research 12:297–306.
Marmot, M.
    1975 Migrants, Acculturation and Coronary Heart Disease. Mimeo, Department of
          Epidemiology, University of California, Berkeley.
Marmot, M., and S. L. Syme
    1976 Acculturation and Coronary Heart Disease in Japanese-Americans. American
          Journal of Epidemiology 104(3):225–247.
Marmot, M., G. Rose, M. Shipley, and P. Hamilton
    1978 Employment Grade and Coronary Heart Disease in British Civil Servants. Journal
          of Epidemiology and Community Health 32:244–249.
Marris, P.
    1958 Widows and Their Families. London: Routledge & Kegan Paul.
Matsumoto, Y.
    1970 Social Stress and Coronary Heart Disease in Japan: A Hypothesis. Milbank Memo-
          rial Fund Quarterly 48:9–36.
McNeil, D. N.
    1973 Mortality Among the Widowed in Connecticut. Yale University, New Haven,
          M.P.H. essay.
Medalie, J., H. Kahn, H. Neufeld, et al.
    1973a Myocardial Infarction Over a Five Year Period. I. Prevalence Incidence and Mor-
          tality Experience. Journal of Chronic Diseases 26:63–84.
    1973b Five Year Myocardial Infarction Incidence. II. Association of Single Variables to
          Age and Birthplace. Journal of Chronic Diseases 26:329–349.

Mitchell, J. C.
  1969 The Concept and Use of Social Networks. *In* Social Newworks in Urban Situations. J. C. Mitchell, ed. pp. 1—50. Manchester: University Press.
Myers, J. K., J. J. Lindenthal, and M. P. Pepper
  1974 Social Class, Life Events, and Psychiatric Symptoms: A Longitudinal Study. *In* Stressful Life Events: Their Nature and Effects. B. S. Dohrenwend and B. P. Dohrenwend, eds. pp. 191—206. New York: John Wiley and Sons.
Nagi, M. H., and E. G. Stockwell
  1973 Socioeconomic Differentials in Mortality by Cause of Death. Health Service Reports 88(5):449—456.
Nuckolls, K. B., J. C. Cassel, and B. H. Kaplan
  1972 Psychosocial Assets, Life Crisis, and Prognosis of Pregnancy. American Journal of Epidemiology 95:431—441.
Oakes, T., and S. L. Syme
  1973 Social Factors in Newly Discovered Elevated Blood Pressure. Journal of Health & Social Behavior 14:198—204.
Ortmeyer, C. F.
  1974 Variations in Mortality, Morbidity, and Health Care by Marital Status. *In* Mortality and Morbidity in the United States. C. F. Erhardt and J. E. Berlin, eds. pp. 159—188. Cambridge, Mass.: Harvard University Press.
Ostfeld, A. M., and D. A. D'Atri
  1977 Rapid Sociocultural Change and High Blood Pressure. *In* Epidemiologic Studies in Psychosomatic Medicine. S. Kasl, ed. pp. 20—37. Basel, Switzerland: S. Karger.
Parkes, C. M.
  1964 Effects of Bereavement on Physical and Mental Health — A Study of the Medical Records of Widows. British Medical Journal 2:274—279.
Parkes, C. M., B. Benjamin, and R. G. Fitzgerald
  1969 Broken Heart: A Statistical Study of Increased Mortality Among Widowers. British Medical Journal 1:740—743.
Price, J. S., E. Slater, and E. H. Hare
  1971 Marital Status of First Admissions to Psychiatric Beds in England and Wales in 1965 and 1966. Social Biology 18:574—594.
Prior, I. A.
  1974 Cardiovascular Epidemiology in New Zealand and the Pacific. New Zealand Medical Journal 80:245—252.
  1977 Migration and Physical Illness. *In* Epidemiologic Studies in Psychosomatic Medicine. S. Kasl, ed. pp. 105—131. Basel, Switzerland: S. Karger.
Ratcliffe, H. L., and M. I. T. Cronin
  1958 Changing Frequency of Arteriosclerosis in Mammals and Birds at the Philadelphia Zoological Garden. Circulation 18:41—52.
Rees, W. P., and S. G. Lutkin
  1967 Mortality of Bereavement. British Medical Journal 4:13—16.
Reid. D. D.
  1966 Studies of Disease Among Migrants and Native Populations in Great Britain, Norway, and the United States. I. Background and Design. *In* Epidemiological Study of Cancer and Other Chronic Diseases. W. Haenszel, ed. National Cancer Institute Monograph 19:287—299.
Robinson, R. V., and J. Kelly
  1979 Class as Conceived by Marx and Dahrendorf: Effect on Income, Inequality and Politics in the United States and Great Britain. American Sociological Review 49:38—57.

Rosenman, R., R. J. Brand, R. I. Sholtz, and M. Friedman
  1976 Multivariate Prediction of Coronary Heart Diseases During 8.5 Year Follow-up in the Western Collaborative Group Study. American Journal of Cardiology 37: 902–910.
Rotter, J.
  1966 Generalized Expectancies for Internal Versus External Control of Reinforcement. Psychological Monograph. 80(1) Whole No. 609.
Satariano, W., and S. L. Syme
  1979 Life Change and Disease: Coping with Change. Paper prepared for presentation to the conference on Biology and Behavior of the Elderly, National Academy of Science, Woods Hole, Mass. June 22–24.
Scotch, N. A.
  1963 Sociocultural Factors in the Epidemiology of Zulu Hypertension. American Journal of Public Health 53(8):1205–1213.
Seligman, M.
  1974 Helplessness. San Francisco: Freeman and Co.
Speck, R. V., and C. L. Attneave
  1971 Social Network Intervention. In Changing Families. J. Haley, ed. pp. 312–332. New York: Grune and Stratton.
Stamler, J., H. Y. Kjelsberg, Y. Hall, and N. Scotch
  1960 Epidemiologic Studies on Cardiovascular-Renal Disease: III. Analyses of Mortality by Age-Sex-Nationality. Journal of Chronic Diseases 12:464–475.
Syme, S. L.
  1974 Behavioral Factors Associated with the Etiology of Physical Disease. A Social Epidemiological Approach. American Journal of Public Health 64:1043–1045.
Syme, S. L., M. M. Hyman, and P. E. Enterline
  1964 Some Social and Cultural Factors Associated with the Occurrence of Coronary Heart Disease. Journal of Chronic Diseases 17:277–289.
  1965 Cultural Mobility and the Occurrence of Coronary Heart Disease. Journal of Health and Human Behavior 6(Winter):178–189.
Syme, S. L., N. O. Borhani, and R. W. Buechley
  1966 Cultural Mobility and Coronary Heart Disease in an Urban Area. American Journal of Epidemiology 82:334–346.
Syme, S. L., and L. G. Reeder
  1967 Social Stress and Cardiovascular Disease. Milbank Memorial Fund Quarterly 45 (entire supplement).
Syme, S. L., and L. F. Berkman
  1976 Social Class, Susceptibility and Sickness. American Journal of Epidemiology 104(1):1–8.
Srole, L., T. Langner, S. Michael, M. Opler, and T. Rennie
  1962 Mental Health in the Metropolis. New York: McGraw-Hill Book Co.
Tyroler, H. A., and J. Cassel
  1964 Health Consequences of Culture Change – II. The Effect of Urbanization on CHD Mortality in Rural Residents. Journal of Chronic Diseases 17:167–177.
U.S. Department of Health, Education, and Welfare
  1973 Adult Use of Tobacco 1970. Publication No. HSM – 73-8727.
Wan, T.
  1972 Social Differentials in Selected Work Limiting Chronic Conditions. Journal of Chronic Diseases 25:365–374.
Ward, A. W.
  1976 Mortality of Bereavement. British Medical Journal 1:700–702.
Wardwell, W., and C. Bahnson
  1973 Behavioral Variables and Myocardial Infarction in the Southeastern Connecticut Heart Study. Journal of Chronic Diseases 26:447–461.

Weiss, N. S.
  1973 Marital Status and Risk Factors for Coronary Heart Disease: The United States
        Health Examination Survey of Adults. British Journal of Preventive and Social
        Medicine 27:41–43.
World Health Organization for the Western Pacific
  1975 The Prevention and Control of Cardiovascular Disease.
Worth, R., and A. Kagan
  1970 Ascertainment of Men of Japanese Ancestry in Hawaii Through WW II Selective
        Service Registration. Journal of Chronic Diseases 23:389–397.
Yeracaris, C.
  1955 Differential Mortality, General and Cause-Specific in Buffalo, 1939–1941.
        American Statistical Association Journal 50(Dec.):1235–1247.
Young, M., B. Benjamin, and C. Wallis
  1963 The Mortality of Widows. The Lancet 2:454–457.
Zurchen, L. A., and C. M. Bonjean
  1970 Planned Social Intervention. Scranton. Chandler Publishing Co.

JOHN B. McKINLAY

4. SOCIAL NETWORK INFLUENCES ON MORBID EPISODES AND THE CAREER OF HELP SEEKING

"Love cannot fill the thickened lung with breath,
Nor clear the blood, nor set the fractured bone;
Yet many a man is making friends with death
Even as I speak, for lack of love alone."

From Sonnet 29 of "Fatal Interview" by Edna St. Vincent
Millay, *Collected Poems*, Harper and Row, 1931. Quoted
in V. R. Fuchs, *Who Shall Live*? Basic Books, New York,
1974, page 52.

INTRODUCTION

Just over a decade ago, Mitchell (1969) presented a timely review of the history
and uses of the concept of a social network. As a metaphor depicting a complex
set of interrelationships in a social system, it has a long history. But he distinguished this purely metaphorical usage "... from the notion of a social network
as a specific set of linkages among a defined set of persons, with the additional
property that the characteristics of these linkages as a whole may be used to
interpret the social behavior of the persons involved". Mitchell traced the emerging popularity of network studies to two main sources: (a) a dissatisfaction with
structural-functional analysis and the consequent search for alternative ways
of understanding social behavior; and (b) the development of mathematical
approaches to social phenomena — particularly graph theory and probability
modeling. Reflecting Mitchell's concerns, Granovetter (1973) argues that a weakness in current sociological theory is its failure to relate micro-level interactions
to macro-level patterns in any convincing way. He suggests, and I concur, that
the analysis of processes in interpersonal networks can provide a fruitful micro-
macro bridge.

In recent years the concept of a social network has been employed (sometimes explicitly but mostly implicitly) in studies seeking to explain the epidemiology of many different problems and the ways in which they are responded
to — both by the afflicted and their families, and the professionals and organizations which attempt to cure or care for them. This chapter will selectively review
some of these studies and attempt to bestow a semblance of order by discussing
them in relation to the notion of a *help-seeking career* — the sequence of stages
typically passed through by a person with a real or perceived problem who is on
the way to treatment, recovery, rehabilitation, or perhaps even death (McKinlay

77

L. Eisenberg and A. Kleinman (eds.), The Relevance of Social Science for Medicine, 77–107.
Copyright © 1980 by D. Reidel Publishing Company.

1971; Goffman 1953). Along with Walker and his colleagues I will use the term "social network" to refer to *that set of contacts with relatives, friends, neighbors, etc., through which individuals maintain a social identity and receive emotional support, material aid, services and information, and develop new social contacts* (Walker et al. 1977).

Those who have employed the notion of a social network usually distinguish certain characteristics as germane to their endeavor. Mitchell (1969:1–50) for example, divides these characteristics into two main classes: the *morphological* — those concerning the relationship or pattern of links in the network with one another (*anchorage, density, reachability* and *range*); and the *interactional* — those concerning the nature of the links themselves (*content, directedness, durability, intensity* and *frequency*). Variations on this original list have been considered by Craven and Wellman (1974) and Granovetter (1973), among others.

Some aspects of social networks of importance for understanding the epidemiology of and responses to particular morbid episodes would appear to be: *anchorage* (the particular individual in a social network whose behavior an observer is attempting to describe or explain); *size* (the number of people with whom an individual maintains meaningful social contact, including any dormant relationships that are or can be activated when particular needs arise); *range* (the distribution of experience, age, ethnicity, attitudes and information within a social network — this is obviously correlated with, but should be considered separately from) size; *strength of ties* (a combination of the amount of time, the emotional intensity, the intimacy (mutual confiding), and the reciprocal services which characterize the tie), *density* (the extent to which the individuals in a network know and have contact with one another independently of a focal individual); *content* (the inferable meanings which persons in a network attribute to their relationships with others); *dispersion* (the ease with which individuals can make contact with, or activate contacts with, others in the network); *frequency* (the amount of contact between individuals comprising a social network); *directedness* (the extent to which contact between individuals associated through the network is unidirectional or reciprocal); *reachability* (the extent to which an individual can use relationships with others to contact other people who are important to him or alternatively, the extent to which people who are important to him can contact him through those relationships).

Further definitional clarity and operationalization of these different morphological and interactional characteristics are necessary if the concept is to have any utility in the explanation of any social behavior. The above list is in no way definitive, nor should it be regarded as exhaustive. There are obvious imperfections and some overlapping. What is presented derives from and is generally consistent with Mitchell's discussion, and is intended as a brief theoretical background to the subject of this chapter: how the concept of a social network can facilitate explanation of the epidemiology of health-related events and much of the social phenomena associated with them.

THE NOTION OF A HELP-SEEKING CAREER

In recent years, some commentators have found it heuristically useful to conceive of the transition from person to patient back to person as a type of career – a sequence of stages typically passed through by an individual with some real or perceived problem, who is on the way to formal treatment, rehabilitation, or perhaps death.

Diagrammatic representation of a typical sequence of stages in help-seeking.

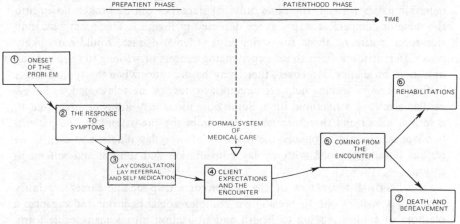

Fig. 1.

A series of stages which may be passed through by individuals with some actual or perceived problem is depicted diagrammatically in Figure 1. It will be observed that this overall career is divided into two main parts: the *pre-patient phase* (comprising the range of behavior and contacts that occur prior to encountering professionals, formal helping agencies and assumption of the sick role); and the *patienthood phase* (comprising those stages passed through subsequent to adoption of the sick role). The transition from pre-patienthood to patienthood is an important point in help seeking for it is the point at which two distinct social networks (the patient's own more or less permanent social network, and the problem-activated formal or professional helping network) intersect. It is here that the formal or "professional" helping network may begin to exert greater social control over an individual's behavior than his/her own social network of friends, relatives, and neighbors. Coping behavior within an individual's social network may parallel, complement or even compete with that offered through the professional helping network. One study by Croog and his colleagues revealed that patients following a myocardial infarction made little use of formal services (other than their physicians) even when relevant services were available, but relied *instead* on friends and relatives (Croog et al. 1972).

Some potentialities and limitations of the notion of a help-seeking career should be highlighted. *Firstly*, the notion should be considered in the context of differences in the definition and distribution of health and illness between and within cultures, social categories and groups, over time. *Secondly*, each stage in the career probably affects, and is affected by, every other stage in the career of help seeking for the problem of concern. What occurs at each stage is likely to shape related behavior during subsequent stages. *Thirdly*, each stage may be considered analytically distinct and amenable to more detailed and separate consideration. *Fourthly*, the career, as depicted in Figure 1 has a direction, a logical beginning (the onset or perception of some problem) and an ending (either rehabilitation or death). *Fifthly*, it is not suggested that all help-seeking behavior passes through the same order of stages, or can be broken down into the same or comparable stages as are depicted in Figure 1. There may be condition-specific careers: those suspecting say, venereal disease, would most likely go a different route from those experiencing cancer, or wishing to terminate an unwanted pregnancy. Moreover, there may be occasions when the typical stages in the process of seeking help are circumnavigated, or are telescoped, as in say, cardiac arrest, or a fractured limb. Some conditions may never be presented to a formal helper and therefore never pass from the pre-patient to the patient-hood phase. Indeed, probably the majority of everyday illness, and even some serious illness, is coped with by lay consultation and referral and self medication.

The heuristic advantages of the notion of a help-seeking career are fairly obvious. It enables one to breakdown complex social behavior and organize a plethora of studies relating to health and utilization into a manageable form, thus permitting one to *both* relate these parts to one another in a systematic way, *and* to bestow a semblance of analytic order on the present chaotic state of knowledge in the field. Therein, however, lies a major disadvantage: it suggests that more order and coherence exist in this area than is actually the case. I shall now selectively review a broad range of literature which relates to some ways in which social networks may influence each stage of the help-seeking career depicted in Figure 1.

THE SOCIAL NETWORK AS AN EPIDEMIOLOGICAL VARIABLE

Evidence from social epidemiology pointing to network characteristics as importantly influencing the etiology of a wide range of problems is now overwhelming. Holmes (1956), for example, has shown that the incidence of tuberculosis in Seattle was highest among people who, because of their "social marginality", lacked significant intimate social contacts. Women lacking social support are known to have more symptoms of tiredness, anxiety, depression and irritability than women with an active support network (Miller and Ingham 1976). Marmot accounts for the high incidence of and mortality from coronary heart disease among Japanese living in California (compared to those in Hawaii or Japan) by the loss of a social support system as these people migrate further from their socio-cultural base (Marmot 1975). Social disorganization has been associated with an increase in mortality from strokes (Neser et al. 1971). People deprived of meaningful human contact or group membership are known to be at higher risk to schizophrenia, accidents, suicide, and respiratory diseases (Kaplan et al. 1977). Various social factors relevant to social networks have been shown by Scotch and Gieger (1962) to be associated with rheumatoid arthritis. Studies over the last several decades, in different parts of the world, have found consistently that populations living in small cohesive societies "insulated" from phenomena associated with Western industrialization have lower blood pressures, which do not differ between the young and the aged (Cassel 1969). When people move from such "protective" societies and have contact with Western culture, they have higher levels of blood pressure and exhibit the essential hypertension characteristic of the Western world. Scotch (1963), in a well-known study of Zulu hypertension, found that blood pressures were higher in urban than in rural dwellers, and that traditional practices (e.g., membership in an extended family, belief in witchcraft, large numbers of children) while seemingly adaptive in a rural setting were non-adaptive in an urban situation. Lower blood pressure was associated with the former condition, while elevated blood pressure was related to the latter setting.

Syme et al. (1964) have shown, in separate studies, that occupationally and residentially mobile people have a high prevalence of coronary heart disease, and that the greater the discontinuity between childhood and adult situations (measured by occupation and place of residence) the higher the risk of such disease. Tyroler and Cassel (1964) in a study of various counties in North Carolina found that over a decade (1950–1960) coronary heart disease increased in relation to the urbanization of the county. In a separate study of two groups of rural mountainers – one composed of individuals who were the first of their family to engage in industrial work while the second comprised workers who were the children of previous workers in the same factory – the first group had more symptoms of illness and higher risk of sickness absence at each age than the second group. Haenzel and his co-workers discovered that death rates from lung cancer in the United States (when controlled for level of cigarette consumption) were considerably higher in the farm-born who migrated to cities, than they were in lifetime urban dwellers (Haenzel et al. 1962).

Hinkle and his co-workers studied groups of men working for the same company and holding similar managerial positions, but differing in their educational background prior to association with the industry. Those who had completed college were mostly fourth generation Americans, sons of managers or white collar workers, had grown up in middle and upper class neighborhoods and experienced significantly fewer of a wide range of illnesses. The group who had not completed college were the sons and grandsons of immigrants, had fathers who were skilled or unskilled workers with less formal education, had grown up in working and lower class neighborhoods and had a significantly greater number of illnesses of all sorts (both physical and emotional) than did the former group (Christenson and Hinkle 1961). Prior and his colleagues, in a prospective study of the health consequences of the migration of Polynesians from the Tokelau

Islands to New Zealand, continue to document the deleterious consequences for health of this marked culture change (Beaglehole 1978).

Only a few studies, derived almost entirely from the seminal work of John Cassel (1969) are considered here. Many others, not only from social epidemiology but related fields, could be cited. Although most of these studies do not explicitly invoke the concept of a social network, it is suggested that their findings and the explanations offered lend strong support to the thesis that the social network structures of individuals, groups and cultures importantly determine the onset of a wide range of morbid episodes, which are reflected as differences in vital statistics.

According to Cassel (1969), some of the most convincing evidence concerning the role of social support systems as determinants of disease comes from animal studies. He reviewed this evidence and suggests that both variations in the size of the groups in which animals interact and involvement in situations where there is confusion over territorial control appear to be important determinants of health. As the number of animals housed together increases, with other factors such as diet, temperature, and sanitation kept constant, maternal and infant mortality rates rise, the incidence of arteriosclerosis increases, resistance to insults (including drugs, micro-organisms and X-rays) is reduced, and there is an increased susceptibility to allexan produced diabetes, convulsions, and certain cancers. Lack of territorial control leads to the development of hypertension in mice, to increased maternal and infant mortality rates, reduced resistance to bacterial infections and decreased longevity. Other studies relating to the ability to electrically induce peptic ulcers depending on whether rats are shocked in isolation (high rates) or in the presence of litter mates (low rates) corroborate the suggestion that support systems are important.

Obviously, the findings of these animal studies cannot necessarily be extrapolated to humans. Nevertheless, as Cassel (1969) suggests, they do provide some evidence pointing to the influence of social support systems in the etiology of a wide range of problems and do permit greater control over complex variables in order to account for most of the variance observed.

The relative importance of social networks (support systems) as against other variables can be illustrated with respect to studies of stress. There is, of course, a vast literature which identifies stress *per se* as an etiological agent in the generation of a broad range of morbidity and mortality (Levine and Scotch 1977; Dean and Lin 1977; Lin 1979). It appears that the existence of a social support network may avert the deleterious consequences of stress by either minimizing the stress itself, or by enhancing the susceptible individuals adaptive resources (Cassel 1974; Cobb 1976; Kaplan et al. 1977). One early study revealed that Allied propaganda to German troops was not effective until the soldier was cut off from his intimate, interpersonal ties — when his own small unit of peers and non-commissioned officers broke up (Shils and Janowitz 1948). Social supports reduce psychological distress following job loss or bereavement (Burch 1972; Gore 1978; Parkes 1972) and the number of psychiatric casualties in combat

(Swank 1949; Reid 1947). Brown and his colleagues found that social support may protect against depression among women confronted with major life events, and that what may be regarded as network characteristics or experiences (number of children at home, early loss of mother, intimacy) act as "amplifying factors" (Brown et al. 1975). Recent studies suggest some interaction between stress *and* social networks in the etiology of a range of illness. Nuckolls and his colleagues found that the absence of social supports was associated with increased complications in pregnancy and delivery, when accompanied with high stress: lack of social support *per se* did not increase risks (Nuckolls et al. 1972). De Araujo and his collaborators found that chronic asthmatics require more medication if they experience high stress *and* have few supporting relationships (de Araujo 1973). The presence of social support networks have also been shown to enhance recovery from severe burns (Hamburg et al. 1953), the coping behavior of Nazi concentration camp survivors (Dimsdale 1974) and afford some protection from severe affective disorder (Brown et al. 1975).

In selectively reviewing this evidence I am suggesting that aspects of social networks *appear* to be implicated, along with other variables, in the etiology of a broad range of morbidity and mortality. Now it is certainly *not* suggested that the contribution or mediating influence of social network characteristics is yet clearly understood, or even that there is general consistency in the findings. Much more conceptual clarification and methodological refinement is necessary before we are at that point. What can be said is that over the last several decades, social epidemiologists, among others, have produced a wealth of evidence relating such phenomena as marginality, cultural discongruity, social integration, social adaption, social conflict, status inconsistency, migration, acculturation and role incongruity to certain patterns of mortality and morbidity. These many disparate studies, taken together, constitute a strong *prima facie* case for looking further at the direct contribution of different network structures to various morbid episodes, and at how they also mediate the influence of other established etiological agents. Having considered the possible contribution of social support networks to the generation of particular illness episodes, we will now look at how social networks may also influence the responses to problems and crises.

THE RESPONSE TO PROBLEMS

The presence of particular problems (or symptoms) may be neither a necessary nor sufficient condition for individuals to begin some search for help. When we say a symptom is a "necessary condition" for help seeking, it is not intended that there is a necessary connection between symptoms and help seeking — although we sometimes say that in order for people to seek some form of care, symptoms must be experienced. In the absence of certain symptoms or states some help seeking may appear absurd (in the absence of a pregnancy, one cannot obtain an abortion). The presence of a symptom or problem can certainly not be regarded as a *logically necessary condition* for help seeking. Other social factors may precipitate help seeking even in the apparent absence of symptoms. Symptoms may be regarded as sufficient conditions for the occurrence of help seeking if, invariably, whenever symptoms arise, help seeking results.

There is still confusion over the importance of symptoms in the process of help seeking. Some hold that most people act on the basis of any symptom, and that the more serious and visible the symptom, the more probable it is that some form of utilization will result. Mechanic (1968) for example, has suggested that "much of the behavior of sick persons is a *direct* product of the specific symptoms they experience; their intensity, the quality of discomfort they cause, their persistence and the like." Elsewhere he suggests that "social factors are considerably less important in help-seeking among those who have severe symptoms than among those who have lesser symptoms," and that few relatives are willing to overlook hallucinatory, delusional, or suicidal behavior, etc. (Mechanic 1969).

There can be no doubting that *severe* symptoms leave the afflicted person little alternative but to recognize that he or she is ill, and that some kind of formal help is required. The examples Mechanic cites (temperature of 105 degrees, fractured leg, broken back, *severe* heart attack, *extreme* psychosis) could hardly be overlooked, and the requisite help-seeking behavior avoided (Mechanic 1969). What proportion of symptoms are we talking about however? Many people – probably a majority – never experience any of these life endangering events, but do experience many non-disabling illnesses and symptomatic episodes. According to one estimate, the average lower middle class American male between the ages of 20 and 45 experiences over a 20-year period, approximately one life endangering illness, 20 disabling illnesses, 200 non-disabling illnesses and 1000 symptomatic episodes. This total of 1221 episodes over 7305 days yields a rate of one new episode every six days (Hinkle 1960). It is to these common everyday vicissitudes that our attention should be directed. While various social factors may be less important in the relatively infrequent *extreme* situations, they may exert considerable influence in the case of non-disabling symptomatology.

Another view of the importance of symptom recognition and the response of help seeking gives emphasis to the role of certain *mediating factors* – events and situations which intervene between presenting symptoms and help-seeking behavior. These events and situations may include the context within which symptoms arise, as well as the characteristics of an individual's or group's social network, which may be mediating factors determining: (a) the relative importance of symptoms, (b) their visibility, and (c) when (or if) help-seeking behavior results.

There are many studies which reveal how the recognition of and response to symptoms varies according to social class, ethnic group, etc. (McKinlay 1972). In addition to these variables, it appears that aspects of social networks may have a distinct influence on which responds to what, when, how, and so on. Zola, for example, has delineated five "triggers" or mediating factors which are likely to influence an individual's decision to seek medical care (Zola 1964).

The *first* he called "interpersonal crisis", in which some situation calls attention to the symptoms and causes the patient to dwell on them. The *second* trigger, "social interference", occurs when symptoms happen to threaten a valued social activity. The *third*, "the presence of sanctioning", involves advice from others to seek care; the *fourth* is a "perceived threat"; and the *fifth*, the "nature and quality of the symptoms", involves similarity of the present symptoms to some experienced previously, or to those experienced by friends or relatives. Notice that the relative importance of symptoms is largely a function of the mediating influence of individuals associated through the network. Zola reported that symptoms, as triggers, have varying degrees of importance in different social strata and ethnic groups. The triggers "interpersonal crisis" and "social interference" were used more often by Italians, while "sanctioning" was the predominant trigger for the Irish. The Anglo-Saxon group apparently responded most frequently to the "nature and quality of their symptoms" (Zola 1966).

The suggestion that social networks have a mediating influence on the perception and relative contribution of symptoms to help-seeking behavior may derive additional support from studies in the area of mental illness. One study, by Eaton and Weil, of the tolerance of deviance within Hutterite communities, provides a useful illustration. Prior to the study it was thought that the prevalence of mental illness was lower in the Hutterite subculture than among comparable groups of non-Hutterites. It was subsequently found, however, that the true prevalence of mental disorder was no different from that in comparative groups, but that its visibility to outsiders was masked by mediating factors in the Hutterite subculture (Eaton and Weil 1955).

In another study of pervasiveness of psychiatric symptomatology, Dinitz and his co-workers pair-matched a group of patients with a non-patient neighbor who lived ten houses away and interviewed them along with another adult person in the household. Interestingly, no significant differences were found between the two groups in the occurrence of many of the "psychiatric" symptoms (Dinitz et al. 1961; Dinitz et al. 1962). As Daniels (1970) points out, many so-called "mental symptoms" are subject to a wide range of commonplace interpretations and, depending on a range of factors, can be understandably excused. Differences between families in the visibility of psychiatric symptoms may be partly explained by findings which show a tendency for family members to normalize neurotic and psychotic symptoms by interpreting such behavior in particular kinds of ways (Yarrow et al. 1955).

In a well-known study of how people define illness, Apple (1960) showed that interference with everyday activities was one of the major criteria used by laymen to define illness. Generally speaking, symptoms which are socially disruptive are more likely to be defined as worthy of some kind of lay or professional attention. Here it is the social disruption that the symptoms cause, and not the symptoms *per se*, which precipitate social action. Moreover, some symptoms or conditions are likely to be differentially disruptive in different social situations. Among professional people, for example, psychiatric symptoms (e.g., verbal incapacity, inability to conceptualize, lack of concentration, memory difficulties) are likely to be immediately detected by both the afflicted and their peers, since much of professional life requires a high level of functioning in these areas. Such functioning does not appear to have the same significance in the everyday life of those in the lower socio-economic categories. These types of symptoms may be disregarded, since they are not as socially disruptive in their consequences. Among manual workers, certain physical symptoms, conditions or accidents (e.g. backache, sprained arm, laceration, etc.) may be more disruptive of social life — especially employment — than among non-manual workers.

The perception of and response to presenting symptoms does appear then to be influenced by networks, along with other social variables. What is regarded as serious and debilitating to individuals in one social network may be only minor and bothersome in another. Moreover, the ability to explain or "understandably excuse" the presence of some symptom or condition probably varies between different social networks.

LAY CONSULTATION, LAY REFERRAL, AND SELF MEDICATION

Having recognized the presence of symptoms, or perceived a need for some form of help, one is typically confronted with several possible courses of action — some of which may be pursued almost simultaneously. A person may, for example, resort to home remedies of proven success in the past, discuss the symptom with relatives and/or friends who may have experienced comparable problems, consult some formally recognized professional, or refrain from any overt social action at all in the hope that the symptom or perceived need will either disappear, or perhaps even make itself more apparent, and hence publicly understandable. It is at this point that people in need may "negotiate" with significant others over *what* possible label should be applied, *how* severe the episode is, *which* help-seeking behavior is most appropriate, and *when* action should be taken. It may also be during this pre-patient phase (i.e., before the adoption of a sick role) that one is most receptive to information from health educators and preventive interventions. During this phase of informal negotiation people are casting around for appropriate "recipes for action" and appear most receptive to suggestions regarding alternative courses of action. Once a specific course has been decided upon, and validated by and with others in the lay referral system, it may be some time before an alternative course can be seriously entertained.

The processes of lay referral and acts of self-medication are seldom separate, and obviously do not always occur in the order depicted in Figure 1. While Freidson (1960) Mechanic (1969) and Coe (1970) appear to give primacy to self-medication in the career of seeking formal care, they would not, I believe, wish to suggest that this sequence is ever immutable. The precise sequencing is presumably situationally variable, and affected by such factors as the background experience of the person or category of people involved, the range and dispersion of informal lay resources, the strength of ties and, of course, the perceived nature and severity of the presenting symptoms.

Perhaps the most well-known study linking social network characteristics to health behavior is that by Suchman (1964) who found that individuals belonging to "parochial" social groups (indicated by ethnic exclusivity, friendship solidarity, and traditional/authoritarian family relations) were less likely to respond to the norms of the medical care system than those affiliated with "cosmopolitan" social groups. In a subsequent re-examination of Suchman's data, some doubts were raised regarding the empirical reliability of his general model as an explanation of utilization behavior (Geersten et al. 1978)

In one study in New York City, Suchman (1964) found that three quarters of his respondents reported discussing their symptoms with some other person (most often a relative) before seeking formal medical care. Zola, it will be recalled, included the influence of others ("the presence of sanctioning") as a key trigger in a person's decision to seek medical care (Zola 1964). Freidson has provided some of the most systematic descriptions of the importance of the diagnostic resources of relatives, friends, neighbors and work-mates, while seeking some form of care. He argues:

Indeed, the whole process of seeking help involves a network of potential consultants from the intimate and informal confines of the nuclear family through successively more select distant and authoritative laymen until the 'professional' is reached. This network of consultants which is part of the structure of the local lay community, and which imposes form on the seeking of help, might be called the 'lay referral structure.' Taken together with the cultural understandings involved in the process we may speak of it as the 'lay referral system.' (Freidson 1960).

Freidson goes on to descriptively classify lay referral systems using the following two characteristics: (a) the *degree of congruence* between the culture of the clientele and that of the professional; and (b) the *relative number of lay consultants* who are interposed between the first perception of symptoms or need, and the decision to see a professional. Considerations of culture are seen as having relevance to the diagnosis and prescriptions that are meaningful to the client and the kind of consultants considered authoritative, while the extensiveness of the lay referral structure is seen as having relevance to the channelling and reinforcement of lay culture, and to the salience of "outside" communication.

These two variables — the content and the structure of the system — are linked to form a typology of lay referral systems which may facilitate the prediction of different types of utilization behavior. Beginning with the most underutilizing category, we have a system in which prospective clients participate in an indigenous lay subculture that is markedly different to that of professionals, and in which there is a highly extended lay referral structure. The *second* type of system has the same indigenous subculture as the first, but varies by having a truncated referral structure which allows the individual to act entirely on his own, or to consult no one outside his immediate family, increasing thereby the use of formal sources. The *third* type of system is one in which lay and professional subcultures are very much alike, and the lay referral structure is extended. The *fourth* type involves a truncated referral structure and a sub-culture similar to that of the professional; Freidson conceives of the process of lay referral as a hierarchical, information-seeking process through which one moves from the less to the more informed and experienced contacts, and beyond that to the formal medical care system. Recently, a useful distinction has been made between the "lay referral network" (the range of informal consultants used by an individual to evaluate symptoms and identify sources of help and courses of action) and the "lay treatment network" (the range of nonprofessional help that is received informally outside the medical care system) (Gottlieb 1976).

Bott has argued that social networks can be conceptualized as being open or closed, as being more or less connected. She suggests:

By connectedness, I mean the extent to which people known by a family (or individual) know and meet one another independently of the family (or individual). I use the word 'close knit' to describe a network in which there are many relationships among the com-ponent units, and the word 'loose knit' to describe a network in which there are few such relationships (Bott 1957).

Granovetter (1973) and Liu and Duff (1972) following Bott (1957) consider the strength of network ties and identify two main types: (a) *Strong ties* (where there is a high degree of interdependence and/or consultation with a relatively small number of persons) and (b) *Weak ties* (where there is little interdependence and/or consultation and the range of consultation contacts is diverse. Evidence from both the United States and Britain reveals that networks characterized by strong ties tend to develop in stable working class neighborhoods (Bott 1957; Gans 1962; Young and Willmott 1957; Fried et al. 1973; Townsend 1957). It has been suggested that the nature of network ties may influence the utilization of services. Protracted lay referral and delayed utilization is thought to be associated with strong tie networks which encourage individuals associated through the network to remain well, and not claim the exemptions derived from adoption of the sick role. Moreover, pressing problems inherent in the network (housing, food) may take precedence over health matters and relegate them to a position of low priority. In contrast, weak tie networks, with their diversity of contacts, may provide information which is confusing or conflicting. In such a situation, individuals may seek professional help earlier than they would if their networks were of the strong tie form (Reeder et al. 1978).

A study of the organization of health and social welfare services and their utilization by lower working class families in Aberdeen, Scotland, considered the apparent role of the family, and its kin and friendship networks, in the seeking of maternity care by a sample of 87 women, divided into two subgroups accord-ing to their use of prenatal services. Differences emerged between the utilizers and underutilizers regarding aspects of the kin and friendship sectors of their social networks, and from questions concerning lay consultation and lay referral for various hypothetical but commonly occurring problem situations. It appeared that *utilizers made greater use of friends and husbands* and less use of mothers or other relatives, and tended to consult a *narrower range* of lay consultants. These findings were consistent with, and perhaps reinforced, observed differences in their network structure. Underutilizers appeared to rely more on a variety of *readily available relatives and friends as lay consultants*. There appeared to be only *one* large *interlocking network* within which the underutilizers obtained the majority of their advice. Utilizers, on the other hand, had separate or *differentiated kin and friendship networks*. There was a lack of reliance on relatives on the part of the utilizers, but no evidence in the data that kin lay consultation was replaced to any large extent by friendship lay consultation. Utilizers appeared to be relatively independent of both kin and friends, and frequently took no prior lay advice from the members of their networks, or consulted only their husbands (McKinlay 1973; Jones and Belsey 1977).

Several studies in Latin America have documented the functional importance of kin ties in terms of such basic activities as economic assistance, help with child rearing, and various other activities (Bryce-Laporte 1970; Hammel 1961; Lewis 1973). Several observers have found that, in sexually segregated societies, women get considerable social support (both emotional and material) from relatives other than husbands (Brown 1975; Lomnitz 1977; Peattie 1968). Conjugal role separation is apparently a common family pattern in Latin America, where men carry out much of their lives away from home and return at mealtimes and to sleep; women's activities, in contrast, are concentrated in the household. One recent study found that social supports other than a woman's partner had no discernible influence on actions the woman took in the case of an unwanted pregnancy. Women who lived with kin, or who visited frequently with relatives outside their households, were no less likely to end the pregnancy than were women with less intense faimly ties (Browner 1979). These results may be explained by the small sample size of the study, the insensitivity of the measurements of network characteristics, or may be accurate but peculiar to Latin America. The study certainly deserves replication.

Salloway and Dillon (1973) found that large *friend* networks tended to precipitate speedy utilization of health services while large *family* networks tended to support delaying behavior. Reeder (1978), following Aday and Anderson (1975), found that the type and structure of the network has less influence on utilization behavior than does the type and content of advice network members give.

A clear distinction between the kin and friendship sectors of social networks may be important for an understanding of help-seeking behavior. Litwak and Szelenyi (1969) suggest that the function of kin is to handle long-term aid and commitments, while friends are more likely to provide affective support, and neighbors help in short-term emergency situations. Adams (1967) argues that the dominant properties of kinship relations involve positive concern, mutual help and constant obligations, while friendships are more concerned with value and attitude concerns and shared social activities. Horwitz (1978) shows that kin and friendship sectors have special spheres of competency. Only advice, which implies no special commitment or knowledge, is a common form of help provided by both sectors. Kin members tended to provide services such as financial assistance and living quarters which imply long-term commitments, permanent ties and invoke a norm of reciprocity. Friends were better suited to provide knowledge of professionals outside the primary group. The general pattern for kin is to attempt to maintain individuals within the informal network, while the tendency of friends is to connect the individual to a wider outside network of professionals. In an earlier study, Kadushin (1958—59), for example, found that friends were more likely than kin to have knowledge of available psychiatric resources.

One study, by Geersten and his colleagues, found that tight-knit social networks tended to facilitate the use of health services (Geersten et al. 1975). Pratt (1972) found that couples with traditional conjugal relationships (unequal power in decision making, strong sex role differentiation and low companionship) display poorer health behavior than do couples with more egalitarian conjugal relations (after controlling for the effect of socio-economic status). Bott (1957) has linked the nature of conjugal role relationships to features of social networks. Salloway and Dillon (1973) suggest that frequent interaction with non-kin (as opposed to relatives) is positively associated with personal health behavior. There can be little doubt that social networks influence self-medication and the seeking of help. But further studies are required before we can be certain of the nature and direction of this influence in particular situations.

Despite Freidson's early attempt to clarify the structures and processes which serve to regulate help-seeking behavior, little empirical work has been conducted in this area. In 1973 I formulated a set of questions which, at that time, were unanswered and generally unformulated. They still remain timely. Is it possible to detect intra-family patterns of help-seeking behavior? Are there certain situations or episodes in which network members play a more important role in defining, consulting, referring, etc., while other conditions involve fewer members? Does the dispersion of the family, as well as related kin and friends, affect the nature of its influence on help seeking? Are kin and friends more important determinants of help seeking than other variables like social class, religion, ethnic group or even regions? Do social network factors play a more influential role in help seeking when only certain age groups are involved, or at different points in the family cycle? Is family involvement in any way related to the particular type of helping agency being utilized? Does the family influence the effectiveness of a program or regimen after a service has been utilized? Does the range of an individual's social network influence the quality and content of the advice received? (McKinlay 1972).

CLIENT EXPECTATIONS AND THE ENCOUNTER

So far the discussion has focussed on how people utilize social network resources *prior* to contact with a formal helper. Attention has been devoted to the role of social networks in the etiology of illness, symptom recognition, self-medication and the process of lay referral and consultation. We can now consider some ways in which social networks also influence what actually goes on during encounters with professionals and formal helping agencies.

It is during the pre-patient phase of the help-seeking career — when individuals negotiate with significant others over labels, symptoms, and possible courses of action — that particular organizations and professionals are identified as the "appropriate" target for help seeking. Moreover, network members may determine *when* some formal service is actually utilized. For example, a friend or relative may initiate contact on an individual's behalf by offering to drive them, coming in to look after the children, making an appointment on their behalf, and so on.

Network members also influence what actually goes on during a formal encounter in at least three main ways. *Firstly*, they shape the nature of an individual's contact with a formal helper during an encounter. Not only do network members identify sources of professional help, but they occasionally also ensure positive encounters by telephoning ahead and requesting "special treatment", by suggesting the use of their name ("tell them that I sent you"), or by instructing the individual to request a particular person. They may also offer instruction in what is likely to be the most effective persuasive appeal in dealing with this particular organization or professional helper (Katz and Danet 1966). In these ways, network members enable the person in need to break through formal channels, by-pass particular categories of workers (who may display negative orientations towards clients), and reach "higher ups", who have a more positive orientation and a broader range of discretion in which to act on the client's behalf (Walsh and Elling 1968). Network members are unlikely to refer a person in need to an organization or profession with whom they have had negative or unfortunate associations in the past. Consequently, when new clients invoke the name of a friend or relative, they are associating their particular case with one for which the professional has already had a positive or successful outcome. The client in this situation has an advantage over those who are "blind referrals", or whose cases are similar to those with unsuccessful outcomes with which the agency has been associated in the past.

Knowledge of and some facility with the intricacies of bureaucracies, or the range of professional services that may be available for a particular problem, appear to be positively correlated with socio-economic status. Middle and upper class network members may be in better position to "pull strings", refer to someone who will "take care of them", or identify people "in the know". The ability of a client to extract some service from an organization or professional has little to do with formal entitlement, but is largely a function of "pulling strings", their repertoire of persuasive appeals and the ability to distinguish and utilize the most effective appeal strategy in particular encounters. Such ability is thought to vary according to social class and ethnic group, among other variables.

Secondly, social network members appear to influence the expectations that clients carry into an encounter. Relatives and friends frequently relate tales concerning what happened when they were in a similar predicament, what they heard happened to others, and so on. They frequently offer predictions as to what is likely to happen to the client, how they will be examined, which questions are likely to be asked, what course of action will be recommended, and so on. Should the actual encounter differ substantially from what the client's network led him/her to expect (e.g., they may not see the person they expected, may not be examined in quite the same way, a different prescription may be given, and so forth) then the client may feel dissatisfied, cheated, or alarmed, at what may be an unexplained departure. Why am I different? How come they didn't do so and so? What were the extra tests for? Is something wrong? (i.e. other than what they expected to be confirmed).

It is sometimes suggested that the level of client or patient satisfaction with a service is less a function of technical expertise than it is the extent to which what goes on during an encounter matches what was expected prior to entering it. If there is a good fit, then the client is more likely to be satisfied; if not, he/she is dissatisfied, or suspends judgement while checking with the network members on what occurred. To some extent, therefore, the social network appears to be integrally involved in the level of client satisfaction with services. Whether or not a client is satisfied may have less to do with the technical content of the professional relationship with the client — how they present themselves, whether things were explained, if the encounter was businesslike, and so forth — than does goodness of fit with expectations, and subsequent evaluations by the network.

Thirdly, the presence of other network members during a formal encounter probably influences the content of the exchange. Coser has described how much of professional medical activity is "insulated from observability", and what this portends for practice (Coser 1961). It is common for nurses to request that intimate relatives and friends "wait outside while the doctor examines Mrs. X". Since what goes on during the encounter may involve the disclosure of nothing of which the relative is unfamiliar, and because it is frequently discussed in detail and at length after the encounter, the exclusion of network observers must serve other functions. Oftentimes, even parents are requested to leave while a child is treated or examined. Such exclusion probably has more to do with the protection of professionals and the organizations which employ them, then it does the protection of a client's privacy. After all, a network member may even be there at the invitation of the client!

The exclusion of observers from professional encounters is seldom bilateral — one network member for one professional aide. It is usually one-sided, the client's social supports removed while the professional's remain in attendance. In this way, the balance of power in the client-professional encounter always remains in the professional's favor. Moreover, by excluding network observers, professionals exclude witnesses of possible incompetence or mistakes. Should something untoward occur, it is effectively one patient or client's word against the professional, and his/her network of helpers, who together present a common front on behalf of the organization. Any information that network members subsequently receive and employ on their clients' behalf derives from the client himself. And of course, knowledge gained from a sample of one (and so emotionally involved an individual as the client) is vulnerable and easily disparaged by the counterclaims of professionals and organizations. It is generally recognized that people perform differently when their work is being observed and evaluated. The presence of friends and relatives during, say, a patient-physician encounter, may encourage more courtesy, and less impersonal treatment of the patient.

The exclusion of network members (whose presence the client or patient may have requested) during professional encounters may be not only an infringement of legal rights, but may represent a high level of insensitivity. When patients ask a relative or friend to accompany them to an encounter with a bureaucracy or professional, they are clearly signalling their apprehension, and are saying, in effect, "will you help by being with me, while I go through this". By excluding the patient's lay support professionals and organizations are, in effect, replying, "your apprehension, or fear, is illfounded or wrong". In essence, it devalues the client's perspective before the encounter actually commences.

The exclusion of network members is wasteful in a number of ways. Anyone who has attempted to elicit information by interview will appreciate that several voices are sometimes more accurate than only one – the patient's or client's. Relatives or friends may correct the client's account by interjecting, "no, that wasn't when it first occurred" or "you always seem to get it after so and so", or "you haven't taken any of those pills for 3 weeks". If present during an encounter, relatives and friends frequently offer corrective amendments to the patient's account, give another perspective on etiology or frequency, point out omissions, and generally add to the accuracy of the history. It is wasteful to exclude what may constitute the most reliable source of verification and perhaps the greatest therapeutically, especially when most accessible. Moreover, network members can be employed by professional helpers to explain a course of action to the patient. "I want you to tell Billy why we have to do this." They can also be involved in the actual treatment ("make sure he doesn't do so and so") and increase the compliance with medical regimens ("make sure he takes these pills 3 times a day until they are finished"; "if you give them to him, he'll take them"; "your husband has to take off 25 pounds"; "Dorothy must quit smoking").

ON COMING FROM THE ENCOUNTER

There is a tendency to limit consideration of the role of social network influences on help seeking to the pre-patient phase of the help-seeking career – that is, up to the point of contact with some professional helper or formal organization. Not only do network associates influence what goes on during, and the outcome of, formal encounters as we have suggested, but also the subsequent course of the problem through the stages of treatment, rehabilitation (in the case of "success") and death and bereavement (in the case of "failure"). Considerable attention has been devoted to the role of networks in going to see the doctor, much less to the role of networks as one comes from the doctor (Stoeckle et al. 1963). Lay consultation and referral, self-medication, etc., should never be regarded as only confined to the pre-patient stage of help seeking. Freidson allows for the possibility of network influences during patienthood when he suggests that a person:

... passes through the referral structure not only on his way to the physician but also on his way back: Discussing the doctor's behavior, diagnosis and prescription with his fellows with the possible consequence that he may never go back. (Freidson 1960).

It has been suggested that, with regard to certain conditions, no lay consultation or self-medication may occur at all prior to contact with a professional, due to a by-passing of, or the inaccessibility of, the lay referral structure. This, however, does not preclude the possibility of such action *after* formal contact with a service or professional.

What goes on during an encounter with a professional helper appears to be subsequently evaluated in discussions with network members against the common stock of knowledge of the network. Such evaluations determine whether the encounter was satisfactory, the prescribed course of treatment "appropriate", or sensible, and so on. During my own field work in Scotland during the late 1960's, I came upon a number of cases where the advice given by professionals was discussed within the confines of the family or friendship network, defined as preposterous, and laughed out of the network "court". It appeared that a client was inclined to comply with the course that was recommended, but was dissuaded from doing so by mothers, sisters, friends, and so on. A number of respondents were literally tired of childbearing and brought back from the formal encounter a sterilization application (to be completed by *both* the woman and her husband). This form was frequently "thrown to the back of the fire" by network members (most frequently by husbands, but also by mothers and fathers).

In some of the cases, the client desired the service, and had accepted the advice of the professional helpers, but her wishes were overridden by the network members. Through constant persuasion, threats, haranguing and so forth, they were often persuaded that the network was "right".

If there is a good fit between the content of a formal encounter and the negotiated expectations clients take into an encounter, then the probability of client satisfaction is increased (Korsch et al. 1968; Francis et al. 1969; Woolley et al. 1977). It also tends to confirm for the client that the experience and knowledge of the network members were correct, thereby further securing the network's position in the help-seeking career. If there is a poor fit between what goes on during the encounter and the expectations, then the client is more likely to be dissatisfied, the professional's actions deemed inappropriate or wrong, and rejected by the client *and* the network. Social network may impose a "heads I win — tails you lose" perspective on the help-seeking career of its members. If experiences during an encounter match expectations, then the input from the network is validated, the client satisfied, and the regimen complied with. If the encounter diverges from expectations, then professional actions are likely to be perceived as inappropriate or wrong, the client dissatisfied, and the recommended regimen dismissed.

While professional helpers must be alert to the ways in which networks may sabotage the regimens offered in what they define as "the client's best interest", there is also potential for involving network members in the regimen. Such involvement is certainly not enhanced by the routine exclusion of relatives and friends during the encounter.

When treatment or rehabilitation takes place on an inpatient basis, clients are somewhat isolated from network resources, control lies with the organization, and compliance is relatively easily assured. Most treatment, however, does not occur in formal organizations, but is "delivered" on an outpatient or ambulatory basis while the client is in the community and subject to the network influences. It is easier to ensure compliance with a regimen in a formal organization or total institution (e.g., weight reduction, bed rest, appropriate exercise, etc.) than it is in the context of the community, when the client is subject to the pressures, temptations and advice of network members. Most treatment does occur in the community, with the client subject to strong network influences. To be effective, therefore, treatment must take account of, and involve, network members.

It is difficult to effect weight reduction, smoking or drinking cessation and the removal of allergens when network members daily engage in, and actually encourage, behavior that is the converse of that prescribed. It is pointless instructing a man to reduce his cholesterol intake when it is his wife or mother who does the cooking. The cook must be involved if the advice is to be effective. What is to be gained from informing an asthmatic patient that he is allergic to animal dander, when the family breeds Siamese cats. Advice to an alcoholic woman to quit drinking is likely to be ineffective if it fails to take account of the fact that her husband arrives home drunk three nights a week. Obviously, he will have to be involved also. Regimens instituted without reference to the network context of the client/patient will be less successful than those which identify and involve network members who can support, reinforce and maintain the prescribed course of action.

Much of the illness that plagues modern man (e.g., cancer, heart disease, accidents, mental illness, alcoholism, etc.,) requires some alteration in "at risk" behaviors (e.g., smoking, diet, exercise, etc.). Our ability to measurably alter the over-all mortality and morbidity rates of these conditions will be largely determined by the extent to which we are able to involve network members in the alteration of behaviors that place people at risk.

REHABILITATION

Aspects of social networks or support systems have been shown to influence the etiology of illness, how problems are responded to and the ways in which services are utilized. In recent times they have also been associated with the process of recovery or rehabilitation (Smith 1979). Research to date, in common with that on the pre-patient stages of help seeking, usually consists of retrospective descriptions (observational studies) of how social network characteristics are, or may be, implicated in behavior that has already occurred.

Although researchers and clinicians remain reluctant to embark on controlled clinical trials, there is strong evidence of the contribution of both personal support networks (Finlayson 1976; Hyman 1972) and more organized support systems (Guggenheim and O'Hara 1976). One illustrative study of the former considered the use of networks by women whose husbands had suffered a heart attack. Those whose husbands had a more successful outcome one year after the attack were more likely to have utilized a larger number of help sources, than did those whose husbands had a less successful outcome. Women whose husbands were non-manual workers were more likely than those with manual husbands to use a wide range of sources. But within each occupational class, the relationship between diversity of the source of emotional support and information, and the outcome for the husband, was observed (Finlayson 1976; New et al. 1968). While these results derive from a relatively small sample of 76, they add further weight to the suggestion that network characteristics are involved at all stages of the help-seeking career — both pre- and post-patienthood. Further studies involving larger numbers and different problems and services are now required.

One such recent study by Berkman and Syme (1979) involved a nine-year follow-up of 4725 adults between the ages of 30 and 69 years in Alameda County, California. Data were collected on the following four aspects of social support: marriage, contacts with close friends and relatives, church membership, and informal and formal group associations. After controlling for initial health status, socio-economic status, various health practices and the utilization of medical services (all of which negatively influenced mortality), the age- and sex-specific mortality rates over the study period showed a strong relationship with the nature of social supports. Specifically, relative risks for those with the fewest social contacts were 2.3 for men and 2.8 for women. A composite social network index correlated negatively not only with overall mortality, but also with the following four separate causes of death: ischemic heart disease, cancer, cerebrovascular and circulatory diseases.

There are an ever increasing number of informal mutual aid or help groups consisting of people who have experienced similar problems or treatments. Well-known examples include: Alcoholics Anonymous, Weight Watchers, Mended Hearts Society (cardiac surgery patients), Reach to Recovery (mastectomy), and so on (Gussow and Tracy 1976). It is not suggested that the activities of those groups are consciously based on social network ideas, but that their activities touch on network structures. Members of such groups receive information, not always provided by the formal helping system, through shared experience. Moreover, they learn that they are not alone or necessarily "abnormal". They can pick up information which they are reluctant to request from the formal system, or for which professionals are considered inappropriate consultants (e.g., when to resume sexual relations after major surgery, suitable coital positions for the handicapped, and so forth). Disabled Vietnam veterans probably received this kind of information from their disabled peers. Roth (1963) has described some ways in which tuberculosis patients obtain information from fellow patients within a hospital. Much of the literature on labeling theory has implicitly assumed that deviant careers are relatively permanent. Trice and Roman (1969), in a much neglected paper, studied the ways in which the activities of Alcoholics Anonymous result in successful delabeling and the replacement of a stigmatized label with one that is socially acceptable.

Aspects of social networks (particularly the negative extreme of social isolation) have been related to the course and outcome of various rehabilitation programs. Litman (1961) found that orthopedically disabled patients who were engaged in little social participation prior to treatment displayed substantially less motivation in a program of physical rehabilitation than did the more socially active patients. Sussman and his colleagues (1964) report that tuberculosis patients who did not live with a family member were significantly less likely, following treatment, to have achieved adequate medical, vocational, economic and social rehabilitation. A similar finding was reported by Bolton and his colleagues (1968) who found that having dependents was conducive to successful vocational rehabilitation. Roth and Eddy (1967) describe the way in which lack of social contacts raises the odds against a successful outcome for patients in a rehabilitation ward of a public hospital. Coser (1962) has shown how patients with a variety of ailments who were socially isolated outside the hospital appeared to resist discharge by suffering relapses when discharge was imminent. Some indirect evidence is also available from studies of treatment for heart disease. Dager and Brewer (1958), for example, found that the more integrated a cardiac patient was with his family, the more his attitudes could be regarded as conducive to rehabilitation. Empathy for a stroke patient on the part of his family was found by Robertson and Suinn (1968) to be conducive to his progress in rehabilitation, thus implying that social isolation impairs rehabilitation. Hyman (1972) has recently added consistent evidence by showing that social isolation impairs stroke rehabilitation by rendering the patient less malleable to the influence of the rehabilitation program.

It is reasonable to assume that certain network characteristics exert considerable influence on the perception of health and well-being. Such an influence is important since, in studies of heart patients, personal perceptions have been found to be predictive of behavioral and rehabilitative outcomes, independently of other factors, such as clinical status. Along with several other factors, Brown and Rawlinson (1976) showed health perception to be predictive of morale after heart surgery. They also showed that the patient's perception of health was significantly and independently related to the tendency to relinquish the sick role after heart surgery (Brown and Rawlinson 1975). Garrity (1973a, b) has shown that perception of one's health after first myocardial infarction is strongly associated with level of morale and return to gainful employment; this study controlled for the effect of all clinical measures of health. In a recent twenty year follow-up of the Midtown Manhattan Study population it was found that self-assessment of health was a strong predictor of mortality (Singer et al. 1976). If perceived health and well-being does exert an independent influence on re-habilitative outcomes, network characteristics may be employed in the future, albeit indirectly, in certain rehabilitative endeavors. Much work remains to be done in this area.

A major challenge in clinical practice is to enlist the support of network members in the process of recovery and rehabilitation. Professional workers must be taught to identify the different types of network structures in which their clients are involved, and encourage members to work along with them towards the patient's recovery. Where social supports are absent, it may be possible to connect the client with the informal mutual aid groups which are thought to influence the recovery process. Medical education generally overlooks the importance of social networks in problem onset, and all stages of help seeking and recovery. Moreover, many health workers are unaware of the range of informal support organizations and groups that are available in the community with which they can ally. Ways must be found to routinely utilize these forms of social support, not just to turn to them when all else appears to have failed.

DEATH AND BEREAVEMENT

Various aspects of social networks have been shown to be importantly involved (in at least two different ways) at what may be considered the final stage of the help-seeking career — death and the process of bereavement. *Firstly*, network characteristics (e.g., size, strength of ties, content, frequency) have been shown to influence the risk of death, independently of such other related variables as social class, sex, age and ethnicity. Here, social networks are employed in epidemiological explanations of the etiology of particular morbid states. Literature pertinent to this usage was discussed earlier in relation to the social epidemiology of problems. A number of studies have pointed to the heavy toll that the death of, or mourning for, a significant other can have on health and longevity. One study by Parkes and his colleagues of the close relatives of 488 persons who died showed that in the first year after becoming widowed, the death rate among surviving spouses was ten times higher than among married people of comparable age and sex (Parkes et al. 1969, 1972). Another study, at the Montefiore Medical Center in the Bronx, revealed that in the first fifteen months after being widowed, older persons with such medical problems as heart disease or diabetes, became much worse and were more likely to seek medical help than those of the same age who were not bereaved (Brody 1979). A further recent study by Somers (1979) revealed high rates of illness and death among persons who are separated or divorced and, in some circumstances, among those who remain single as well. It appears that being married and residing with one's spouse (without regard to the quality of the relationship) is the healthiest of all marital states (Brody 1979).

A *second* way in which social networks may figure during this final stage in the help-seeking career is through their mediation of the consequences of bereavement. Here, the concept of a social network is employed to understand not the etiology of the death, but the response to a death. In an extremely useful review, Walker and his colleagues suggest that "bereavement is especially relevant to social networks since it constitutes a major disruption of the surviving spouse's intimate network and severely tests the supportiveness of that network" (Walker et al. 1977). They quote from Boswell's work on the way in which networks affect the response to crisis:

At any one time the members of the social network are in the potential position of being mobilized to deal with a problem situation. Depending on the gravity and type of the latter, links long dormant may be brought into an instrumental relationship again. An understanding of the ways in which the set of relationships, analyzed as the social network, may be used is crucial to the understanding of how problems are met and solutions reached. (Boswell 1969).

Perhaps more than any other variable, social networks may determine how the crisis of death is responded to or coped with by particular individuals and groups.

Several researchers have noted that Western industrialized cultures lack clear prescriptions for how to mourn the dead, with the result that people in grief have few acceptable channels for the social expression of their loss (Gorer 1965; Blauner 1966). In nonliterate cultures, however, one often finds rituals that permit the public expression of anger, sadness, loss, fear, and the many other feelings associated with death, which it is apparently desirable to express. Many non-Western cultures also have clear prescriptions concerning the appropriate length of the mourning period, in whose presence one should mourn, from whom various kinds of support can be expected, how grief should be expressed, and so forth (Averill 1968; Volkard 1959). The church appears to have been a major institutional support for the bereaved in Western societies. However, a number of studies over the last decade or so reveal that the bereaved are not now utilizing this particular support system. It has been suggested that mutual help groups have emerged to substitute for the absence of appropriate rituals and support systems in Western culture. Widow to widow programs, for example, appear to provide opportunities for the bereaved to learn to live as a widow, or single parent, and seem to enhance the quality of life (Walker et al. 1977). One can hardly be impressed by the many studies associated with the general areas of death and bereavement. Many of them are impressionistic, methodologically defective, and evidence a kind of social work avuncularity. Still, they are suggestive, and argue for properly designed and executed studies which could shed light on the relationship between social support systems and the process of bereavement.

A number of authors have found it useful to view bereavement as a passage through several distinct phases and suggest that social networks have a differential influence at each phase (Gorer 1965; Parkes 1972; Vachon 1976). Research to date has tended to focus on the bereavement experiences of women whose husbands have died, and point to the ambiguous position such women find themselves in within the social system. There are reports that they lack a social identity acceptable for membership in a network, that they are stigmatized, and that married couples feel threatened and uncomfortable in their presence (Walker et al. 1977).

The concept of a social network has been shown to be of considerable utility in explaining behavior at earlier points in the help-seeking career, and in many other areas as well. It is frequently suggested that different social classes, age categories, cultural groups respond to the crisis of death differently. Now it is likely that these differences may be explained, in large part, by the different network patterns known to be associated with different classes, age categories and ethnic groups. In other words, network influences on the bereavement process may be masked by the different network structures found among the various groups that are thought to respond to death in different ways. Once the precise nature of network influence can be specified, it may be possible to deliberately manipulate network structures in order to "maximize the tranquilizing influence of human companionship" (Lynch 1977). Some movement in this direction may result from the work reported by Walker and his colleagues who, along with some others, are training and organizing a group of widows as widow contacts to provide social support, and are evaluating the outcome (Walker et al. 1977). It appears that there is often a lack of fit between the social and psychological needs of people involved in grief work, and their own social support system. This lack of fit is probably exacerbated in Western cultures with their characteristic high rates of geographic mobility, attenuated extended family systems, and the instrumentalism attending many personal relationships.

Appropriate intervention by the so-called "helping professions" in the future may involve the routine assessment and perhaps the modification/mobilization of the active and dormant support structures of those experiencing crisis-induced stress. Before social networks can be routinely utilized as therapeutic aides however, there must be considerably more operational clarity of the concept. Despite the plethora of observational studies which suggest that social networks may be useful therapeutic aids, it will only be through properly designed and conducted prospective studies that their actual effectiveness will be placed beyond dispute and the findings form a basis for some social policy concerning the allocation of resources in this particular area. From the available literature it is impossible to tell whether it is the influence of particular network structures, or something else entirely, which produced the results claimed for the social support system. Death and bereavement remain the stage in the help-seeking career where the least is known about the precise influence of social support systems. And yet, it is at this point that the concept, as a basis for effective interventions, may have the greatest potential.

In this chapter I have attempted to illustrate the potential of the concept of a social network for understanding the etiology of particular morbid episodes, how they are responded to, recovery from them, and so forth. The overall emphasis has been on a person in some kind of need. The picture I have been painting is, necessarily, incomplete. Cutting across the career of the person seeking, receiving and benefiting from help is the encounter with the formal system of helping (depicted in Figure 1 as vertical broken line). This formal system comprises the army of professionals, paraprofessionals, semiprofessionals, agencies, organizations and institutions which are also variously involved in the delivery of help. The concept of social network offers as much for the understanding of this formal or professional helping behavior as it does the understanding of client help seeking. These various helpers and institutions may also be usefully viewed in network terms and aspects of social networks have already been shown to influence the uptake of new drugs, patterns of referral, clinical decision making, career choices, etc. Limitations of space alone preclude a consideration of this body of data.

REFERENCES

Adams, B.
  1967   Interaction Theory and Social Network. Sociometry 30:64–78.
Aday, L. A., and R. Anderson
  1975   A Framework for the Study of Access to Medical Care. Robert Wood Johnson Foundation, University of Chicago.
Apple, D.
  1960   How Laymen Define Illness. Journal of Health and Human Behavior. 1:219–225.
Averill, J. P.
  1968   Grief: Its Nature and Significance. Psychological Bulletin. 70(6):721–748.
Beaglehole, R., et al.
  1977   Blood Pressure and Social Interaction in Tokelauon Migrants in New Zealand. Journal of Chronic Diseases 30:803–812.
Berkman, L. F., and S. L. Syme
  1979   Social Networks, Host Resistance, and Mortality: A Nine Year Follow-up of Alameda County Residents. American Journal of Epidemiology 109(2):186–204.
Blauner, R.
  1966   Death and Social Structure. Psychiatry 29:378–394.
Bolton, B. F., A. J. Butler, and G. N. Wright
  1968   Clinical Versus Statistical Prediction of Client Feasibility. Madison: University of Wisconsin Regional Rehabilitation Research Institute.
Boswell, D. M.
  1969   Personal Crises and the Mobilization of the Social Network. *In* Social Networks in Urban Situations. J. C. Mitchell, ed. Manchester: Manchester University Press.
Bott, E.
  1957   Family and Social Network. London: Tavistock.

Brody, J.
    1979 Marriage is Good for Health and Longevity, Studies Say. New York Times, Tuesday, May 8.
Brown, G. W., M. N. Bhrolchain, and T. Harris
    1975 Social Class and Psychiatric Disturbance among Women in an Urban Population. Sociology 9:225–254.
Brown, J. S., and M. Rawlinson
    1975 Relinquishing the Sick Role Following Open-Heart Surgery. Journal of Health and Social Behavior 16:12–27.
    1976 The Morale of Patients Following Open-Heart Surgery. Journal of Health and Social Behavior 17:135–145.
Brown, S. E.
    1975 Love Unites Them and Hunger Separates Them: Poor Women in the Dominican Republic. In Toward an Anthropology of Women. R. Reiter, ed. New York: Monthly Review Press.
Browner, C.
    1979 Abortion Decision Making: Some Findings from Columbia. Studies in Family Planning 10(3):96–106.
Bryce-Laporte, R. S.
    1970 Urban Relocation and Family Adaptation in Puerto Rico: A Case Study in Urban Ethnography. In Peasants in Cities: Readings in the Anthropology of Urbanization. W. Mangin, ed. Boston: Houghton Mifflin.
Burch, J.
    1972 Recent Bereavement in Relation to Suicide. Journal of Psychosomatic Research 16:361–366.
Cassel, J.
    1969 Physical Illness in Response to Stress. Unpublished manuscript. University of North Carolina at Chapel Hill, pp. 1–30.
    1974 Psychosocial Processes and 'Stress': Theoretical Formulation. International Journal of Health Services 4:471–482.
Cassel, J. and H. A. Tyroler
    1961 Epidemiological Studies of Culture Change, I. Health Studies and Recency of Industrialization. Archives of Environmental Health 3:25–39.
Christenson, W. N., and L. E. Hinkle, Jr.
    1961 Differences in Illness and Prognostic Signs in Two Groups of Young Men. Journal of American Medical Association 177:247–253.
Cobb, S.
    1976 Social Support as a Moderator of Life Stress. Psychosomatic Medicine 38:300–314.
Coe, R.
    1970 Sociology of Medicine. New York: McGraw-Hill.
Coser, R. L.
    1961 Insulation from Observability and Types of Social Conformity. American Sociological Review 25:28–39.
    1962 Life in the Ward. Lansing: Michigan State University Press.
Craven, P. and B. Wellman
    1974 The Network City. In The Community: Approaches and Applications. M. P. Effrat, ed. New York: Free Press.
Croog, S. H., A. Lipson, and S. Levine
    1972 Help Patterns in Severe Illness: The Roles of Kin Network, Non-Family Resources and Institutions. Journal of Marriage and the Family 34:32–41.
Dager, E. Z., and D. L. Brewer
    1958 Family Integration and the Response to Heart Disease. Proceedings of the Purdue Cardiac Seminar, Purdue University, pp. 62–64.

Daniels, A. K.
  1970 Normal Mental Illness and Understandable Excuses. American Behavioral Scientist
        14:167–184.
Dean, A., and N. Lin
  1977 The Stress-Buffering Role of Social Support: Problems and Prospects for Sys-
        tematic Investigation. Journal of Nervous and Mental Disease 165:403–417.
de Araujo, G., et al.
  1973 Life Change, Coping Ability and Chronic Intrinsic Asthma. Journal of Psycho-
        somatic Research 17:359–363.
Dimsdale, J.
  1974 The Coping Behavior of Nazi Concentration Camp Survivors. American Journal of
        Psychiatry 131:792–797.
Dinitz, S., et al.
  1961 Psychiatric and Social Attributes as Predictors of Case Outcome in Mental Hospi-
        talization. Social Problems 8:322–328.
Dinitz, S., et al.
  1962 Instrumental Role Expectations and Performance of Mental Patients. American
        Journal of Sociology 68:248–254.
Eaton, J. W., and R. J. Weil
  1955 Culture and Mental Disorders. Glencoe, Illinois: Free Press.
Finlayson, A.
  1976 Social Networks as Coping Resources: Lay Help and Consultation Patterns Used
        by Women in Husband's Post-Infarction Career. Social Science and Medicine
        10:97–103.
Francis, V., et al.
  1969 Gaps in Doctor-Patient Communication. New England Journal of Medicine 280:
        535–540.
Freidson, E.
  1960 Client Control and Medical Practice. American Journal of Sociology 65:374–382.
Fried, M., et al.
  1973 The World of the Urban Working Class. Cambridge, Mass.: Harvard University
        Press.
Gans, H.
  1962 The Urban Villagers. New York: Free Press.
Garrity, T. F.
  1973a Social Involvement and Activeness as Predictors of Morale Six Months After First
        Myocardial Infarction. Social Science and Medicine 7:199–207.
  1973b Vocational Adjustment After First Myocardial Infarction: Comparative Assess-
        ment of Several Variables Suggested in the Literature. Social Science and Medicine
        7:705–717.
Geersten, R., et al.
  1975 A Re-Examination of Suchman's Views on Social Factors in Health Care Utiliza-
        tion. Journal of Health and Social Behavior 16(2):226–237.
Goffman, E.
  1953 The Moral Career of the Mental Patient. Psychiatry 22:123–142.
Gore, S.
  1978 The Effect of Social Support in Moderating the Health Consequences of Unem-
        ployment. Journal of Health and Social Behavior 19:157–165.
Gorer, G.
  1965 Death, Grief and Mourning in Contemporary Britain. London: Cresset.
Gottlieb, B. H.
  1976 Lay Influences on the Utilization and Provision of Health Services. Canadian
        Psychological Review 17:126–136.

Granovetter, Mark S.
    1973 The Strength of Weak Ties. American Journal of Sociology 78:1360–1380.
Guggenheim, F., and S. O'Hara.
    1976 Peer Counselling in a General Hospital. American Journal of Psychiatry 133:
          1197–1199.
Gussow, Z., and G. S. Tracy
    1976 The Role of Self-Help Clubs in Adaptation to Chronic Illness and Disability.
          Social Science and Medicine 10:407–414.
Haenzel, W., D. B. Loveland, and M. G. Sirken
    1962 Lung-Cancer Mortality as Related to Residence and Smoking Histories. Journal
          National Cancer Institute 28:947–1001.
Hamburg, D., B. Hamburg, and S. deGoza
    1953 Adaptive Problems and Mechanisms in Several Burned Patients. Psychiatry 16:
          1–20.
Hammel, E. A.
    1961 The Family Cycle in a Coastal Peruvian Slum and Village. American Anthropol-
          ogist 63:989–1005.
Hinkle, L. E., et al.
    1960 An Examination of the Relation Between Symptoms, Disability and Serious Ill-
          ness in Two Homogeneous Groups of Men and Women. American Journal of
          Public Health 50:1327–1336.
Holmes, T. H.
    1956 Multi-discipline Studies of Tuberculosis. In Personality, Stress and Tuberculosis.
          P. J. Sparer, ed. New York: International University Press.
Horwitz, A.
    1978 Family, Kin, and Friend Networks in Psychiatric Help-Seeking. Social Science and
          Medicine 12:297–304.
Hyman, M. D.
    1972 Social Isolation and Performance in Rehabilitation. Journal of Chronic Diseases
          25:85–97.
Jones, R. A. K., and E. M. Belsey
    1977 Breast Feeding in an Inner London Borough – A Study of Cultural Factors. Social
          Science and Medicine 11:175–179.
Kadushin, C.
    1958 Individual Decisions to Undertake Psychotherapy. Administrative Science Quar-
    –1959 terly 3:379–411.
Kaplan, B. H., J. Cassel, and S. Gore
    1977 Social Support and Health. Medical Care 15 (Supplement to No. 5): 47–58.
Katz, E., and B. Danet
    1966 Petitions and Persuasive Appeals: A Study of Official-Client Relations. American
          Sociological Review 31:811–822.
Korsch, B. M., et al.
    1968 Gaps in Doctor-Patient Communication. Pediatrics 42:855–871.
Langlie, J. K.
    1977 Social Networks, Health Beliefs, and Preventive Health Behavior. Journal of
          Health and Social Behavior 18:244–260.
Levine, S., and N. Scotch
    1970 Social Stress. Chicago: Aldine.
Lewis, O.
    1973 Some Perspectives on Urbanization with Special Reference to Mexico City. In
          Urban Anthropology: Cross-Cultural Studies of Urbanization. A. Southall, ed.
          New York: Oxford University Press.

Lin, N., et al.
1979 Social Support, Stressful Life Events, and Illness: A Model and an Empirical Test. Journal of Health and Social Behavior 20(2):108–119.
Litwak, E., and I. Szelenyi
1969 Primary Group Structures and Their Functions: Kin, Neighbors and Friends. American Sociological Review 34:465–481.
Litman, T. J.
1961 The Influence of Concept of Self and Life Orientation Factors Upon the Rehabilitation of Orthopedic Patients. Ph.D. dissertation, University of Minnesota.
Liu, W. T., and R. W. Duff
1972 The Strength of Weak Ties. Public Opinion Quarterly 36(3):361–366.
Lomnitz, L. A.
1977 Networks and Marginality: Life in a Mexican Shantytown. New York: Academic Press.
Lynch, J. J.
1977 The Broken Heart: The Medical Consequences of Loneliness: New York: Basic Books.
McKinlay, John B.
1971 The Concept 'Patient Career' as a Heuristic Device for Making Medical Sociology Relevant to Medical Students. Social Science and Medicine 5:441–460.
1972 Some Approaches and Problems in the Study of the Use of Services – An Overview. Journal of Health and Social Behavior 13:115–152.
1973 Social Networks, Lay Consultation and Help-Seeking Behavior. Social Forces 51(3):275–292.
Marmot, M.
1975 Acculturation and Coronary Heart Disease in Japanese Americans. Ph.D. dissertation, University of California, Berkeley.
Marris, P.
1958 Widows and Their Families. London: Routledge and Kegan Paul.
Mechanic, D.
1968 Medical Sociology. New York: Free Press.
1969 Illness and Cure. In Poverty and Health. J. Kosa, A. Antonovsky, and I. K. Zola, eds. pp. 191–214. Cambridge, Mass.: Harvard University Press.
Miller, P., and G. Ingham
1976 Friends, Confidants and Symptoms. Social Psychiatry 11:51–58.
Mitchell, J. Clyde, ed.
1969a Social Networks in Urban Situations. Manchester: The University of Manchester Press.
1969b The Concept and Use of Social Networks. In Social Networks in Urban Situations. J. C. Mitchell, ed. pp. 1–50. Manchester: Manchester University Press.
Neser, W., H. Tyroler, and J. Cassel
1971 Social Disorganization and Stroke Mortality in the Black Population of North Carolina. American Journal of Epidemiology 93:166–175.
New, P. K., et al.
1968 The Support Structure of Heart and Stroke Patients. Social Science and Medicine 2:185–200.
Nuckolls, K., J. Cassel, and B. Kaplan
1972 Psychosocial Assets, Life Crisis and the Prognosis of Pregnancy. American Journal of Epidemiology 95:431–441.
Parkes, C. M.
1972 Bereavement: Studies of Grief in Adult Life. New York: International Universities Press.

Parkes, C. M., B. Benjamin, and R. G. Fitzgerald
    1969 Broken Heart: A Statistical Study of Increased Mortality Among Widowers.
          British Medical Journal 1:740–743.
Pearlin, L. I., and C. Schooler
    1978 The Structure of Coping. Journal of Health and Social Behavior 19:2–21.
Peattie, L. R.
    1968 The View from the Barrio. Ann Arbor: University of Michigan Press.
Pratt, L.
    1972 Conjugal Organization and Health. Journal of Marriage and the Family 2:85–95.
Reeder, S., A. C. Marcus, and T. E. Seeman
    1978 The Influence of Social Networks on the Use of Health Services. Unpublished
          paper, U.C.L.A.
Reid, D.D.
    1947 Some Measures of the Effect of Operational Stress on Bomber Crews. In Psycho-
          logical Disorders in Flying Personnel of the R. A. F. London: H. M. SO.
Robertson, D. K., and R. M. Suinn
    1968 The Determination of Rate of Progress of Stroke Patients Through Empathy
          Measures of Patients and Family. Journal of Psychosomatic Research 12:189–191.
Roth, J. A.
    1963 Information and the Control of Treatment in Tuberculosis Hospitals. In The
          Hospital in Modern Society. E. Freidson, ed. pp. 293–318. Glencoe: Free Press.
Roth, J. A. and E. M. Eddy
    1967 Rehabilitation for the Unwanted. New York: Atherton Press.
Salloway, J. C., and P. Dillan
    1973 A Comparison of Family Networks and Friend Networks in Health Care Utiliza-
          tion. Journal of Comparative Family Studies 4:131–142.
Scotch, N. A.
    1963 Sociocultural Factors in the Epidemiology of Zulu Hypertension. American
          Journal of Public Health 52:1205–1213.
Scotch, N. A., and H. J. Geiger
    1962 The Epidemiology of Rheumatoid Arthritis: A Review with Special Attention to
          Social Factors. Journal of Chronic Diseases 15:1037–1067.
Shils, E. A., and M. Janowitz
    1948 Cohesian and Disintegration in the Wehrmacht. Public Opinion Quarterly 12:
          280–315.
Singer, E., et al.
    1976 Mortality and Mental Health: Evidence from the Midtown Manhattan Re-study.
          Social Science and Medicine 10:517–525.
Smith, R. T.
    1979 Disability and the Recovery Process: Role of Social Networks. In Patients, Physi-
          cians and Illness. E. G. Jaco, ed. pp. 218–226. New York: Free Press.
Somers, A. R.
    1979 Marital Status, Health, and Use of Health Services. Journal of American Heart
          Association. 241:(17):1818–1822.
Stoeckle, J. D., I. K. Zola, and G. E. Davidson
    1963 On Going to See the Doctor: The Contributions of the Patient to the Decision
          to Seek Medical Aid. Journal of Chronic Diseases 16:975–989.
Suchman, E. A.
    1964 Sociomedical Variations Among Ethnic Groups. American Journal of Sociology
          70:319–331.
Sussman, M. B., et al.
    1975 Rehabilitation and Tuberculosis. Cleveland: Western Reserve Press.
Swank, R. L.
    1949 Combat Exhaustion: A Descriptive and Statistical Analysis of Causes, Symptoms
          and Signs. Journal of Nervous and Mental Diseases 109:475–508.

Syme, S. L., M. M. Hyman, and P. E. Enterline
    1964 Some Social and Cultural Factors Associated with the Occurrence of Coronary
          Heart Disease. Journal of Chronic Diseases 17:277–289.
Townsend, P.
    1957 The Family Life of Old People: An Enquiry in East London. London: Routledge
          and Kegan Paul.
Trice, H. M., and P. M. Roman
    1969 Delabeling, Relabeling and Alcoholics Anonymous. Presented at Southern Socio-
          logical Society, New Orleans.
Tyroler, H. A., and J. Cassel
    1964 Health Consequences of Culture Change: The Effect of Urbanization on Coronary
          Heart Mortality in Rural Residents of North Carolina. Journal of Chronic Diseases
          17:167–177.
Vachon, M. L. S.
    1976 Grief and Bereavement Following the Death of a Spouse. Canadian Psychiatric
          Association Journal 21:35–44.
Volkard, B., and S. T. Mitchell
    1959 Bereavement and Mental Health. In Exploration in Social Psychiatry. A. Leighton,
          et al., eds. New York: Basic Books.
Walker, N. K., A. MacBride, and M. L. S. Vachon
    1977 Social Support Networks and the Crisis of Bereavement. Social Science and
          Medicine 11:35–41.
Walsh, J. L., and R. H. Elling
    1968 Professionalism and the Poor: Structural Effects and Professional Behavior.
          Journal of Health and Social Behavior 9:16–28.
Woolley, F. R., et al.
    1977 The Effects of Doctor-Patient Communication on Satisfaction and Outcome of
          Care. Social Science and Medicine 12:123–128.
Yarrow, M., et al.
    1955 The Psychological Meaning of Mental Illness in the Family. Journal of Social
          Issues 11:12–24.
Young, M. and P. Willmott
    1957 Family and Kinship in East London. London: Penguin Books.
Zola, I. K.
    1964 Illness Behavior of the Working Class: Implications and Recommendations. In
          Blue Collar World. A. B. Shostak and W. Gomberg, eds. pp. 350–361. Englewood
          Cliffs, N.J.: Prentice-Hall.
    1966 Culture and Symptoms: An Analysis of Patients Presenting Complaints. American
          Sociological Review 31:615–630.

SECTION 3

ILLNESS BEHAVIOR

ANDREW C. TWADDLE

5. SICKNESS AND THE SICKNESS CAREER: SOME IMPLICATIONS

In the past two decades sociologists have become interested in questions of illness and sickness beyond the search for social factors associated with diseases. The work in this area has led to the concept of sickness as a form of deviant behavior, the identification of distinctive "sick roles", and investigation of the decision making processes associated with the experience of sickness from the standpoint of the patient. This work has been recently summarized using the heuristic concept of a "sickness career".

No attempt will be made in this paper to add substantially to this literature from either a theoretical or an empirical point of view. For the interested reader, I have made summary statements elsewhere (Twaddle and Hessler 1977:96–136; Twaddle 1979). Rather, the focus will be on how these concepts may be of use to the health professional in two roles, clinician and citizen. In the first sense, the health professional is concerned with the problems of identifying the nature of health problems and in devising effective means of intervention directed at solving those problems. In the second, (s)he is concerned with keeping people well, reducing health hazards and organizing the delivery of health related services.

Toward this end, we will begin with an important set of distinctions among disease, illness and sickness. While these terms are often used interchangeably in everyday life, they are here distinguished to focus attention on three quite different modalities by which "non-health" can be experienced. The confusion of these modes can result in great difficulty, especially in communications between patients and professionals. Second, we will address the question of *why* the sickness career is important to the clinical and citizenship interests of health professionals by reviewing trends in the physician-patient relationship. These trends have led simultaneously to great professional autonomy on the part of physicians and great alienation among patients which is reflected in, among other things, a spectacular rise in malpractice litigation in recent years. Only then will we deal with the question of *how* the sickness career model can be used to (1) improve the accuracy and efficiency of diagnosis and treatment and (2) to design more effective and humane systems of responding to health needs of both individuals and populations.

DISEASE, ILLNESS, AND SICKNESS

Health is increasingly being recognized as having psychological and social dimensions in addition to the biological ones. The term *"disease"* is used to indicate the biological dimension of nonhealth, which has come to be the focus of

111

L. Eisenberg and A. Kleinman (eds.), The Relevance of Social Science for Medicine, 111–133.
Copyright © 1980 by D. Reidel Publishing Company.

medicine in the past two centuries. Disease is an "objective" phenomenon that can be measured through laboratory tests, direct observation, or other "signs". It is what happens to indivduals when their physiological functioning departs from "normal" or they become hosts to other organisms which limit life expectancy or capacities. "*Illness*" refers to the more subjective or psychological dimensions of non-health that are generally of more immediate concern to the people experiencing them. These include pain, weakness, dizziness, numbness, or some other "symptom" that has them worried either because of immediate discomfort, its effects on capacities for social functioning, or what they think it may portend. "*Sickness*" refers to the social dimension: the ability to meet obligations of group living. It is the result of being defined by others as "unhealthy". It generally results from having one's failure to meet social obligations defined by others as the result of disease or illness.

In addition to the implications of this distinction for the discussion below, there are three points that should be of practical concern to clinicians.

First, *the question of who is healthy and who is sick is a matter of great inherent ambiguity that is actively negotiated between symptomatic people and other people* ranging from members of the immediate family to friends and neighbors to people presumed to know about health matters because of personal experience, special training, or connections with the medical care system. As will be described below, prior to seeing a health professional decisions have been made by the symptomatic individual and others that (s)he has a problem that falls within the domain of that particular professional. There has been no "delay".[1] Rather, a lay diagnosis has been made. The ill person is judged by others to be sick. This is a social fact that the professional must accept whether or not any underlying disease is identified.

Second, *almost no patient comes to the health professional with a disease.*[2] Instead they come with symptoms that involve how they feel and what they can do and how they are viewed by others. These symptoms are almost invariably "real"[3] and it is the duty of the professional to respond to them. However, it is not only disease that can be the "cause". Through interviewing, laboratory tests and observation, the health professional "makes a diagnosis". That is to say, (s)he converts the sickness from one based on illness into one based on disease or, failing to make the conversion, rejects the designation of the patient as sick. In the former case, the medical process makes little common sense unless the connections between the symptoms and the disease are explained to the patient in a way that (s)he can accept. In the latter case, the patient is left still suffering from the problem brought to the professional's attention and experiences either a sense of rejection or a conviction that the professional does not "know what (s)he is doing". For these reasons, health education should be a central role, if not *the* central role, of all health professionals.

Third, *to understand the causes of the complaints brought to health professionals one must focus attention on a wider range of variables than the biological ones*. All of the symptoms and many of the signs of illness and disease can be brought about by social and psychological factors in ways partly recognized in the concept of "functional" illness. Increasingly, it is recognized that these same factors can bring on the diseases themselves. An adequate medical history must encompass not only physical symptoms but also the patient's interpersonal relationships, recreational activities, work activities, living conditions, and the like. Adequate therapy must often involve intervention into these areas of life as well as the more traditional biochemical and surgical interventions. As the papers by McKinlay and Zola describe, these more traditional interventions have treated only the symptoms of disease from an epidemiological point of view. Effective intervention requires action in areas that have been heretofore set aside from medical concerns as "political". The historically recent narrowing of medical attention to disease has produced some benefits in our knowledge about the human body. It has done so at a tremendous cost. To be relevant to health, medical concerns must include illness and sickness as well.

TRENDS IN THE PHYSICIAN-PATIENT RELATIONSHIP

The distinction between disease, illness and sickness also calls attention to changes in medical practice that have fundamentally altered the physician-patient relationship. Certainly prior to the 19th centrury the focus of the medical practitioner was directed to the patient's environment both in the search for causes of illness and for cures. A social epidemiological approach was to be found as late as the middle of the 19th century in Europe, when Virchow wrote in the first issue of the journal, *Reformed Medicine*, "medicine is a social science and politics are nothing else than medicine on a large scale". With the early successes in applying the germ theory of disease, however, the concern with the social and personal qualities of the patient receded from the central concerns of medicine, displaced by an almost exclusive focus on disease (c.f. Bohlin et al. 1978).

With the Flexner Report in the United States in 1910, the basic medical curriculum was built around the biological and physical sciences. Social, psychological and environmental concerns were all but eliminated from training of physicians, and nurses were trained in providing support services to medicine. Nevertheless, well into the 20th century medicine was practiced in relatively small towns and the practitioner tended to be a generalist who knew his patients well. Hence, he had a good intuitive grasp of many of the important social factors affecting diagnosis and treatment.

Subsequent to the Flexner Report, however, many changes became evident. Changes in the population, the rapid increase of biophysical knowledge and increasing demand escalated the work pressures on the medical care system at a time when the number of qualified practitioners was declining. The scale of organization increased as medical practice shifted from the home to the hospital, both because of the need for greater productivity and the need to accomodate expensive technological developments. Medical practice became highly specialized, coordination became an issue, and care, from the standpoint of the patient, became fragmented, disorganized and expensive.

The professional autonomy of the physician, which, as Freidson (1975) showed, developed prior to any demonstrable benefits of medicine, was enhanced along at least four dimensions. A body of specialized knowledge about disease and treatment, not shared by the lay public, increased the *clinical* autonomy of the physician. The concentration of practice in settings controlled by physicians increased their *organizational* autonomy. *Economic* autonomy increased with the limitation of payment to a fee-for-service system that gives total control over charges to medical practitioners. Finally, the increased prestige of medicine and the enormously high incomes of physicians provided both power and authority and allowed practitioners to chose their own lifestyle and to set the terms of interaction with patients, a form of *class and interpersonal* autonomy.

The other side of the development of autonomy for practitioners was the development of alienation among patients along the same four dimensions: *clinical*, in that patients could not assume they knew either the true causes of disease nor did they have access to drugs without medical prescription; *organizational*, in that they had to seek medical services on the "turf" of the professional rather than in the familiar setting of the home; *economic*, in that the elimination of barter or payment "in kind" meant that patients had to accept the financial terms dictated by medicine or do without service;[4] and *class and interpersonal*, in that deference was required to a greater degree and they were seen not as persons but as "cases" (Twaddle and Stoeckle, MS).

One result of increasing professional autonomy and patient alienation is that there are several challenges to the power and autonomy of medicine in political terms. In the United States these can be diffusely felt as the movement for the development of health care teams in which the physician will be expected to relate as an equal with nurses and other professionals, a movement particularly strong in nursing (Mauksch and David 1972); and in the unsteady movement toward a national health insurance system, if not a national health service. The trends are much more apparent in a country with more developed social services, such as Sweden. There, the organization of medicine as a super-specialized, hospital-based service in which physician-patient and physician-other relationships are authoritarian is under attack not only by leftist politicians (Ågren 1978) and radical students (Janlert 1978) but by researchers (Gustafsson 1978), planners for the county governments (Landstingssektorns Framtidsstudieverksamhet 1978), and practicing physicians (Jersild 1978). The result is a shift in national policy toward primary care of symptomatic people as the dominant form of sickness care (*Sjukvård*) (Hessler 1978). Equally important in discussions among health planners is the shift toward prevention of disease by focusing on the environment (*hälsovård*) and in the positive promotion of good health (*friskvård*) through nutritional improvements, exercise programs and the like. Berglind et al. (1978) report a paradigm shift from treatment to prevention, from cure to care, from disease to behavior producing disease, from the individual to the population as the unit of treatment, from illness as a concern of medical professions to health as the business of everybody, from right to treatment to the duty to remain healthy (c.f. Tibblin 1978). Clearly the effort is being made to reduce the autonomy of medicine and the alienation of patients along all of the dimensions we have listed.

At a more individual level in the United States there has been an escalation of malpractice litigation. Both the number of lawsuits alleging injury resulting from inept or ignorant practice and the size of awards have increased substantially in recent years. Malpractice insurance premiums have reached astronomical figures and physicians are clearly worried about the future. There is a widespread belief that it is not the elderly, out-of-date, isolated practitioner who is likely to be sued, but rather the highly trained, superspecialized, hospital based, university physician who is practicing state-of-the-art medicine.[5] This has been taken by physicians as evidence that the public is ignorant of what constitutes "good medicine", reflecting a feeling that such suits are gratuitous and capricious. Yet, it is just such a physician who would have the most alienated patient. And the phenomenon is not limited to the United States. In Sweden the National Board of Health and Welfare has an office where patients can make complaints about the quality of their medical services. There too, the rate of complaint filing has escalated, and disproportionately the complaints are about treatment in the large, highly specialized, high technology, hospital care. It seems safe to conclude that malpractice suits in a highly developed medical care system with no national health program and complaints in a highly developed medical care system with a national health program are equivalent phenomena. Both reflect frustrations of the public in dealing with autonomous professionals. To use our distinctions by analogy, malpractice litigation is an illness, and perhaps a sign. The disease is the Alienation-Autonomy Syndrome.

The issues that we have identified — complex organization, the organization of work, the impact of technology, alienation, interaction and the like — are the classic themes of sociology. From the standpoint of citizenship, if only at the level of identifying problems and protecting one's own interests (another central sociological theme), it is required that the health practitioner be sociologically informed. To institute changes that provide meaningful improvements to the public is a task that cannot be done, I would submit, without careful sociological investigation.

At the clinical level of the encounter between professional and patient there is yet another implication of this analysis. As medical practice became specialized and hospital based, physicians more frequently found themselves dealing with patients who were not personally known to them, about whom they knew nothing beyond what could be gathered in a short interview or observed during the course of treatment. While conventional medical wisdom has it that more than 90% of a diagnosis comes from the interview, it has become more difficult to assess the information gained. How much weight can one give to the description of a symptom? What inferences can be made about the impact of symptoms on the lives of the patients? What kinds of treatment would best fit the lifestyle of the patient and would be followed? Because information taken by interview is difficult to assess without training, more weight is given to the use of laboratory tests in making diagnosis, and communication between physician and patient tends to be task-specific and often seems to be "cold". Clearly such a situation is less humane than one in which the physician and patient are friends who have a long personal history of relating to one another and where there can be more personal reciprocity in the provision of services. Equally clearly, we will not, even in the moderately long run, return to a society organized around small towns and medicine organized around general practice. What is needed is some substitute for the diagnostic and therapeutic "intuition" that comes with person-oriented as opposed to disease-oriented medicine. Here I submit that the social and behavioral sciences have become indispensable to competent practice. I further submit that one specific area of social science knowledge of primary importance is that subsumed under the concept of the sickness career, to which we now turn.

THE SICKNESS CAREER

The concept of a sickness "career" focuses attention on the decisions made by and/or for a person as (s)he becomes symptomatic, defined as sick, a patient, etc. As with other careers (occupational, aging, fraternal, etc.) sickness is something a person goes through over a period of time. There are definable stages and a goal (Roth 1963). The sequence of decisions that constitute a sickness career takes place for any individual in specific *settings* in interaction with *other people*, who in accordance with their assessment of the problem and taking into account their own needs and the *opportunities* for alternative courses of action which are available, apply the *social norms* of their particular group and set *expectations* for behavior. The individual must then assess (or have assessed for her/him) the range of opportunities and the rewards and costs associated with each option and *negotiate* whatever conflicts exist in the expectations upheld by others. This must be done for each of several more or less distinguishable decisions, which we discuss below. First we require some clarity on the concepts.

Social norms are expectations for behavior shared by groups of people. In a broad and general sense, a large and complex society such as the United States may be said to have norms, at least at the level of broad values. In a smaller country such as Sweden, these norms may be more intensely felt and dynamically important in guiding behavior. One such example important to the present discussion is the *sick role*, a set of expectations developed to distinguish sick from well people and analytically to distinguish those who voluntarily reject social norms from those who are unable to live up to them. The sick person (as compared with a criminal or a well person, for example) is expected to be exempt from normal activities, to be defined as unable to conform to norms without help from others, to "want to" get well, and, given symptoms of a certain duration and severity, to seek a treatment agent defined as competent by her/his group and to cooperate with that treatment agent in the attempt to re-establish good health. While of great analytical utility for sociological theory, this formulation is of limited utility to a practitioner because of the great variations found in the ways in which different groups uphold the central norms and the ways in which they "fill in the blanks" by specifying, for example, the degrees and kinds of exemptions, the kinds of help that are appropriate, the kinds of treatment agents regarded as "competent", what constitutes "cooperation", and the like. There are aggregates in the population that can be distinguished primarily by their values and norms. These are often associated with differences in nationality and religion and are identified as *ethnic groups*.

The concept of opportunities refers to the resources available to pursue alternative courses of action. All behavior requires resources. These include a functioning body, a degree of intelligence, various tools, money, freedom to plan the use of time, knowledge, and access to other people, to indicate only a few items. What kinds of resources are required will depend on the kinds of behaviors being demanded or sought. It is important to recognize that to conform to the demands of being sick and to claim the privileges thereof requires certain resources, some of which we will discuss below. Also, all disease and illness alters the resources available for behavior. In every instance, to state the minimal case, disease and illness reduce the efficency of the most basic resource, one's own body. They also almost invariably affect the kinds of interpersonal relationships of the sick person and of those who surround her/him. They usually affect income, intellectual resources, work, authority and power. When we describe the resources available to aggregates of people within societies, the groups differentiated are referred to as *social strata or classes*.

To understand the behavior of individuals requires an appreciation of the fact that they belong to groups. People have many social indentities. As the holder of any *one*, they are encircled by their relationships with other people who have an interest in that aspect of their behavioral potential. Each of those others will exert influence by holding expectations that focus on that particular relationship. The individual in question will be faced with conflicting expectations in most cases and will have to make choices, negotiate solutions and make compromises according to the inherent unpleasantness of the expected behaviors, the power of the others involved, the valuation of the tasks, the availability of resources, and the need to take into account the energies and resources needed for other social indentities, including similar bargaining with other people with interests in those identities. This is an existential reality of social life. It is one too often overlooked by health professionals. This "circle of others" is involved in all of the decisions that constitute the sickness career. Their influence is what leads people toward or away from contact with health professionals and they also influence the degree to which a patient will "cooperate" with treatment. Effective work on the part of health professionals requires that this aspect of the patient's social situation be kept in mind. It is a most important therapeutic resource.

Within this framework, then, what are the decisions that sick people must make, or have made for them, and how are those decisions made?

(1) All decisions about health matters take place against the background question of what it means to be "well". Being healthy means different things to different people. In different populations health may mean:

— a feeling of well being,
— absence of symptoms, or identifiable medical conditions,
— ability to carry on normal activities,
— the ability to recover from serious disease,
— not expecting to get sick, or
— being told by a physician that one's health is good.

In each case it is important to get some idea of what the patient means by being well, as this is, from the perspective of that patient, likely to be the goal of treatment. It is both a norm upheld by his or her group and a set of expectations brought to the therapeutic encounter.

(2) Against the background of being well, some change from normal is judged to have occurred. Virtually any change in a person's life may raise the question of changes in health status. People differ in the kinds of symptoms they are likely to notice. Among the most dramatic are changes in capacities, where a person becomes unable to do certain things (s)he is used to doing. This may be noticed by the individual or by others. More frequently the change is in the form of how people feel. They have pain, dizziness, weakness, numbness or some other symptom that is subjectively experienced. If such symptoms affect the appearance or behavior of the individual in question it may also be noticed by others. Least frequently, the change noticed may be in a form that involves neither feeling states nor capacities. This can be unusual lumps, changes in skin color or texture, unusual bleeding and the like. There are two important points in relation to being well. First, cultural groups differ in the importance they attach to interpersonal relationships, enduring suffering, self monitoring, and group survival. These differences influence the likelihood of any given change being noticed as a possible symptom. Noticing capacity changes is more frequent in groups placing a value on achievement and work, for example. Feeling state changes are more likely to be important in groups placing a high value on interpersonal relationships, etc. Secondly, the kinds of capacities required to meet the expectations for normal behavior varies by position in the social structure. The relative importance of physical strength, manual dexterity, visual acuity, or clear thought, for example, varies with the kind of work one does and hence with social class. In general, the more centrally a change affects a valued activity, relationship, or goal, the more likely it is to be noticed.

(3) A decision must be made that the change is or is not significant. Frequently, the first step is to regard the symptoms as "normal" or transient: something that comes with age, or is the result of some unusual activity, or is otherwise within the range of changes that "mean nothing". A symptom is more likely to be regarded as significant when:

— it interferes with normal activities or characteristics, as discussed above;

— the symptoms are clear — they are obvious to others and are already defined as meaning sickness in the group;

— they excede the tolerance threshold of the individual and/or (s)he expresses the symptoms to others — features that vary with ethnic identity, social class and the particular interactions in question;

— the symptom is unfamiliar and regarded as threatening to the individual or to others;

— it is seen as being caused by an underlying serious problem;

— it is thought to lead to serious incapacities or death, or it is expected to last for a long time;

— there are other crises in the life of the individual and attention to the symptoms can alleviate some stress; and

— other people think they are serious.

A core point is that symptoms are *always* negotiated with others. This negotiation starts in the household, in the typical case, and expands to less intimate relationships until social support is developed for some course of action. In several studies in which patients have been interviewed in detail about events leading them to medical care, not one case has been developed in which there was not an agreement between the patient and someone regarded as authoritative — either because of experience with similar symptoms or presumed technical expertise — that the symptoms were important and needed treatment.[6]

(4) A decision must be made that help of a particular type is or is not needed. The others with whom the individual interacts guide the individual toward or away from the health professional. In most instances, it is decided that the individual is competent to treat himself using remedies known within the friendship group or family. Sometimes the advice of a pharmacist is sought, especially in countries such as the United States with a loosely regulated trade in medications.[7] Only a minority of illness episodes result in seeking the advice of a professional treatment agent. Consultation with a professional is more common when the "lay culture" is compatible with the professional culture and a large number of others, in what Freidson (1961) called the "lay referred system", are consulted. Different cultures have different traditions for healing that may lead them instead to faith healing, herb healing or some other alternative to medicine. Also, the higher the social class of a group, the more likely they will consult with physicians, although this relationship seems to be weakening in recent years.

(5) A particular treatment agent must be selected. For people without previous contacts a referral is generally made by a family member, friend, neighbor or co-worker to a practitioner known to her or him. There is some evidence that this selection will be made more often than not within ethnic groups. If available, the patient will select a physician who is of the same ethnic identity as himself.[8] The exception may be when the selection may bring contact with a higher status group in the community. Once "in the system" referrals tend to be

from one physician to another through friendship networks. The physician should be aware that many decisions have been made about the health problem before (s)he is consulted. Furthermore, the patient has quite strong support for the consultation. Both the patient and a circle of others think that something is wrong and that the physician should do something about it. Furthermore, the odds are good that they have an image of how the physician should procede, what kinds of "tests" or "treatments" are to be expected, etc. To work effectively with the patient the physician needs to know not only the nature of the signs and symptoms of disease, but also the nature of the expectations brought by the patient to the encounter. If these are not agreeable to the physician, they need to be explicitly negotiated. Failure here leads more often to a failure of treatment than does failure in the diagnosis of disease or the identification of efficacious therapy.

(6) A decision must be made regarding the degree and type of cooperation to be offered to the treatment agent. This is not an either-or proposition in which patients can be divided into those who are and are not cooperative. It has been found that if one lists all treatment instructions in detail and asks in each instance whether a patient has conformed to all aspects, a totally cooperative patient is not to be had. Rather, there are differences in the degree to which patients follow instructions and in the kinds of instructions they will or will not follow. Variations are found with ethnicity, social class, the kinds of treatment involved and in the interaction contexts, both patient-physician and patient-other. Every treatment has a cost, not only in monetary terms, but also in terms of discomfort, degradation, and the sacrifice of alternative pursuits. If this cost is higher than the corresponding benefits, at least as perceived by the patient, the likelihood of cooperation is reduced. In fact, this is a most difficult point for many health professionals to grasp precisely because health is such a core value for them. Relative to health professionals, the value placed by others on health is something that must compete with other values. At times careful education of the patient is required to alter her or his perceptions. At time those values must simply be respected. In general, however, cooperation is higher when:

— the treatment involved is passive (the patient must allow the professional to do something) rather than active (the patient must do something),

— among Northwest European populations, when the active treatment focuses on dietary restrictions rather than the taking of medications,

— among Southeast European populations, when the active treatment focuses on the taking of medications rather than dietary restrictions,

— the treatment seems to be working,

— the patient has a rather low work orientation, is less educated and has a more formal relationship with the physician (in a rural population with heart disease),

— the duration of symptoms is longer,

— the treatment program fits the expectations of the patient (this is especially important with respect to the use of diagnostic tests, as most who discharge themselves from the hospital against medical advice do so because they are convinced they have become subjects of medical experiments),

— the treatment program does not interfere with other important activities and goals of the patient,

— the treatment does not interfere with important activities and goals of those who interact with the patient daily, and

— communication between the physician and patient is such that each understands how the other defines the problem, they share a common language (not just nominally, but they attach the same meanings to words) and they respect one another's goals in the relationship between them.

Again it should be emphasized that neither the patient nor the physician comes to the relationship free of other commitments. The physician is bound to the norms of good practice and must meet the professional expectations of his or her colleagues. Hence, (s)he is not free to provide whatever the patient desires whatever the consequences. It tends to be less recognized that the patient comes bound to the norms of her or his social class, ethnic group, family and friends regarding the ways in which symptoms are to be presented, the kinds of treatments that are acceptable, the ways in which (s)he should relate to the physician and so forth. (S)he is not free either to take whatever the physician offers. Failure to conform to group norms brings sanctions, often literally a fate worse than death. It is my view that appreciation of this fact alone would do much to improve the relationships between health professionals and patients. There are other implications for health professionals, however, both as clinicians and as citizens.

SOME CLINICAL IMPLICATIONS

For the practicing clinician there are several implications of this formulation of a "sickness career", although to my knowledge none has yet been explicitly investigated. In what follows, it is fair to interpret the statements I present as explanations and conclusions to be hypotheses for applied sociomedical research.[9] In my view, the implications for the professional are most clear with reference to improving the speed and accuracy of diagnosis, improving the effectiveness of treatment planning, improving the professional-patient relationship by sensitizing the professional to the situation of the patient, and reducing patient complaints about service and malpractice litigation.

It is axiomatic among experienced physicians that the single most important source of information leading to a diagnosis is the interview (or "history") with the patient. Estimates vary, but it is held widely that more than 90% of the skill in making a diagnosis comes from the interview. Laboratory tests and observation serve only to confirm the diagnosis or to help select among a few alternative possibilities.[10] It would be expected that considerable attention would be given in the medical curriculum to the skills of interviewing. Yet this is not the case. Instead, medical schools emphasize the laboratory skills, and attention to interviewing is limited to a partial list of items that should be asked about. Few pay any attention to the necessary interpersonal skills.

There is reason to believe that the clinician who becomes familiar with the sickness career model and with the evidence for it and the method on which it is based will become more skilled at making diagnoses by interview. Several years ago I was involved with a research project at a large teaching hospital in which we were interviewing patients admitted to the medical ward. The interviews were done by a young woman with a recent undergraduate degree in psychology and no medical training. They focused on the experiences of the patient prior to hospitalization with special attention to the social situation and interpersonal influence patterns that we later characterized as the sickness career. Transcribed interviews were reviewed by a study physician, who was board certified in internal medicine. The purpose of the review was to assess the quality of medical service prior to hospitalization. The interesting thing was the physician was able to make diagnoses on the basis of the interviews. These diagnoses were confirmed by a review of the medical record to ascertain laboratory findings; and in a large proportion of cases the diagnosis was reached by the research physician, who had not seen the patient, before the staff physicians on the ward! In two instances experiences with medical students pointed in the same direction. In one, a small number of third year students were given systematic exposure to the concepts behind the sickness career (social class, ethnicity, interaction, etc.). They felt that as a result they were able to outperform the students who had not had such exposure in both speed and accuracy of diagnosis. In the second instance, students were provided with similar exposures, this time in the first year. They were then sent to observe in a number of settings in a teaching hospital (clinics, emergency ward) where medical histories were taken. They reported with great sensitivity that the interviews they witnessed were defective. Physicians failed to hear what the patient was telling them; by their conduct they blocked certain kinds of information from being provided. The result was that the interviews did not generate the data needed for accurate diagnosis. These same students were then able to interview the same patients; while they lacked the technical knowledge needed to make the diagnosis themselves, they did generate better quality of information so that on the basis of their reports a diagnosis could be made. These were both training exercises and not part of a research protocol. They are suggestive leads, however, which point toward the possibility that knowledge of the sickness career can improve a core aspect of medical practice.

A second area in which the sickness career has implications for the health professional is with respect to treatment planning. The success of treatment critically depends upon an appreciation of what it means to the patient to be well, what kinds of symptoms (s)he has noticed and why they are important, how well (s)he understands what the treatment consists of and why, and the degree to which (s)he believes the professional takes an interest in her or him. Again, the sickness career model provides a sensitizing tool, a checklist, if you will, of the kinds of questions that need answers. To be successful, a treatment plan needs to be followed. This requires an effort on the part of the professional to see to it that there is a correspondence of goals with the patient and that there is mutual understanding regarding the nature of the means and how they relate to goals. In other words, education of the patient must be a core role of the professional, and the sickness career model calls attention to content areas for that education process. This, of course, means that the nature of the physician-patient relationship must move away from an activity-passivity model (in which the physician is active and the patient passive) toward a guidance-cooperation or a mutual participation model (Szaz and Hollender 1956) in which the patient is seen as legitimately having an active role in the treatment process. Cassee (1975) has shown that improved therapeutic outcomes among hospital patients are facilitated by open communications between nurses and patients. Skipper and Leonard (1968) have shown that when the parents of children admitted for surgery are provided with a brief description of the normal course of events that might be observed in the immediate post operative period this has little effect on expressed attitudes, but almost all the important physiological parameters of post-operative recovery are significantly improved. The issue, then, is not simply one of more humane treatment of patients (although that is itself a worthy goal) but of technical competence as well. An understanding of the issues raised in the sickness career model affect therapeutic outcomes directly. Little research effort has been directed toward measurement of such impacts. As investigators develop this area there is no doubt that knowledge of the materials covered by the sickness career model will be basic to good practice in the future.

A third area of clinical implications is with reference to the alienation of patients. One expression of this alienation in the U.S. is the lawsuit for malpractice. It will be recalled that there are at least four dimensions of alienation: clinical, organizational, economic, and class/interpersonal. Not all of these are equally reducible and of those that are, the sickness career is not relevant to all. In the individual professional-patient encounter, for example, the degree to which either organizational or economic alienation can be reduced is marginal, although both are amenable to political action as we will discuss below. The implications of the sickness career are not zero, however. While, the *objective* control over organizational settings remains with the professional, the *subjective* feelings of alienation on the part of the patient can be reduced by providing information on how to manipulate the system to his or her own ends. To some degree, the individual professional can subvert the system by lowering charges, refusing to charge the poor and otherwise directly attacking economic alienation. The system, however, would remain in professional hands, making such an attack not only politically risky for the individual professional, but also one that provides more of a "safety valve" than a real force for change (c.f. Waitzkin and Waterman 1974). In both instances, reduction of these forms of alienation must be seen more in the citizenship than in the strictly clinical roles of professionals and will be discussed below.

Clinical alienation is more difficult. With the tremendous growth of knowledge about the human body and intervention in disease processes, medical knowledge has become more and more removed from "common sense". There is no way in which the lay public can become equally expert with the professionals. In an aggregate sense, clinical alienation is inherent in the situation of having health professionals who have a real knowledge base. This will not be reduced by any action on the part of individual practitioners. The health education movement to the contrary, I have doubts that any collective actions will have much impact either. With reference to the single patient with a single health problem, however, a great deal can be done to see that there is a real understanding of the disease process and its relationship to the signs and symptoms that are of immediate concern. Alternative treatment possibilities can be presented and the patient can be allowed to make an informed choice about which ones to pursue. This would lead to greater cooperation and reduce feelings of alienation on the part of the patient. For that individual it might also reduce objective alienation.

The greatest impact of the sickness career model is in its potential to reduce class/interpersonal alienation. In the typical encounter with health professionals, the patient is caught in one or more "double binds".[11] Mutually exclusive expectations for behavior are simultaneously held by the professional or among members of the groups with whom the patient interacts. For example, Bloor and Horobin (1975) have shown that it is inherent in the typical expectations physicians hold for patient behavior that the patient is simultaneously expected to not present with "trivial" complaints and to accept the authority of the physician once the relationship has been initiated. In the first instance, the patient is presumed to have enough expertise to distinguish between important and trivial symptoms, to judge when medical care is needed and to select an appropriate treatment agent. In the second, (s)he is expected to have no knowledge and to passively accept what the physician offers. This applies with special clarity to the issue of delay. One repeatedly sees patients derided both for presenting with symptoms that do not indicate serious disease processes ("wasting the time" of the professional with "trivia") *and* for taking too much time to decide that symptoms are important enough to seek medical attention. In the first instance the patient is presumed to have the necessary knowledge to judge the severity of symptoms; in the second, (s)he is presumed to have failed to recognize the need for expert opinion early in the disease process. There may also be a double bind between the expectations of the professional and those of the others with whom the individual interacts. With respect to rehabilitation of stroke patient, for example, New et al. (1968) have shown that in the typical case the rehabilitation center staff expected that the patient would pursue an active program of special exercises and that (s)he would be assisted by other members of the household. The members of the household, however, expected that the patient would follow a treatment program in conjunction with the rehabilitation center staff in such a way as to minimize the disruption of their lives. Not explored, but highly likely is that the staff put the household members in a double bind in which they could not meet the treatment obligations the staff wanted them to assume and their other social committments. Freidson (1975) has indicated another problem in that diseases that are unique and of great concern to the patient are often *ordinary* to the physician, who sees many such "cases". He gives as an example the fact that upper respiratory infections are common to a medical practice, but not necessarily to an individual patient. "And in so far as they are considered ordinary it is not legitimate for the patient to make a great fuss about the suffering they involve. His subjectively real pain is given little attention or sympathy because it is too ordinary to worry about." Thus the professional often seems to the patient to be callous or indifferent while the patient seems to the professional to be overwrought. Knowing this, the patient is caught in the double bind of wanting relief from suffering while not wanting that concern dismissed as trivial. The perspectives of both the patient and physician will be supported by their respective groups. The sickness career model calls attention to the range of other people who are influential in the behavior of patients and to the variety of expectations they can hold for behavior. By consciously seeking information in this area, the professional can help to avoid many a double bind for the patient and to help her or him negotiate a way out of those that are present. In short, the sickness career model has the potential of helping to avoid placing unreasonable expectations on patients. Such expectations are alienating, produce anger and frustration, and lead to reduced cooperation with treatment.

There is reason to believe that attention to the issues raised by the sickness career can reduce the likelihood of lawsuits against the practitioner for malpractice. As outlined at the beginning of this chapter, such lawsuits are an American expression of the alienation of the patients from the health care providers.[12] While there are objective aspects to this alienation that the individual practitioner can do little about, it is the subjective aspect that leads to action against the practitioner. The patient who sues is one who has experienced the encounter with the professional as one which is unfeeling, uncaring and mechanical; one where the patient as a person feels that (s)he has been reduced to a disease, in short, dehumanized. We have noted that it is in the settings where such a disease oriented, high technology practice is the rule that such lawsuits seem the most frequent. The obvious remedy is to interact with the patient in such a way as to communicate interest, caring and involvement beyond the disease process. I suspect that it would be the rare case where a professional who showed an active interest in the content of the sickness career and who took that information into account in interacting with and treating the patient would ever be sued.[13]

From the clinical standpoint, then, the sickness career model can provide a means for improving diagnosis, treatment, and therapeutic effectiveness.

SOME IMPLICATIONS FOR THE CITIZEN-PROFESSIONAL

In the developed world the alienation of patients and the associated autonomy of professionals is a political issue, much more apparent, we have noted, in countries with systems more organized than in the United States. Even in the United States, however, there is a considerable literature now on the problems of developing a health care system. While not the primary social knowledge that leads to solutions of such problems, the concept sickness career can make some essential contributions to problems that affect all professionals, even though not all are concerned. Some form of nationalized system of health care is now inevitable. The problem is to shape it in ways that the real needs of people are met.[14]

In the United States in recent years there has been much discussion of designing a system of health care "delivery" that meets several criteria.

— *availability of service*: services provided in allocation where it is possible for people to reach them. There has been discussion of the fact that adequate availability differs with the type of service under consideration, most importantly the frequency with which it is used and the speed with which it is needed. The distribution of (wo)man power is here a major issue.

— *accessibility of service*: the ease with which people can avail themselves of the services that are available. Here there has been discussion of plant architecture, charges for services, personnel attitudes, working hours and screening procedures.

— *acceptability of service*: the services should be of types that seem reasonable to people and that they want; they should be provided under conditions which preserve the dignity and self respect of patients and which help to solve their problems rather than worsen them.

— *relevance of services*: services provided should be of a type that meets the needs of the people they are intended to serve and that are appropriate to the kinds of health problems they have.

— *affordability of service*: in that the society can absorb the costs. The system of health care must be designed so as to not bankrupt the larger systems it ostensibly supports.

To this list we should add one feature not discussed so frequently

— *flexibility of service*: the ability of services to adapt to individual needs, local conditions, and changes in the population being served.

That the system in the United States, and in most of the world, fails to meet such criteria is obvious enough to allow us to omit extensive documentation of that point. Different societies, however, have confronted different aspects of these criteria with different degrees of success. Availability, for example, has been addressed most effectively in the United Kingdom and Denmark, where a system of general practitioners puts primary care within walking distance of almost every home. This has been accomplished in both countries by a system of incentives and disincentives for the location of practice.

Accessibility has been best addressed in countries with highly developed social welfare systems (such as Sweden).[15] Acceptability, however, seems low in Sweden where people complain about the cold, impersonal irrelevant treatment delivered in tertiary care centers and the absence of general practitioners in many areas. Flexibility is high in the United States, where there are numerous different kinds of practice organization, financing schemes, etc. The discussion of this point must be deferred to another place, simply being noted here.

Throughout the world health care is a political concern. The issues raised here cannot be resolved by the simple application of technology nor by the development of support systems, such as a national health insurance program, that leave questions of power unresolved. No system that has left the medical power structure in control has survived the threat of impending bankruptcy. Some increased public authority is inevitable in countries which, like the U.S., have left medical care organization in a 19th century liberal mode. The task is to see to it that public authority is designed to meet the criteria listed above. Toward this end, attention to the sickness career may help to provide some guidelines.

If we start with the baseline state of being well we can identify some key problems involved in maintaining health. It has been well established that keeping well and its converse, getting sick, have little to do with medical care. McKeown (1976) in the United Kingdom and the McKinlays (1977) in the United States have shown that only a small part of the historical decline in the death rate is the result of medical intervention. Instead, the most important factor in the decline has been improvements in nutrition followed by environmental changes (most importantly in creating a clean water supply) and changes in personal behavior. For the future the same factors will be important in a somewhat different order: behavioral changes with reference to tobacco consumption and exercise will be most important, followed by environmental changes associated with the control of pollution and nutritional improvements. To be relevant, a national *health* system must provide services directed toward these issues, finding means that meet the listed criteria. This will involve programs in health information, the provision of access to adequate food, strong disincentives to the manufacture and distribution of tobacco products and the like.[16] It will mean a vast expansion of resources in the area of what have been called "welfare services": providing work, controls over the health standards of work environments and the like. Some of the cost of this expansion can be gained back through the consequent reductions in morbidity.

The requirements of the next two steps of the sickness career can also be met for the most part with services that are less expensive than medicine. The greatest need is for people to have someone to turn to who is not as awesome as a physician in making the judgements that some change has occurred and that it may or may not be significant. Health stations at the neighborhood and workplace level, for example, might be staffed on a part-time basis with someone trained in first aid. That person could be a first contact who might be able to help decide whether a more sophisticated consultation is needed and who the appropriate source might be. Such a person could in many instances be a source of direct help. While this would increase the total utilization of the system, it could cut back on the use of the more expensive tertiary care services. How such services are organized, however, must be variable at the local level. The same kind of initial referral source is not likely to be equally acceptable in a middle class suburb of Northwest Europeans and a rural community of Native Americans. It needs to take account of the social class and ethnicity of the population and the kinds of interactions patterns typical of the community. To as great a degree as possible the initial contact people should be accessible as part of the circle of others involved in the decision making. Health education emphasis needs to be placed on the symptoms of locally occurring disease, etc.

The types of help sought by people should be available in the community at the level where they are needed. This means that primary care providers need to be located near the places of work and residence. For more esoteric services it may be that having one location in the world where a particular procedure is carried out might be adequate. In between there may be some skills that are required at one location in a city, etc. People should be able to approach the primary care system without excessive cost or physical barriers and at times when it is most convenient. Such providers should be able and willing to treat the wide range of health problems, including illness and sickness, not just disease. To be acceptable, care must be personal in ways so defined by the community concerned. Specialists should be located so as to be available where and when needed by referral. Overall *the emphasis must be on keeping the services no more sophisticated than necessary at each level.* Further, *the provision of unsophisticated services that meet major health needs should take priority over more sophisticated services meeting the needs of a few.* The several cardiac intensive care units in Addis Ababa, for example, do little to meet the needs of a country that suffers from severe nutritional and parasitic disease. Such services, in fact, divert badly needed resources from the more pressing problems.

Cooperation with treatment will be enhanced in general when the patient is accepted as having legitimate complaints, even when those are not ones of primary interest to the provider, when (s)he has easy access to readily available services, when the services make sense and take his or her needs into account. This has more to do with how the services are provided than with the way in which they are organized, except that a referral system that involves considerable waiting cannot be tolerated.

Obviously this is only one approach and it is intended for illustration alone. The essential points are that any system of health care needs to be planned, created and monitored with the following in mind. It has to provide an emphasis on solving problems that are important in the community; it must deal with health, illness and sickness as well as with disease; the services must be provided at times and places that facilitate their use; they should emphasize keeping services as unsophisticated as practicable; they should be provided without cost or other barriers at the point of delivery; they should be flexible, adapting to changing local conditions; and they should be cost conscious, not bankrupting the larger system. It is my judgement that to allow specialized medical interests to control the planning and implimentation and/or to "fossilize" the present system with insurance coverage of a "fee-for-service" economy will lead to a crisis such as that now being experienced in Sweden. There, a great achievement has been the creation of a system that provides virtually equal access to services for everyone in the society, at least within geographic regions. Cost is not an important issue in the decision to seek medical care. At the same time, the physician-run, hospital-based, tertiary-care system, which dominates medical care in the country, has increased in cost to the point where medical care threatens to bankrupt the system. The country is being forced to reorganize health care by putting the emphasis on the development of primary care services which, especially in the urban areas, are scarce indeed. There is some question as to whether this can be done quickly enough to avoid major disruptions in service.

CODA

In this paper I have attempted to suggest some ways in which the concept of the sickness career might be used by health professionals. We began by distinguishing the concepts of disease, illness and sickness, noting that physicians are trained in the first of these while patients present complaints involving the second or third. Hence there is an immediate problem in the physician-patient relationship in establishing a universe of discourse. Next, we took a very brief look at trends in the physician-patient relationship that have led on the one hand to increased professional autonomy on the part of physicians and increased alienation on the part of patients, a situation with inherent pressures for change. The sickness career is then presented as a model for organizing information about patients with a focus on the decisions they make about their health in response to symptoms. This information can substitute for the direct experience and observation of the older small town practitioner and focus questions that can lead to a more humane and relevant encounter for the patient. It also provides some orientations that can be useful as we move inevitably toward a national system of health and medical care.

The concept of the sickness career itself, however, was not elucidated in detail. It is hoped that students and practitioners will be provoked or enticed to follow up this chapter by becoming more familiar with the findings of social science research and in developing the skills needed to keep current with the literature in this area. Maybe a few will begin to wonder about the potential applications suggested here and develop an interest in applied sociomedical research. While it will not gain them enormous prestige among their colleagues in the near future, nothing could be more important as a contribution to health.

NOTES

1. There is a literature that suggests that patients with a symptom that is threatening (e.g. a lump that might be cancer) will avoid seeking help lest their fears be confirmed. Undoubtedly such cases exist, but I have doubts that they are frequent. None of the

hospitalized patients in any of my studies can be said to fall into such a category. Yet the "diagnosis" of "delay" is commonly found in conversations with physicians and in medical records. Usually all that is being observed is a time period between onset of symptoms and contact with a treatment agent. Delay is inferred (c.f. Sweet and Twaddle 1969).

2. In commenting on an early draft of this paper, Leon Eisenberg suggested that this statement does not hold when the patient is referred by another professional. I partly agree. The professional often refers the disease to another colleague. The patient, however, will likely still present with symptoms. Depending on the amount and type of communication between the patient and the referring professional (s)he may be sensitized to the fact that it is the disease that is being referred.

3. By "real" is meant simply that the patient is not feigning symptoms in most instances, not that the symptoms necessarily mean a disease. Out and out fraud is to be found occasionally here as in any other area of life, but with no greater frequency.

4. Leon Eisenberg has suggested that patients have always had to meet the price demanded by the physician. To a degree this is true, but there has been an important historical shift in that degree. On the one hand there has been a shift in the economic situation of medical practice. At the turn of the century there were relatively more physicians per capita, a larger number of competing healing systems, and a relatively greater public service orientation to medical practice. Fee schedules were frequently relaxed or ignored and services or goods were often accepted in lieu of fees. The more modern bureaucratized system does not allow for such flexibility. Also, in small towns patients and physicians were often well known to one another in a variety of roles other than that of physician-patient. This made the relationship more multidimensional and allowed for the direct exchange of services in more of a gift relationship than an economic one.

5. A careful search has failed to turn up any reliable data on malpractice suits, although several papers present figures of unknown origin. This statement represents the conventional wisdom of my medical colleagues.

6. As I write this I can use myself as a case example. For about a week I have been aware of a skin lesion on my neck. I am aware that there is a 99% chance that it is "nothing", but it has characteristics such that there is a small chance that it is very serious. If I were at home I would have no problem in asking a friend, who is also a dermatologist, for an opinion. However, I am on a sabbatical leave in another country and it is between Christmas and the New Year. I have mentioned the condition to my wife, but while expressing some concern she has not suggested any course of action. I am unable to get opinions from my colleagues. After all, I am a *medical* sociologist and they would not presume to give advice in an area they see as one in which I am expert. My work has brought me in contact with a large number of health professionals, but only one I know well enough to ask for advice on the basis of friendship. This being the holiday season, he is on vacation. I am aware of the overburdened primary care system, and while I think I could find a way to be examined quickly, I am not a taxpayer and feel reluctant to make such a claim for service. In short, I think I want to get an expert opinion but I have not yet mobilized the social support that I need. Hence, I wait until the end of the holiday season.

7 This may or may not be a pharmacist depending on the society in question. Also, what it means to be a pharmacist varies with the society. In Sweden, for example, the *Apotek* dispenses almost exclusively prescription drugs. Only twelve items are available for "over the counter" sales and these can only be sold if specifically requested. If someone askes for advice about symptoms they must be referred to a physician.

8. This is based on studies which focused on religious and nationality identities. It is not known whether the data would hold for racial identities.

9. Work in this area has until now been focused on the development of sociological

knowledge rather than its applications. Applications will require more attention to sociology on the part of health professionals and institutional arrangements for secure employment of sociologists in medical settings.

10. Leon Eisenberg commented on an aspect of laboratory tests that I had not considered and which merits direct quotation. ". . . a laboratory test which may be quite useful when the history (e.g. interview data) suggests that the patient is likely to have the disease can be quite misleading if it is used on a random basis. That is, even if a test has only a five percent false positive rate but when the disease it tests for is rare, then the false positives on a random community sample will far exceed the true positive. Contrariwise, if history suggests that the patient is very likely to have the disease, then the test will be strongly confirmatory. Consider the following case. Disease X occurs in one in a thousand people. Test Y for disease X is accurate 95% of the time. Then, in a sample of 1000 people, it will produce 50 false positives for each true positive. On the other hand, if the history makes the given person tested a presumptive case, then a positive test makes it 95% likely he has the disease."

11. The concept of double bind is presented in this volume in the chapter by Alexander. A different dimension is to be found in Twaddle (1979) where seeking a physician is presented as inherently a double bind situation where the symptomatic person must seek the alienation of the physician-patient relationship in order to reduce the alienation imposed by the symptoms themselves.

12. Each society will have different mechanisms available for patients to express alienation and to redress grievances. It is very much in the American tradition to handle conflict through litigation. The size of the settlements may be influenced by the fact that lawyers often work on a contingency fee basis, often benefiting more than the patient from the settlement. In Great Britain, where there is a tradition of general practice, greater use of physicians for smaller complaints, and an effective disciplinary system for physicians, the rate of malpractice litigation is infinitesimal. In Sweden, where there is no provision for malpractice suits, there is an office at the National Board of Health and Welfare which has responsibility for receiving complaints. The rate of such complaints has escalated rapidly in recent years paralleling the American experience with malpractice litigation. The experience in Denmark is reported to be similar to that of Great Britain, although I have no direct knowledge of the situation there. Denmark also has a national health service based on general practice. It seems plausible that countries with a well developed system of primary care have patients who are less alienated and hence less likely to file complaints or sue.

13. Eisenberg notes that physicians who are incompetent from the biophysical point of view are sometimes protected from legal action by cultivating the confidence of their patients. He cites the case of a charlatan who claimed to have a cancer cure and who caused hepatitis in a number of patients by failing to sterilize his needles. At a hearing to consider revocation of his licence, dozens of "cancer cures" showed up to protest the suspension.

14. Some countries, such as Sweden, have developed national health care systems that have left control of the system in the hands of the physicians. Predictably, such systems are organized in the interests of the professionals. They are highly specialized and built around large, high technology, tertiary care hospitals. They are intellectually exciting to physicians, extremely expensive and largely irrelevant to the health needs of the population. P. C. Jersild (1978), a physician-novelist, has characterized the political role of the physician in Sweden as ". . . dessa vitrockade strutsar som stod med huvudena nerkörda i halsen på patienten, blinda och döva för omgivningen". (". . . these white coated ostriches who stood with their heads pushed down the throats of patients, blind and deaf to their environs.") As his story unfolds, it is the working of a system that ignores sickness careers toward its own destruction that we witness in this novel set in a major hospital.

15. Especially for students in the health professions a distinction needs to be drawn between social welfare and socialism. The two are often confused. Social welfare refers to the provision of services that provide support to the population by placing a lower limit on the degree to which people are allowed to suffer deprivation. Pensions, sickness insurance, family support services, food subsidies, and health care itself are part of this system. Socialism, on the other hand, is an economic system in which industrial workers are the owners of the places in which they work and in which occupational decisions are reached democratically. Sweden, for example, is a capitalist country, with 80% of industry in private (e.g. nongovernmental) hands and a highly developed welfare system. The United States is a capitalist country without a highly developed welfare system. The Soviet Union is a capitalist country that has concentrated capital in the hands of the state. China, under Mao Tse-tung seemed to be developing a socialist economy, but recent events have apparently reversed that trend. Indeed, the biggest problem with the study of socialism is that of the "empty cell". There is no national case example to be studied. There are, however, some cases of individual firms organizing along socialist lines. Schumacher (1973) provides a case example. Far from being socialist, welfare systems support the stability of capitalistic organization.

16. Eisenberg objected to a statement in the earlier draft that we need "strict controls" on the production and distribution of tobacco by referring to the experience with prohibition. His point may be a good one, but it may be that the failure of prohibition has been inadequately interpreted. For example, Sweden is a country with a large amount of public drunkenness. Alcohol is very much part of the culture and no attempt has been made to prohibit consumption (although *Systembolaget*, the state-run company for distribution of alcohol products has almost continuous advertising campaigns against excessive drinking). A strict prohibition, however, has been issued against driving after any alcohol consumption whatsoever. This seems to have worked well. It is strictly enforced and has strong penalties.

REFERENCES

Berglind, H., et al.
  1978 Sjukvård i tillväxt: en Problemöversik. Lund: Liber Läromedel.
Bloor, M., and G. Horobin
  1975 Conflict and Conflict Resolution in Doctor/Patient Interactions. *In* A Sociology of Medical Practice. C. Cox and A. Mead, eds. pp. 271–284. London: Collier-MacMillan.
Bohlin, A., et al.
  1978 Recent Trends in Medical Sociology in Sweden. Paper presented at Research Committee 15: Sociology of Medicine, Session 3; World Congress of Sociology, Uppsala, Sweden.
Cassee, E.
  1975 Therapeutic Behavior, Hospital Culture and Communication. *In* A Sociology of Medical Practice. C. Cox and A. Mead, eds. pp. 224–234. London: Collier-MacMillan.
Cox, C. and A. Mead
  1975 A Sociology of Medical Practice. London: Collier-MacMillan.
Freidson, E.
  1961 Patients' Views of Medical Practice. New York: Russel Sage.
  1975 Dilemmas in the Doctor/Patient Relationship. *In* A Sociology of Medical Practice. C. Cox and A. Mead, eds. pp. 285–298. London: Collier-MacMillan.
Gustafsson, R.
  1978 Bot och Omvårdnad eller Vårdproduktion? Stockholm: Prisma.

Hessler, R.
    1978 Sweden's Crisis in Medical Care: A Shift in the Welfare Paradigm. Unpublished
        manuscript, University of Missouri, Columbia.
Janlert, V.
    1978 Sjukvård Efter Kriget. Motpol 56(3–4):5–8.
Jersild, P.
    1978 Babels Hus. Stockholm: Bonniers.
Landstingsektorns Framtidsstudieverksamhet
    1978 Läkarbristöverskottet: Debattunderlag. Stockholm: Landstingsförbundet.
Mauksch, I. and M. David
    1972 Prescription for Survival. American Journal of Nursing 72:2189–2193.
McKeown, T.
    1976 The Role of Medicine: Dream, Mirage or Nemesis? London: The Nuffield Provin-
        cial Hospital Trust.
McKinlay, J. and S. McKinlay
    1977 The Questionable Contribution of Medical Measures to the Decline of Mortality
        in the United States in the 20th Century. Health and Society. The Milbank
        Memorial Fund Quarterly 55.
New, P., et al.
    1968 Hope and Reality. Mimeograph, Tufts Medical School.
Roth, J.
    1963 Timetables. Indianapolis: Bobbs-Merrill.
Schumacher, F.
    1973 Small Is Beautiful: Economics as if People Mattered. New York: Harper and Row.
Skipper, J. and R. Leonard
    1968 Children, Stress and Hospitalization: A Field Experiment. Journal of Health and
        Social Behavior 9(4):275–287.
Sweet, R. and A. Twaddle
    1969 An Exploration of Delay in Hospitalization. Inquiry 4(2):35–41.
Tibblin, G.
    1978 Aktiv Egenvård. In Nytt Från Läkaresällskapets Riksstämma 1977. SPRI Rapport
        3:171–177.
Twaddle, A.
    1979 Sickness Behavior and the Sick Role. Boston: Schenkman-Hall.
Twaddle, A. and R. Hessler
    1977 A Sociology of Health. St. Louis: C. V. Mosby.
Twaddle, A. and J. Stoeckle
    MS Autonomy, Alienation and the Physician-Patient Relationship, manuscript sub-
        mitted for publication.
Waitzkin, H. and B. Waterman
    1974 The Exploitation of Illness in Capitalist Society. Indianapolis: Bobbs-Merrill.

6. THE SICKNESS IMPACT PROFILE:
THE RELEVANCE OF SOCIAL SCIENCE TO MEDICINE

The past decade has been a period of rapid growth in the representation of social sciences in the curriculum of medical education. The social ferment of the 1960's precipitated an enormous interest in the health of disadvantaged individuals and social groups. Awareness of the importance of social and economic factors as determinants of the health levels of individuals and groups became acute. Further, the discrepancies of access to health care associated with social, economic and cultural factors became clear. Students were outraged that these injustices had not been previously recognized and corrected. Curriculum "reform" became the by-word of the day and an important part of the reform was to consist of enhancement of the role of social, especially behavioral, sciences in medical teaching and practice. New faculty members were recruited, new courses were developed, and whole new departments sprang into being. Students and faculty alike were urged to view the patient as a "whole person" and terms such as holistic medicine, comprehensive care, continuity of services began to appear frequently in medical literature. Simultaneous with the increased awareness of social factors as determinants of health in disadvantaged groups came an awareness of many unsatisfactory aspects of the health care system for all segments of society. Increased specialization and fragmentation of medical care as it was delivered by many specialists and sub-specialists to a single individual led to the conviction that no one was keeping an overall eye on the health problems of any one person. The concept of a new type of health care provider, the family physician, grew rapidly; (s)he was to be a felicitous combination of the attributes of the old general practitioner and the skills of the most common aspects of internal medicine, pediatrics, obstetrics-gynecology, and psychiatry. Great emphasis was placed on the physician's understanding of individual and family behavior. Increased recognition was given to the restoration or maintenance of individual and family function as a legitimate product of the process of medical care.

If health and disease are seen as entities placed on a continuum ranging from excellent health at one end to severe disease at the other it is clear that most physicians function at the disease end of the spectrum. The one notable exception is the family physician who is likely to function anywhere along this continuum. He shares the patients who cluster at the disease end of the continuum with the specialist and the sub-specialist. But, as he moves into the health end of the continuum he is working more and more in the exclusive area of family practice. This is clearly less developed territory; territory in which we believe there is expectation of disease prevention. Further, this is territory that is populated principally by younger and more recently educated physicians. They have

L. Eisenberg and A. Kleinman (eds.), The Relevance of Social Science for Medicine, 135–150.
Copyright © 1980 by D. Reidel Publishing Company.

tended to push their practice towards the health end of the spectrum and with that have moved away from the unquestioned acceptance of the biomedical model.

The biomedical model and the biomedical definition of disease assumes that all illness has a biological origin with corresponding biologic (i.e., physical) symptomatology. This orientation tends to develop and rely on measures of medical care that are biochemically or physiologically based. Underlying this orientation is an assumption that non-physical symptomatology has a non-physical origin and therefore lies outside the purview of traditional medical care. Hence, the specialty of psychiatry often has seemed to have developed at arm's length from the rest of medical care. The "new curriculum" of the late 1960's and 1970's recognized the exclusions and the assumptions and placed emphasis on inclusion of the social sciences, in particular the behavioral sciences, in medical education.

The behavioral aspects of health and sickness might have received earlier attention if the first important medical curriculum reform movement (Flexner 1910) had not placed exclusive emphasis on the sciences of anatomy and physiology as the basic sciences in medical education. Recognition of the importance of psychology, sociology, anthropology and economics to the study of medicine might have led toward developments in medical care and health services that were quite different from what did occur. As it happened, concepts of health and disease and the whole process of medical education has focused on the biomedical model of disease.

The newly growing prominence of social sciences in medical education does not necessarily represent a rejection of the biomedical model but rather a suggestion that the model be broadened in concept and in application. If this is to occur we must ask what factors would facilitate earlier identification of disease than is now possible. Is it increased knowledge of the earliest processes? Is it more sensitive tests to document the processes? Or is it more complete knowledge of the high risk factors that undoubtedly precede many of the earliest processes? There are of course many diseases that may be and are detected far in advance of signs and symptoms perceived by patient or physician. Hypertension, diabetes, glaucoma, and many neoplasms are among them. Yet, there are other conditions that are preceded by physician visits for what are seemingly non-specific and undiagnosable complaints. The family physician often has such individuals under his care and finds himself faced with a patient who has diffuse and all-encompassing problems. Often, it is possible to analyze these problems in terms of the individual's functioning as a participating and productive member of society. Function then becomes a focal point around which the physician may follow individuals or family units long before they become patients. Such a focus provides a unique opportunity to explore the relationship between social functioning and biochemical and physiologic functioning. Crucial to investigating this relationship is the incorporation of measures of behavioral function in the clinical practice of medicine. Ideally, the measuring instrument should be at least as reliable and credible as the biomedical measures that are characteristically used in assessing patient progress.

The remainder of this chapter will discuss the conceptual development and some applications of such a measure, the Sickness Impact Profile (SIP).

The development of the SIP was an interdisciplinary effort including the work of physicians, social scientists, health administrators and lay users of health services. The basic concept originated from physician observations that most health care is delivered for the purpose of reducing sickness or modifying the impact of sickness on a person's behavior and general life pattern. This view of the purpose of health care is particularly appropriate for the care of patients in the ambulatory setting, especially the minimally disabled and chronically ill. It was reasoned that a sensitive measure of changes in sickness impact would provide a way to assess the outcome of changes in health services and medical care (Gilson et al. 1975; Bergner et al 1976a).

Three important concepts underlie the SIP. First, a very deliberate decision was made to confine this measure of sickness impacts to behavior. This decision was not intended to deemphasize the impact of sickness on emotions, feelings, and beliefs but rather indicates the researchers' convictions that such impacts are reflected in an individual's performance. Second, a deliberate effort was made to confine measurement to performance, what the person does, rather than potential ability or capacity for a behavior. The concept of performance has several attributes that make it potentially useful as a basis for development of an outcome measure of health care: performance may be affected by medical treatment even though the underlying disease process or capacity to perform may be unaffected; performance or behavior may be reported directly by the individual under consideration; performance of the individual under consideration can be observed and reported by another respondent; performance can be measured when the individual is not receiving medical care; a measure based on performance or behavior permits relating diverse definitions of disease and sickness by uncovering common patterns of behavioral dysfunction. The adherence to behavioral performance, while imposing some limitations, provides for a sounder, more reliable and valid instrument than one based on a combination of behaviors, emotions, feelings and beliefs or a combination of performance and capacity. The third concept underlying the development of the SIP is the measurement of sickness rather than health or wellness. Health-related behavioral change or dysfunction is a concept both familiar and relevant to the individual. As a basis for health status assessment, health-related behavioral change assures measurement of significant events from the point of view of the individual, society, and the health care system. Individual behavior in society is often defined within the context of fulfillment of that individual's social role. One's importance to society may be considered in relation to one's level of function within a social role. Many factors may influence functional level, including amount of sleep, parental training, personal habits and expectations, and societal habits and expectations. Health and sickness undoubtedly affect behavior and role performance. An injury as insignificant as a sprained finger may impair functioning in one's role as a parent (feeding, playing), student (writing), musician (piano playing), lover (sexual relations), and so forth.

The healthy individual may be thought of as behaving without limitation and therefore functioning optimally. The sick individual may be thought of as behaving with limitation and therefore exhibiting dysfunction. Health sickness and function-dysfunction can each be conceived of as a single continuum parallel to one another. Presumably there are levels of positive health ranging from maximally healthy to minimally healthy, just as there are levels of positive function ranging from maximally functional to minimally functional. At some point, however, the continuum moves toward the negative side — not healthy (sick), not functional (dysfunctional). The medical care process is usually concerned with this negative side. Rarely does it promulgate new programs, develop new techniques or plan new health systems in order to maximize the health or functioning of an individual or group. Even so-called preventive programs aimed at examining the well, are often directed toward detection and treatment of sickness. Thus, the behaviorally based measure of health status should measure sickness or dysfunctional behavior since it is most relevant to the process being assessed. A final reason for the concept of measuring sickness instead of health may be derived from the fact that in any complex system it is easier to measure an aberration from the norm than it is to measure the normality of the whole or of each factor contributing to the complexity of the system. If health is compared to a piece of fabric composed of a complicated network of interwoven threads it may be easily understood that the identification and measurement of a few aberrant or broken threads is a much simpler proposition than a total description of all threads in the fabric.

The SIP contains 136 statements (or items) about health related dysfunction which may be administered by an interviewer in 20 to 30 minutes or may be self-administered. In completing the SIP the subject is asked to respond to or check only those statements that he is sure describe him on a given day and are related to his *health*. Sample statements drawn from each category of the Sickness Impact Profile are shown in Figure 1.

HOW THE SIP WAS CONSTRUCTED

In constructing the instrument the aim was to obtain as comprehensive a sample of the impact of sickness on a person's behavior as possible. As a starting point statements were gathered directly from a broad sample of individuals. An open-ended request form was used to solicit specific statements that described sickness-related changes in behavior. Those individuals sampled included ambulatory patients in doctors' offices, patients in the hospital, the apparently healthy, and health care providers. Over 1000 completed request forms were collected. In addition, the scientific literature on health measurement was reviewed and additional statements were gathered from previously developed instruments

Category	Items Describing Behavior Related to	Selected Items
SR	Sleep and Rest	I sit during much of the day
		I sleep or nap during the day
E	Eating	I am eating no food at all, nutrition is taken through tubes or intravenous fluids
		I am eating special or different food
W	Work	I am not working at all
		I often act irritably toward my work associates
HM	Home Management	I am not doing any of the maintenance or repair work around the house that I usually do
		I am not doing heavy work around the house
RP	Recreation and Pastimes	I am going out for entertainment less
		I am not doing any of my usual physical recreation or activities
A	Ambulation	I walk shorter distances or stop to rest often
		I do not walk at all
M	Mobility	I stay within one room
		I stay away from home only for brief periods of time
BCM	Body Care and Movement	I do not bathe myself at all, but am bathed by someone else
		I am very clumsy in body movements
SI	Social Interaction	I am doing fewer social activities with groups of people
		I isolate myself as much as I can from the rest of the family
AB	Alertness Behavior	I have difficulty reasoning and solving problems, for example, making plans, making decisions, learning new things
		I sometimes behave as if I were confused or disoriented in place or time, for example, where I am, who is around, directions, what day it is
EB	Emotional Behavior	I laugh or cry suddenly
		I act irritable and impatient with myself, for example, talk badly about myself, swear at myself, blame myself for things that happen
C	Communication	I am having trouble writing or typing
		I do not speak clearly when I am under stress

Fig. 1. Sickness impact profile categories and selected items.

containing references to behavioral dysfunctions. Finally, a total of 1250 statements was submitted to rigorous screening procedures. Statements or items were phrased so that each described a behavior or activity and specified a dysfunction. From these statements a standardized and structured interview form or prototype instrument was developed and administered to diverse groups of individuals. Over a four-year period a series of field tests and revisions reduced the number of statements from 312 to 136 which are grouped into 12 categories (Figure 1).

DEVELOPING, SCALING AND SCORING THE SIP

One of the objectives of developing the SIP was to assess a wide range of sickness-related impacts varying from minor to very severe dysfunctions. Special importance was attached to the need to evaluate the provision of routine medical care to the mildly sick. Such medical care often occupies large numbers of health professionals during a substantial part of their working day, and accounts for a sizeable portion of health care expenditures.

For the instrument to be useful in measuring outcomes, a method of scoring the responses of an individual to the SIP statements was needed. Obviously, the difference between a minor impact of sickness such as walking shorter distances, and a major one, such as not walking at all, had to be recognized in the scoring process in order to convey useful information in a quantitative way. For this reason procedures were developed to scale, or attach weights to statements and categories. During the development of the instrument a total of 133 judges rated the relative "severity of dysfunction" of each statement so that scale values could be assigned. The judging group was composed of 108 health care consumers and 25 health care professionals and pre-professional students. They were asked to rate each statement in terms of severity without regard for who might be experiencing it, what might be causing it, or future implications. Agreement among the judges was very high (Carter et al. 1976).

A score for the overall SIP instrument is computed by summing the scale values of all statements checked by a respondent and dividing that sum by the grand total of all statement scale values. This ratio is then multiplied by 100 to convert it to a simple percent. Similarly, scores can be computed for each SIP category.

As part of the developmental process, the interrelationships among SIP category scores were examined using cluster and factor analytic techniques. The results of these analyses indicated that two groups of categories consistently clustered together across all field trial samples. Categories A (ambulation), BCM (body care and movement), and M (mobility) constitute a Scoring Dimension that reflects physical dysfunction; categories SI (social interaction), C (communication), AB (alertness behavior), and EB (emotional behavior) constitute a Scoring Dimension that reflects psychosocial dysfunction. The remaining SIP categories, SR (sleep and rest), RP (recreation and pastimes), E (eating), W (work), and HM (household management) are scored individually. Percent scores for the Scoring Dimensions may be calculated in the same manner as the category and overall scores. The SIP format permits rapid manual scoring of individual results or transfer to a machine readable medium for computer scoring.

RELIABILITY TESTING

Reliability is evidenced if an instrument yields similar results when it is repeated at different times in similar circumstances and if responses are internally consistent with each other. Test/retest procedures were carried out with many subjects in the initial period and repeatedly in various field trials as an ongoing "quality control" of each study. Reliability was tested in several ways: in comparability of total scores each time the SIP was repeated, in comparability of category scores and in comparability of the specific items checked on test/retest trials.

Twenty-four hour test/retest reproducibility was assessed in 1974 using a modified Latin square design controlling for interviewer, type of administration, and type and severity of subject illness (Pollard et al. 1976). Further tests of reliability in 1976 showed: (1) test/retest reliability in terms of score was high and was not affected by administration or subject-related variables; and (2) test/retest reliability in terms of agreement in items checked was moderately high and showed considerable subject variability not accounted for by administration and subject-related variables (Table 1). Internal consistency was measured by Cronbach's Alpha (Cronbach 1959) and is moderately high across all SIP categories (Table 2).

TABLE 1

Reliability of SIP by category
1976 sample

Category	Test/retest Score correlations	Test/retest item agreement
SR	0.87	0.64
E	0.62	0.56
W	0.89	0.50
HM	0.79	0.56
RP	0.81	0.52
A	0.92	0.49
M	0.88	0.54
BCM	0.77	0.38
SI	0.82	0.53
AB	0.84	0.38
EB	0.72	0.50
C	0.79	0.47

TABLE 2

Spearman-Brown adjustment of alpha coefficients
to describe internal consistency for each category
in 1976 random sample

Category	α'
SR	0.79
E	0.50
W	0.73
HM	0.86
RP	0.79
A	0.76
M	0.78
BCM	0.58
SI	0.79
AB	0.83
EB	0.82
C	0.67
Overall	0.94*

N = 468.
$\alpha' \equiv \alpha$ that would be obtained if the number of items in each category was equal to 20.
* not adjusted.

In summary, very high levels of reliability were found with different administrations by the same interviewer to the same subject, different interviewers to the same subject, and between interviewer and self-administered forms taken by the same subject. Also, the internal consistency of individual categories and the instrument as a whole has been demonstrated.

VALIDITY

Validity is the ability of an instrument to measure the particular set of characteristics it claims to measure. Validity is tested by observing how well the instrument relates with other measures of the same characteristics.

Studies of validity are important not only to establish that the instrument measures what it purports to measure, but also to identify those parts of the instrument which overlap or duplicate existing measures. Especially important is the need to identify those portions of the instrument which provide information not previously available and to define the extent to which more accurate predictions can be made than with existing instruments.

Broad validation of a new instrument also aids in its acceptance among a wide group of potential users. If SIP scores are valid and if they provide desirable new information, the SIP will provide a valuable and useful measure of health status. An important first step in this validation research addressed the question of agreement among various instruments purporting to measure health status or some specific aspects of it. The study of these relationships assesses the correlation of the new instrument with existing instruments administered to the same subjects. Two further validation efforts involved comparing the new instrument with judgments of appropriate observers assessing roughly the same concept, i.e., the patient's judgment of his own health or sickness, and the clinician's assessment of the patient's health and clinician assessments of dysfunction (Bergner et al. 1976b).

In studies of the relationship between the SIP and a measure of activities of daily living, and between the SIP and a measure of activity limitation (National Health Interview Survey), correlations were high. The relationship between the SIP and subject's assessment of sickness and dysfunction were high and between the SIP and clinician's assessments of sickness and dysfunction, were moderately high. The SIP was consistently more highly related to self-assessments than to clinician assessments. Though correlations varied among physician groups, the category scores that correlate most highly with physician ratings are the same across groups. For all physicians, those categories describing dysfunctions in ambulation, mobility and confinement and sleep and rest are the best predictors of the physician's rating of the patient's dysfunction (Table 3).

TABLE 3

Correlations between other health measures and SIP
percent score 1976 Sample (N = 230)

Activities of daily living index*	0.46
NHIS (National Health Interview Survey)**	0.55
Self-assessment of sickness	0.63
Self-assessment of dysfunction	0.69
Clinician assessment of sickness	0.40
Clinician assessment of dysfunction	0.50

* These data were obtained during the 1974 field trial on a selected group of patients being treated by a Rehabilitation Medicine Service (N = 67).
** An ongoing interview survey of the National Center for Vital Statistics.

A further group of criteria against which a new instrument may be measured and assessed includes "objective" clinical findings (laboratory, x-ray or other paraclinical measures). Such objective criteria clearly associated with progress or retrogression of clinical disease prove to be almost as hard to come by as a clear definition of health or sickness. Nevertheless, short of such validation, it is unlikely that health status indicators will be used where they are needed: to provide an outcome measure and planning tool to assist in a variety of ways, which range from evaluating therapeutic regimens to planning health care facilities.

In order to assess the validity of the SIP in relation to laboratory and/or other clinical data that are used to diagnose and follow patients, three diagnostic categories were selected that met the following criteria: (1) the clinical test data were considered valid and reliable indicators of the patient's course; (2) the clinical test data could be expected to reflect patient functioning; (3) tests were repeated at regular intervals that coincided with expected changes in patient's condition; (4) the patient's condition would change in an expected direction during the course of the study; and (5) a sufficient number of cases could be expected during the study period. Few diagnostic groups meet these criteria. Patients undergoing total hip replacements, newly diagnosed hyperthyroid patients, and arthritics enrolled in a double-blind drug study, were selected because they covered a range of types of conditions and met the criteria better than other groups considered. Patients in each diagnostic category were tested at least three times with both the clinical test(s) and the SIP. The type of clinical data varied from tests of range of motion for hip patients, to thyroxin levels for hyperthyroids, to grip strength and joint assessment for arthritics. The study design included assessments of SIP test/retest reliability for each subject, completion of surrogate SIPs by family members and clinicians, clinician ratings of dysfunction and sickness and subject ratings of his/her own level of dysfunction and sickness.

As a general statement it may be said that the SIP showed a high correlation with the established and accepted tests in all three disease conditions and at all the stages of the diseases that were tested. Also, except for arthritis patients, the SIP predicted each set of criteria better than self or clinician assessments of dysfunction, and for all three groups it provided more sensitive descriptions of characteristic patterns of dysfunction than the criterion measures did. A characteristic pattern of SIP category and dimension scores across all hip patients and across all hyperthyroid patients was found, and characteristic and unchanging patterns were found for individual arthritic patients. These characteristic patterns permitted differentiation among diseases and among patients. A detailed description of the clinical validation of the SIP, including simultaneous clinical tests, is in progress in a paper to be published separately.

The validation of the SIP assures its usefulness as a health status outcome measure in a variety of circumstances. It may be used at the level of (1) small groups, (2) individual patient, and (3) general populations:

1. Small Groups. The SIP may be useful especially for therapeutic trials: testing new therapies in controlled clinical trials of drugs; medical procedures; surgical methods; prosthetic devices and implants; physical and social and environmental manipulations, e.g., in long-term care of terminal illness. Two hypothetical examples based on data we have collected will illustrate the potential for clinical use. Patient A (Figure 2) who underwent total hip replacement for osteoarthritis

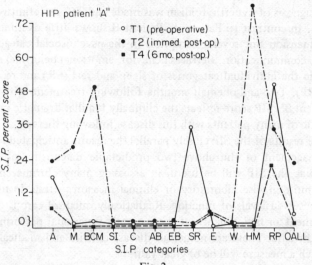

Fig. 2.

during the course of the SIP studies shows a characteristic pattern before surgery of dysfunction mainly in the physical dimension categories (ambulation, mobility, and body care and movement) with relatively small impact shown on the psychosocial and individual categories. As might be expected during the immediate postoperative period, SIP scores mirror even greater dysfunction; however, scores taken six months after surgery reflect the remarkable recovery often noted in this condition.

Patient B (Figure 3) is an individual whose first SIP was obtained immediately

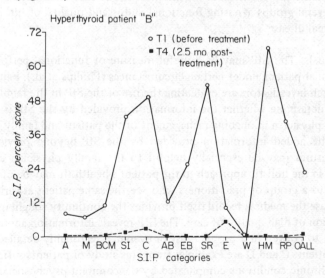

Fig. 3.

after the diagnosis of hyperthyroidism was made and before definitive treatment was started. In contrast to Patient A, Patient B shows little dysfunction in the physical dimension but severe disruption in the psychosocial categories (social interaction, communication, alertness behavior, emotional behavior) and marked aberration in the individual categories of sleep and rest (SR) and recreation and pastimes (RP). Two-and-one-half months following treatment with radioactive iodine, Patient B's SIP score reflects the clinically familiar dramatic improvement characteristic of many patients with this disease following therapy.

Since the results of the SIP closely parallel the results anticipated by clinicians in the management of the above two predictable diagnostic categories, it is expected that the SIP will be useful in assessing many chronic conditions in which the most precise laboratory or clinical measures often do not correlate well with observed levels of function. Realistically, medical care is often aimed at improvement or maintenance of the patient's functional performance rather than outright cure. There are numerous disease entities and medical care issues in which such a measure will be of great value.

The SIP is being used by investigators at St. Thomas' Hospital Medical School in London where it is being administered to the handicapped in order to determine long-term care needs, an increasingly important issue in the United States. The SIP is one of several assessment measures being used by the National Heart and Lung Institute in its evaluation of nocturnal oxygen therapy for patients with chronic obstructive pulmonary disease. The Seattle/King County Department of Health is using the SIP to assess the health status of patients who have survived for six months after resuscitation from a cardiac arrest. In this study patients are being compared on the basis of which of two types of mobile manpower aid units assisted them at the time of their cardiac arrest. The SIP is being used by several groups assessing functional status and quality of life in patients with terminal disease.

2. Individuals. The SIP may be a useful measure of functional performance in the individual patient under certain circumstances (Phillips et al.). Family physician research investigators are evaluating the use of the SIP in the family practice setting to determine whether the information provided by the SIP is helpful to the family physician in ongoing management of the patient and family in chronic disease. The added information provided by the SIP beyond previous health status measures may be especially helpful to the family physician and others interested in the holistic approach to the patient's health. It may be of particular assistance to a group of practitioners who see the same patient at various times, in which case the medical record itself provides the continuity sought unceasingly as a criterion of high quality of care. The SIP reveals information about function impossible to convey in a problem list or even in a reasonably detailed narrative history. Patients C and D are examples from this study of patients suffering from multiple chronic conditions complicated by concomitant psychosocial problems or reactions. Patient C is a 50 year old black female under care for several years

in a family medical center for hypertension, asthma, hemorrhoids, cervical adenopathy and headaches. SIPs completed in 1974 and in 1979 are shown in Figure 4. The attending physician expressed interest and some surprise at the

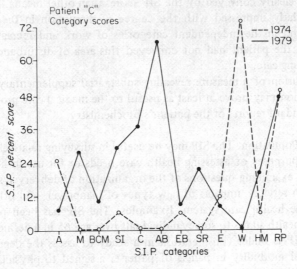

Fig. 4.

increasing disruption in the psychosocial dimension shown by the second SIP and felt able to suggest more specific interventions than had been possible with this patient previously.

Patient D (Figure 5) is a 44 year old Greek-American with chest tightness,

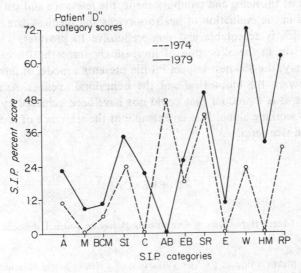

Fig. 5.

degenerative arthritis, obesity, adult onset diabetes mellitus, hyperlipidemia, and first degree A-V block. SIPs done in 1974 and repeated in 1979 reveal a persistent and worsening pattern of dysfunction which his physician felt was much more clearly conveyed by the SIP scores than other means. The physician was particularly impressed with the degree of disruption in the psychosocial categories and in the independent categories of work and recreation and pastimes, since the patient had not conveyed this area of disturbance adequately during ongoing care.

The inclusion of a measure revealing substantial supplementary information about function may prove at least as useful to the medical care provider as some types of standard reports of the patient's biochemistry.

3. General Population. The SIP may be useful in surveying relatively large populations for purposes of assessing health care needs or for use in health services research for examining questions of the organization of delivery systems, financing of health services, impacts of new types of manpower, and other rearrangements in the health care system. Examples: The SIP has been proposed as a measure of health status to survey individuals over age 65 in a defined geographic area. The SIP is under consideration in a study to assess the degree and types of functional morbidity in panels of patients assigned to physicians in a large prepaid health care plan where it is desirable that physicians carry comparable patient loads. Since patients may vary greatly in their degrees of morbidity and demands on the system, the SIP may prove a useful tool in studies to address equitable distribution of patients among physicians.

With growing national pressure for increased access to health services and new mechanisms of financing and reimbursement, the relevance and sensitivity of the SIP may aid in the evaluation of health services and medical care. The use of a measure which is acceptable and comprehensive to providers and consumers alike may assist in the allocation of increasingly scarce health care resources.

In summary, the Sickness Impact Profile presents a model of interdisciplinary research between the biomedical and the behavioral sciences. As a measure of health status, it is a product that could not have been achieved by either group of scientists working alone. It is an example of the relevance of social science to medicine and vice versa.

REFERENCES

Allport, F. H.
    1934 The J-curve Hypothesis of Conforming Behavior. Journal of Social Behavior 141:
        183.
Bergner, M., et al.
    1976a The Sickness Impact Profile: Validation of a Health Status Measure. Medical Care
        14·57

1976b The Sickness Impact Profile: Conceptual Formulation and Methodology for the Development of a Health Status Measure. International Journal of Health Services 6:393.

Bobbitt, R. A., et al.
1966 Development and Application of an Observational Method: Continuing Reliability Testing. Journal of Psychiatry 63:83.

Campbell, D. T., and D. W. Fiske
1959 Convergent and Discriminant Validation by the Multitrait-multimethod Matrix. Psychology Bulletin 56:81.

Carter, W. B., et al.
1976 The Validation of an Interval Scaling: The Sickness Impact Profile. Health Services Research. Winter 1976:516–528.

Cronbach, L. J.
1951 Coefficient Alpha and the Internal Structure of Tests. Psychometrika 16:297.

Cronbach, L. J. and G. C. Gleser
1953 Assessing Similarity Between Profiles. Psychology Bulletin 50:456.

Ekwall, B.
1960 Method for Evaluating Indications for Rehabilitation in Chronic Hemiplegia. Acta Medica Scandinavica, Suppl 450.

Flexner, A.
1910 Medical Education in the United States and Canada; A Report to Carnegie Foundation for the Advancement of Teaching, Bulletin Number Four. New York.

Gilson, B. S., et al.
1972–73 Development and Application of the Sickness Impact Profile: A Pilot Study. Department of Health Services, University of Washington, Seattle, Washington, xerox.
1973–74 Revision and Test of the Sickness Impact Profile, Department of Health Services, University of Washington, Seattle, Washington, xerox.
1974–75 Further Tests and Revision of the Sickness Impact Profile, Department of Health Services, University of Washington, Seattle, Washington, xerox.
1975 The Sickness Impact Profile: Development of an Outcome Measure of Health Care. American Journal of Public Health 65:1304.

Gillo, M. W. and M. W. Shelly
1974 Predictive Modeling of Multivariable and Multivariate Data. Journal of the American Statistical Association, September 646–653.

Gleser, G. C.
Undated Quantifying Similarity Between People. In The Role and Methodology of Classification in Psychiatry and Psychopathology, USDHEW, PHS.

Haataja, M.
1975 Evaluation of the Activity of Rheumatoid Arthritis. Scand. J. Rheum. 4:Supp. 7.

Harris, W. H.
1973 Preliminary Report of Results of Harris Total Hip Replacement. Clinical Orthopedics and Related Research 95:168.

Katz, S., et al.
1963 Studies of Illness in the Aged: The Index of A.D.L. Journal of the American Medical Association 185:914.

Meltzer, J. W. and J. R. Hochstim
1970 Reliability and Validity of Survey Data of Physical Health. Public Health Reports 85:1075.

Phillips, T. J., et al.
In Progress. "The Value of Functional Health Assessment in Patient Management by the Family Physician."

Pollard, W. E., et al.
  1976 The Sickness Impact Profile: Reliability of a Health Status Measure. Medical
        Care 14:146.
  1978 Examination of Variable Errors of Measurement in a Survey-based Social
        Indicator. Social Indicators Research 5:279.
Sokal, R. R. and P. H. A. Sneath
  1963 Principles of Numerical Taxonomy. San Francisco: W. H. Freeman & Company.
Tryon, R. C. and D. E. Bailey
  1970 Cluster Analysis. New York: McGraw-Hill.
U.S. Department of Health, Education and Welfare
  1972 Interviewing Methods in the Health Interview Survey. Vital and Health Statistics:
        Series 2, No. 48.
  1975 Publication No. (HRA) 76–1776.
  1976 Publication No. (HRA) 77–1539.

7. CULTURAL INFLUENCES ON ILLNESS BEHAVIOR: A MEDICAL ANTHROPOLOGICAL APPROACH

Ideas about illness and what to do when ill vary with culture. That is obvious. A doctor might find the special interests of the medical anthropologist most helpful to him in work with patients from different cultural backgrounds from his own. Mixture of social class and ethnic origin is common in cities. But there are some aspects of an anthropological approach to illness behavior which have, I think, more general interest than just the appeal of the exotic. These aspects derive partly from the particular character of anthropological research and the way it may provoke us to question or reflect on what we accept as normal or natural behavior. We may see that it is customary rather than natural to behave in that way. We become concerned to discover the social reasons for such customary acts or responses.

Most anthropologists work in surroundings they were not brought up in. Direct observation of another community by living in it for about a year or more is the common way in which data are collected in the first place. Anthropologists usually have to learn a new language for their work, have to accommodate to unfamiliar customs and to material conditions of life they are not used to. This style of field study brings firsthand practical experience of how people in a community live. It provides the chance of following longer sequences of behavior and more complicated events at a personal level. A small number of people may become well-known to the observer. He is in a position to find out about people's ideas and opinions on some subjects in detail: he can see how closely what people say they would or should do in certain circumstances corresponds with what they actually do. The local community and the home setting is more likely to be the place where the anthropologist observes the sick than in the hospital or the clinic or the consulting room. Professional medical people are not so likely to have the time or opportunity to see their patients at home. The home visit and care given in the patient's home are dwindling features of a doctor's work in most industrialized societies. Without opportunities to see patients at home, a doctor may have small chance of imagining very accurately the conditions in which they live or the settings in which most illness is played out. It is easy to attribute one's own assumptions, outlook and background to others, but it is often mistaken to do so.

Lay people perceive illness differently from a doctor. The doctor has spent a long time learning which features he must look for to diagnose and treat illness well. His patients do not share that knowledge; they have not had his daily contact with sick people extending over years to bring them a comparable experience of illness observed. The name of a particular sort of illness or symptom does not necessarily have the same associations for the lay person and the doctor, even

151

L. Eisenberg and A. Kleinman (eds.), The Relevance of Social Science for Medicine, 151–162.
Copyright © 1980 *by D. Reidel Publishing Company.*

when they both use the same term correctly. They refer to the same thing, perhaps, yet give it different significance. But it will often be the case that the doctor professionally classifies an illness differently from his patients and their relatives, though in talking to them he must use ordinary language and non-specialist terms. The names of Greek and Latin fancy, which weigh down the classification and description of disease in medicine, were introduced so as to try to keep clear, and be clear about, what was referred to. A doctor has to learn the definitions and discriminations: using them correctly will show another doctor that he has a proper medical education in the high culture of 'cosmopolitan medicine'. Terms in common usage such as 'stroke,' 'heart attack,' 'nervous breakdown,' 'tummy ache,' 'lumbago,' are part of a lay classification of illness. The two classificatory systems, one specialist, the other lay, are not in competition as to whether one is right and the other wrong: each may be right when used in its proper context. They differ in precision and discrimination, in how and where they draw the boundaries between kinds of illness and in the information they convey. It is possible for the doctor to use his technical terms to impress, confuse or bewilder his patient, but he is more likely (and more sensible) to want to make his meaning plain to his patient by using intelligible language. Translation between lay and technical medical terms can present the same sort of problems as those which face the anthropologist at work in a foreign culture, except that there the problems show up perhaps more clearly.

An example may bring home how the classification of illness is relative to culture. The divisions of one classificatory system need not be drawn in parallel, or correspond, to those found in another. It is easy to make the mistake of assuming they are. My example comes from New Guinea.

Palu lived in a village in the north of New Guinea. He was about 50 years old and was seriously ill. His belly and legs had swollen; he felt weak. He decided to try to walk to the Mission Hospital, but the path along the ridge leading to it passed through the nearest neighboring village. When he came to this village, the people there would not let him pass through because they were frightened that his illness would infect them. They said he had *sik lepro*. That is the Pidgin English for 'leprosy.' He was turned back. Some time later he died in his own village, his belly grossly swollen. The body was buried with special haste for fear of the illness jumping to someone else. I was told of these events about two years after they had happened when I returned to the village where I had worked before. A complicated chain of misunderstandings lies behind them.

It is probable that leprosy was introduced in this inland part of New Guinea as a result of contact with coastal people and Europeans. These contacts became more frequent in the 1950s. After a few cases of leprosy had been diagnosed, the health department arranged for some health education patrols to tell people about leprosy, its dangers, and the need for prompt treatment. A special treatment house for lepers was established at the Mission Hospital. It was set apart from the rest of the hospital. People had to stay there a long time for supervised treatment. When they absconded, police were sometimes called to fetch them back from their villages. *Sik lepro* was a serious matter: that was quite clear to the villagers.

The education patrols showed people how to recognize the early skin signs of leprosy and tried to impress on them the need to come for treatment. In order to impress this on them, they emphasized the risk of disfiguring and destructive changes later on if they did not come. They showed them pictures of the horrible effects of the disease. They also stressed the dangers of contagious spread to others: if you harbor the leper, you may yourself fall victim; if you hide your illness, you may infect your children. What stood out to the people was the new name *sik lepro*, the stern attitude to treatment, threats of disfiguring swelling, the possibility of spread to others. But none of the local lepers was obviously disfigured or deformed. Most could show only some skin blemishes; one or two had slight thickening of their earlobes. There was little that seemed to justify so much concern. On the other hand, occasionally people were seriously sick with swellings when there had been no injury to account for them. Some people would recall the warnings about *sik lepro* and suggest that as the diagnosis. With it went fear of spread to others.

I think it quite probable that Palu died from liver failure: I had examined him about three years before his last illness and found him then to have a much enlarged liver and spleen as well as the past story of a severe illness in which he had vomited for a long time, his urine went dark, and he had pains in his right side. His final illness was considered by some people in his village to have been a case of *sik lepro* because he had swelled up. That was what counted for them for a diagnosis of *sik lepro*. They gave that sense to the term and chose to use it so. They also grasped its seriousness and the risk of catching it from someone else. They had learned from the health educators that there were special horrors to leprosy. They were not convinced of them by the skin blemishes of early leprosy, but they granted them to what they took to be the bad *sik lepro* where there was swelling. The pressure put by health personnel to persuade people to take treatment, the isolation of a *haus lepro* (leper house) set aside for lepers, contributed to single out the disease as a special kind of sickness.

They were learning an attitude to leprosy that has a long history. The sources for it go back to the Book of Leviticus in the Bible which sets out the rules for recognizing the leper, for his exclusion from society, and for his cleansing if the leprosy should leave him. In medieval times the leper was said to be 'dead to the world' (by Rothar's edict: *il est mort quant au siécle*), he was separated from society and denied the right to his estate, to own or inherit goods, or to make a will (Brody 1974:80–5). For the early Christian view came to be that leprosy was an emblem of sin, the external revelation of internal evil, a symbol of the many vices which defile mankind (ibid. 119–33). Leprosy has not wholly lost that taint despite the changes in our knowledge of the disease. The stigma associated with leprosy and the disproportionate horror of it have lasted into our times to add to the misery of those afflicted by it (Gussow and Tracy 1968, 1970).

The bitter irony behind this story is that the condition described in the Bible is not leprosy as we know it. The name of 'leprosy' got attached to the condition discussed in Leviticus when the Hebrew Bible was translated into Greek. The Septuagint translators used the Greek word *lepra* for the condition called *zara'at* in Hebrew. Contemporary Greek medical descriptions of the skin condition then called *lepra* do not remotely resemble modern leprosy. *Lepra* was used in the first and second centuries for a circular, superficial, scaly eruption of the skin. The word underwent a radical change of meaning and application in the centuries that followed (Macalister 1904). A change occurred then rather like the one now taking place on a tiny scale in the region of New Guinea where I worked. The name endures as *lepro* or *sik lepro* only to give the illusion of stable reference. *Lepro* (to a few New Guineans at least) can refer to any serious swelling that appears without trauma, and is accompanied by general malaise. The special concern and fear accompanying the name of *lepro* is misapplied by them to a new range of states now brought within its compass. *Sik lepro* may mean one thing to the doctor or the health educator, and something else to the man or woman he is talking to. They share a common vocabulary but they use it differently. They do not have the same medical education or experience.

Special attitudes towards a kind of illness may hold fast to a name, and a name that was intended first as a neutral label or description may become tainted by moral or emotional associations. Use of the name then may arouse fears or shame in someone's mind and alter the behavior of others towards him or her. The actions of the villagers who would not let Palu walk on the path through their village, of his kin who buried him so hastily, show that power of a name to influence behavior towards the sick. It is a particular example of the general tendency for ideas about cause and effect to color attitudes taken to illness, and to guide or prejudice actions taken in response to it. It is difficult to detach evaluation from description. Sometimes doctors use mystifying jargon explicitly to try to escape from the unpleasant associations of a name: for example, they speak of 'strabismus' when they mean a squint, of 'Hansen's disease' when they mean leprosy, etc. They hide a name in the hope of neutralizing moral associations which, though not necessary or intrinsic to the illness, are yet so firmly stuck to it. The artificial Greek and Latin of technical terms in medicine may sometimes also serve to disguise nasty, distressing or shaming facts.

Behind every classification of illness there are purposes which may be more or less clearly formulated, or left implicit. The example of leprosy draws attention to the way in which stigma may become wrongly or unfairly attached to a particular disease name. But the association of disease names with particular ideas about cause and effect is a common principle used in the classification of diseases, and a would-be helpful one. The purpose is to sort out illnesses according to the kinds of problem they present for prevention or treatment. It would be misleading to point out the occasional stigmatizing associations of some kinds of disease without also stressing that most names for diseases are intended to help guide appropriate action in response to them.

The people I worked with in New Guinea, for example, did not give close attention to clinical signs and symptoms, and did not have an elaborate classification of the clinical syndromes of illness. Reference to the clinical feature of swelling in the new *sik lepro* was odd in terms of their customary practice. In their view, remedial action and the prevention of illness depended on knowing the cause for illness. They did not think that the cause of serious illness was likely to be detectable from close attention to the clinical signs and symptoms of the patient. It was more relevant, they thought, to know about what the patient had been doing recently. One of their recognized causes for illness might make one patient vomit, but another cough, and a third have an aching knee. There could be common features about the circumstances of the patients' recent lives which might enable them to identify the same cause at work in all three illnesses, but these common features could not be discovered through physical examination of the three sick people (Lewis 1975:128–54, 244–67). It was therefore relevant for them to ask about someone's recent social and personal history when he fell ill, but not appropriate to go to examine his body and physical functioning. In contrast, our understanding of the links between symptoms, physical signs, correct diagnosis and correct treatment makes it necessary for the doctor to be granted certain privileges of intimate access to the patient. Our assumptions about the things relevant to treatment determine what we pay attention to. What a doctor judges most relevant or pertinent may not coincide with the expectations of his patients. When his questions or actions fail to match their expectations, or seem to them irrelevant, he risks losing some of their goodwill and confidence in him.

Illness may be classified in medical textbooks in various ways: compare, for instance, a general textbook of medicine and one of pathology, a handbook guide to differential diagnosis, a first aid manual, a compendium of emergency medicine, a monograph on the diseases of an organ or a system. They provide examples of how the same phenomena may be sorted out differently depending on the purpose in view — there are books organized according to the presenting complaint, the chief physical signs, the part of the body or the functional system affected, the underlying pathology, the divisions of cause, etc. The New Guinea people I worked with would find little in such classifications to correspond with their views of the relevant and necessary information. They would want to see much more about the social circumstances of the affected person, and his social relations with the people round him, brought in and related to the diagnosis of the different kinds of illness. But such information is ignored in our usual medical classifications.

We, just as they, circumscribe what we consider relevant, and neglect much else. For the most part we tend to constrict the field of our medical focus to the individual patient, his body and its functioning. Big advances in the control and treatment of some diseases have come through intensive study limited in this way. But it is not always satisfactory to confine our vision so.

There is the practical aspect: we may know what organism causes tuberculosis, what its various effects are and how to treat them. But questions of trying to explain the patterns of incidence of tuberculosis in particular populations or communities, or of finding how to persuade people to come for treatment, are not answered if we confine our view of illness to what takes place inside the body. If we change our sights to ask why do those people then and there fall ill, there is much more to answer, for poverty, bad food, bad housing, poor education, laws on the marketing of milk or on the holding of land or jobs, may all have played their part to make them vulnerable to the illness, or to expose them to it and reduce the likelihood of them receiving treatment or seeking it (Jansen 1973:147–97).

In the *Health Book for the Tailor Trade*, Alfred Adler, who was later to become famous as a psychiatrist, wrote about the social and economic conditions of the small tailor in Austria and Germany in 1898. Technical progress, which gave advantages to the clothing manufacturers, was less beneficial for him:

He uses only the sewing machine, he works only for a small local market, and is much more exposed to economic fluctuations. The worst calamity is the uneven distribution of work through the year: there are five or six months of intensive overwork, during which the tailor labors sixteen, or eighteen hours a day, if not more, assisted by his wife and children. And during the remaining part of the year there is almost no work at all ... The living conditions of the small tailor are miserable in every regard. His lodging and working space, which are one and the same and are situated in the cheapest and unhealthiest part of the town, are damp, airless and overcrowded ... They work in a stooped sitting position, breathing in the dust of the cloth. Pulmonary tuberculosis is twice as frequent among them than in the average of the other trades ... The peculiar stooped sitting position determines deformations such as scoliosis, kyphosis, rheumatism and arthritis of the right arm ... Because of needle pricks, they often suffer from abscesses on fingers ... (Ellenberger 1970:599–601).

For certain medical purposes it might be just as relevant to classify illnesses according to the social attributes of the people affected (age, wealth, education, religion, occupation, distance from and access to a health center), or by social effects of the illness (stigma, interference with obligations at work, in the home, job performance, chronic or fleeting social inconvenience). Such features as these may correlate better with differences in the behavior of people ill (for instance, delay in seeking advice, readiness to comply with treatment, liability to relapse after discharge) than features that are intrinsic to the kind of disease they suffer from.

One may contrast two approaches to a person's illness: one generalizing, the other individualistic. One is to attempt to classify it because it conforms to some typical pattern, then it can be assigned to a category; the other is to look on someone's illness as an event, as a patch of personal biography, to be understood rather than classified. It is only by ignoring most of what is individual in people's illnesses that common types or categories can be recognized.

The classification of disease in scientific medicine aims to define categories of disease in terms of fact and evidence that will be observable, public and explicit. The desire to make categories that can be applied universally and will allow like to be compared with like, requires the choice of biological criteria. This is because mankind everywhere has the same basic biological nature but differs greatly in regard to his social arrangements, ideas and values. By setting up exclusively biological criteria to define the kinds of disease, we may make it possible for an observer to decide objectively whether some disease, specified strictly in these terms, is present or not. The criteria in principle should be independent of culture. But such a biological classification of types of disease must necessarily fail to identify most of the individual, social and subjective aspects of the experience of illness. Any attempt to grasp and understand people's behavior in illness demands that we concern ourselves with these subjective aspects.

All people perceive the world selectively and give it meaning by relating what they perceive to themselves and to their past experience. The intensity of the sensation of pain, for example, does not follow automatically from the extent and nature of an injury. Fear of implications for the future may intensify awareness of pain in the surgical patient, or, by contrast, the hope and likely chance of escape from deadly risks of battle may diminish the injured soldier's sense of pain and his complaints, though the injury be similar in both cases. Beecher's (1959) studies on pain and its relief have shown the power of ideas about the meaning of a situation to modify experience of it. Zborowski (1952) described the different responses of people of Jewish, Italian, Irish and 'Old American' extraction to pain and related them to different cultural attitudes and expectations — concern with immediate relief of pain or rather desire to know its cause and what implications it might hold for future illness; desire for sympathy and company; values set on silent fortitude, self-reliance and so on. Pain, like fear and anxiety, is open to the influence of culture. The subjective reality of pain or fear is not to be denied or contraverted by some dogmatic reference to objective fact. The reality of illness as experienced by the sufferer depends also on the assumptions of that person set in his cultural milieu which affect how he pays attention to himself. To understand his behavior we must go beyond the narrow focus on the biological features of his illness.

Montaigne wrote in 1588:

"in regard to bodily health no man can furnish more useful experience than I, since I offer it unadulterated, quite uncorrupted by art and theory. In the realm of medicine experience is, so to say, a cock on his own dunghill, since reason must entirely give way to it" (Montaigne 1927: Bk III, 556).

"These years" he wrote,

"have been so generous as to make me familiarized with the stone in the bladder . . . Of all the misfortunes of old age it is just the one I dreaded most . . . And yet, when formerly I dimly foresaw (these bodily and really essential sufferings), with a sight enfeebled and mollified by the enjoyment of the happy and prolonged health and repose that God had given me, for the best part of my life, I conceived them in imagination to be so unbearable that in truth my fear of them was greater than my present suffering. Wherefore I am ever more confirmed in this belief, that most of the faculties of the soul, as we exercise them, disturb the peace of life more than they promote it. I am at grips with the worst, the most sudden, the most painful and most irremediable of all diseases. I have already experienced five or six very long and painful attacks of it. And yet, unless I flatter myself, even in this condition there is something endurable for a man whose soul is free from the fear of death, and free from the menaces, conclusions, and consequences which the doctors keep dinning into our ears" (ibid: Bk II, 209–10).

"In my opinion that faculty (the imagination) is all-important, at least more so than any other. The most grievous and the most common ills are those that fancy puts upon me. I like this Spanish saying from several points of view, *God defend me from myself*" (ibid: Bk III, 566).

"How many people have not been made ill by the mere force of imagination ... But even though knowledge could really do what they say, blunt the point and lessen the bitterness of the misfortunes that attend us, what more does it do than what ignorance does, much more simply and manifestly? The philosopher Pyrrho, in peril of a great storm at sea, could offer his companions no better example to follow than the serenity of a pig, their fellow-traveler, which was looking at the tempest with perfect equanimity" (ibid: Bk II, 585).

Montaigne stresses the power of ideas about illness to affect experience of it. The imagination fed by fears about it can make the suffering worse. We learn these fears from others. And we also learn how we should behave when ill. Montaigne's stoicism is tempered and humanely understanding when he discusses the conventions of his time regarding the expression of pain:

"I have always regarded as affectation that precept that so sternly and precisely tells us to put on a good face, a disdainful and indifferent mien, when suffering pain ... What matter whether we wring our hands, as long as we do not wring our thoughts? ... In so extreme a calamity it is cruelty to expect so composed a bearing. If we play the game it is no great matter that we make a wry face. If the body finds a relief in lamenting, let it lament. If agitation pleases it, let it tumble and toss at its pleasure ... We have enough to do to contend with the evil, without laboring over these superfluous rules. I have said all this in excuse of those we generally see raging and storming under the shocks and attacks of this disease. For my part I have hitherto suffered them a little more patiently (and I stop short at groaning, without braying)" (ibid: Bk II, 211–12).

Apart from what is instinctive in the moves to ease, escape or cry out the pain, there is a voluntary element in response which may well not seek to hide what is felt, but rather seek to alert and reveal how it does hurt. Given the privacy of pain, the sufferer must express it to make it known. He needs and wants help. The ways to convey this information or to gain sympathy are subject to particular conventions which vary with the standards of fortitude in pain, differing in expectation according to age, sex, and status, and the extent to which loud calls for help are approved. The conventions serve to make the behavior less open to misunderstanding. The conventions vary by culture, as does response to them.

For instance, what I had supposed to be a natural way of showing sympathy only made matters worse for Dauwaras, a man suffering much pain, whom I knew in the village where I worked in New Guinea. His joint pains were understood by himself and others as the sign of attack by an afflicting spirit and accordingly he withdrew from normal social life, abstained from certain foods and chat. He lay apart from others, dirty with ashes and dust on his skin. He hardly answered if spoken to. The pain persisted and got worse, so he moved to a small dark hut in which he stayed alone most of the time. His illness was understood to be severe. People came to spend the day sitting with his family and hamlet neighbors. They chatted; they ate a meal. The visits took place on many days during his long illness. Almost no one went to see him or to talk to him, except for those who went explicitly to treat him. I pitied him in his pain and isolation. I passed much of one day chatting to him in a well-meaning effort to cheer him up in what I imagined was a miserable solitude in the dark of the hut. That night his pains came on redoubled. We had talked about many things – about his illness, possible reasons for it, what the others were doing, about past times, warfare, his spells of contract labor at the coastal plantations. Next day the senior man in his family, his eldest brother, asked me not to visit him to talk like that; such talk brought on his pain and added to the risk of the spirit continuing to afflict him, for it saw that he behaved as a normal man would, and disregarded the warning threat of death it gave him in the pain.

In this brief illustration, I would point out first, the stereotyped social withdrawal with dirt and griming used to indicate to others, not verbally, but by behavior, what the patient felt. Additional marks of the severity of his pain and his perception that he was seriously ill came later – in the things he refused to eat, his silence. his abandonment of all body covering, even his penis-covering, his self-neglect and dirt. Secondly, the behavior was responded to by the demonstration of sympathy in terms appropriate for that society – they came to visit, as they said, "to sit around him," called by the sense of affection as well as duty. His appeal was clear. Later when he got much worse, some slept the night in his hamlet to show concern for him – still they did not talk or sit with him, but only towards the end, some came to weep over him. They came into the doorway of the hut and squatted down to weep or wail at the sight of him. Dauwaras, the man, realized how many people had come, and on so many days, to show him sympathy (he was worried at the work it meant for the women of his extended family and the drain on his brothers' food resources) but he was touched by their sympathy; for their tears he said he would repay them, as custom expected.

With Dauwaras, the diagnosis of the spirit attacking played a part in the later attention he gave his pain. The spirit was concerned with the successful growth of certain plants, especially bananas and yams. Of course he avoided these foods, but he still found that he had pain and it got much worse when people passed near where he lay carrying bananas or yams. So barriers were put at a distance round him to keep people off lest the influence of the spirit following its foods renew his suffering. These measures relieved him a little. The spirit then began to trouble him in his dreams, appearing in its dream-form as a great black pig, and he woke to agony following such dreams. The attention he gave his pain stemmed from the pain itself, but also his suffering reflected the significance he attached to his pain, what it meant to him in terms of the spirit cause, its power and his knowledge of those he had known in the past who had died by it. In his case, though they tried to heal him by performing the great rites of the spirit, they failed; his pain persisted. Then they and he realized that there must be some additional cause, yet undiscovered and malignant, seeking his ruin.

In every society there are some conventions about how people should behave when they are ill. In every culture there are ideas about the significance of different signs or symptoms of illness. The extent to which such conventions and expectations can determine how someone behaves when ill varies with the disease he suffers from. There will be some diseases which impose their effects so severely or so suddenly that there is little chance for the sufferer to adjust or modify his response to them. His behavior is largely involuntary. But in most illness there is some interplay of voluntary and involuntary responses in the expression of illness. The patient has some control of the way in which he shows his illness and what he says about it. How he acts is influenced by the setting in which he finds himself and his appreciation of the situation and the people about him. The social costs or benefits, like loss of time at work, the effects of an open declaration of disability or impairment, the possibility of evading unwelcome duties or obligations because of illness, all may complicate how and when someone decides to seek advice or treatment. How we behave when ill may well vary according to whether we are alone, at home, at work, or in the street among strangers, because we have all learnt to recognize that there are social constraints and rules which govern the conditions for which we can expect sympathy, ridicule or help. Reciprocally, the readiness of others to show concern and give assistance is conditional on their view of their obligations to the sick person, their understanding and evaluation of his state, and on considerations of time, money, urgency and capacity to help. We should not neglect, in favor of sole concentration on the sick person, the responses of other people to someone ill, as though they were not cultural aspects of illness behavior. Social behavior in illness is by definition an interaction with others: to forget the others leaves us blind to influences that may have shaped and motivated much of what someone did when he was ill.

Illness is no respecter of person, time, place or convention, and that contingency intrinsic to illness can be most inconvenient and give it great power to disrupt social plans. The responses made to illness depend on much more than just what kind of illness strikes. The responses also depend on who is struck and when. The segregation and distribution of social roles within a network or an organization of institutions are critical here: they may act to make the illness have severe social repercussions though these consequences are not specific to the kind of disease. From that point of view any illness severe enough to prevent the person from carrying out his or her duties may have a severe impact if it occurs at the wrong time. It may affect others within the system of which that person is a part, and determine the urgency with which they act to do something about it.

The behavior of married women in the New Guinea village I worked in, when they were ill, reflected the constraints of their domestic duties. The wife with a young family to feed is the central figure in providing for her family's daily needs. I found that men paid more attention to their own trivial or mild illness, and more readily took time off to stay home ill than women. They could afford to indulge in indisposition. Young married women, on the other hand, sometimes put on an exaggerated display of being ill: they seemed to me to overact how sick and miserable they felt. This conspicuously ill behavior was not confined to women, but when I compared the men with the women who showed it, I found that the behavior in men was more often associated with some particular explanation or fear about the implications of what they had noticed in themselves whereas with women such behavior, unattached to any elaborate explanation, made it rather seem an end in itself, as though the young married woman having greater pressures on her not to stop work for mild illness, and needing to justify abandoning her domestic duties, did so in part by making very clear to others just how ill she felt to gain some sympathy.

Possibilities of care, of sympathy, the allocation of responsibility for sickness in others, affect how people show their illness. In a small-scale society, such as a New Guinea village community, the obligation to show concern at the serious illness of one member is distributed widely within the community, according to acknowledged bonds of kinship and coresidence. The illness of one member may have effects on many. Experience of general upset when someone is ill may go a little way towards explaining why people in many small-scale societies lay stress on the social and moral causes and effects of illness. In complex industrialized societies illness has become a more private matter, its treatment is confined more within the family, or else turned over to medical experts in clinical offices or hospital settings. It may be hard for the doctor who has little opportunity to see his patients in their homes or work-places to assess some of the social forces that may have influenced and shaped their attitudes to their illnesses and their responses to them.

REFERENCES

Beecher, H.
  1959 Measurements of Subjective Responses. New York: Oxford University Press.
Brody, S.
  1974 The Disease of the Soul. Ithaca: Cornell University Press.
Ellenberger, H.
  1970 The Discovery of the Unconscious. London: Allen Lane
Gussow, Z., and G. Tracy
  1968 Status, Ideology, and Adaptation to Stigmatized Illness. Human Organization 27:316—25.
  1970 Stigma and the Leprosy Phenomenon. Bulletin of the History of Medicine 44: 425—49.
Jansen, G.
  1973 The Doctor-Patient Relationship in an African Tribal Society. Netherlands: van Gorcum.

Lewis, G.
    1975 Knowledge of Illness in a Sepik Society. London: Athlone Press.
Macalister, A.
    1904 Leprosy. *In* The Dictionary of the Bible. J. Hastings, ed. Edinburgh: Black.
Montaigne, M.
    1927 The Essays of Montaigne (Translated by E. J. Trenchmann). New York and
          London: Oxford University Press.
Zborowski, M.
    1952 Cultural Components in Responses to Pain. Journal of Social Issues 8:16–30.

SECTION 4

CULTURE, MEANING, AND NEGOTIATION

8. THE MEANING OF SYMPTOMS: A CULTURAL
HERMENEUTIC MODEL FOR CLINICAL PRACTICE

INTRODUCTION [1]

Any good doctor knows ... that the patient's complaint is more extensive than his symptom, and the state of sickness more comprehensive than localized pain or dysfunction. As an old Jew put it (and old Jews have a way of speaking for the victims of all nations): "Doctor, my bowels are sluggish, my feet hurt, my heart jumps — and you know, Doctor, I myself don't feel so well either." (Erikson 1964:51)

It is commonly recognized by clinicians, especially those who practice in ethnically mixed settings, that a patient's culture affects the experience and expression of symptoms. "Old Jews" have a special "way of speaking" that is rooted in a particular history and culture of suffering. The same might be said for Frenchmen, Puerto Ricans in New York City, Down East folks in Maine and other peoples. Members of diverse cultural groups experience and express pain differently. Communication of these experiences may be through somatic, psychological, or interpersonal idioms, with symptoms narrowly limited or encompassing many organ systems. In addition, societies differentially lavish attention on bodily parts — the French on the liver, Iranians on their hearts, others on the stomach or the blood.

Cultural differences in symptom expression are familiar to the clinician and have been verified by years of sociological research. In clinical practice, however, knowledge of such differences often seems to have little practical value. A patient's "medical folklore" may be of intrinsic interest to the anthropologically inclined, and illness attributed to such causes as hexing or witchcraft may require a special therapeutic response. In general, however, cultural or "ethnomedical" information often seems irrelevant to the basic diagnostic and therapeutic tasks of the clinician. Even in psychiatry, where definitions of abnormality are recognized to be culturally conditioned, one often hears a grand rounds case presentation begun with a disclaimer: "I know there are important cultural dimensions to this case, but since I am no specialist in Puerto Rican (native American, Pentecostal, Pakistani, etc.) culture, I will focus here on the psychodynamic (biological, pharmacological) aspects of the case."

The lack of apparent clinical relevance of the cultural patterning of symptoms results from the employment of very narrow biomedical models in clinical practice, models fraught with epistemological and practical difficulties. The dominant mode of clinical reasoning interprets symptoms as "manifestations" (Feinstein 1973) of an underlying biological reality. While it may be recognized that culture can systematically distort this manifestation, it is generally assumed that complaints may be mapped directly onto sensations and pathological processes. The

165

L. Eisenberg and A. Kleinman (eds.), The Relevance of Social Science for Medicine, 165–196.
Copyright © 1980 by D. Reidel Publishing Company.

primary tasks of the clinician, then, are to "decode" the patient's complaints —
"a process of converting observed evidence into names of diseases" (Feinstein
1973:212) — and to carry out "rational treatment" (Kety 1974), based on
knowledge of a causal chain at the biological level. This mode of clinical reasoning narrowly limits the relevance of social and cultural data. If we were to base
this paper on such an approach, we could attempt to provide the clinician with
a "cultural code" for various subcultures that would account for systematic
"distortion" of symptoms and aid the physician in remapping complaints and
symptoms onto appropriate disease entities. In some limited cases, such an
approach might be feasible. However, even though it would bring cultural data
into the diagnostic schema, this model would fail to take into consideration the
degree to which symptoms are grounded in the social and cultural realities of
individual patients. It would also inherit the limitations of the predominant
biomedical understanding of clinical practice. A more fundamental reconceptualization of clinical practice — of clinical models and the process of clinical
judgment — is required if anthropological and sociological insights are to be
introduced into clinical reasoning.

Although more than two decades of sociological research has demonstrated
clearly that patterns of symptoms and care-seeking vary systematically by medical subcultures (e.g., Zola 1966; Zborowski 1952; Mechanic 1972; Lin et al.
1978), alternative models for clinical practice have not been forthcoming.
Sociological research, even when undertaken in clinical settings, has focused on
characteristics of *groups* (ethnic, class, gender, religious, etc.). In order for
findings of such research to be made relevant for practitioners, new clinical
models will have to be developed that seriously face the clinician's imperative —
to interpret symptoms of *individuals* and to make appropriate therapeutic
responses in limited clinical encounters. Scattered throughout the medical
literature are case studies and clinical accounts of difficulties in treating ethnic
patients who believe themselves to be affected by rootwork, hexing, or other
traditional illness causes, each with clinical suggestions for the physician. With
few exceptions, however (e.g., Maduro 1975; Kleinman and Mendelsohn 1978),
these accounts treat such cases as clinical oddities. The basic challenge to an
empiricist model of clinical practice posed by the sociological findings and the
clinical anecdotes has not been adequately faced nor met with a reconceptualization of clinical transactions.

We suggest that *a meaning-centered approach to understanding clinical practice* provides a basis for reconceptualizing clinical transactions and for translating
findings of the social sciences into models that can be used by clinicians and
taught in medical education. Anthropological research on illness and healing
shares a common "clinical" interest with medical research: while seeking general
knowledge, both attend to individual persons, illness episodes or clinical encounters. (In addition, medicine and anthropology share a fascination with the
exotic.) In the past decade, extensive work by medical and psychiatric anthropologists has combined with a new interest in language and symbolic systems to

provide a framework for a meaning-centered medical anthropology. This approach first *recognizes all illness realities to be fundamentally semantic* (B. Good 1977). Whatever the biological correlates or grounds of a disease, sickness becomes a human experience and an object of therapeutic attention as it is made meaningful. Folk illnesses and symptoms of ethnic minorities do not represent the exception or a cultural distortion. *All* illness realities are meaningfully constituted. Explanatory models and networks of meanings, grounded in medical subcultures, are employed in all medical systems to construct and interpret experience. Second, a meaning-centered approach *recognizes all clinical transactions to be fundamentally hermeneutic or interpretive.* All clinicians routinely engage in translating across medical subcultures or systems of medical meanings and interpreting patients' experiences. A healer or physician abstracts from a sufferer's complaints information considered relevant and interprets the complaints as resulting from an underlying pathology. This reality is communicated to the client and becomes the object of therapeutic efforts. Because the patient's symptoms and the identified pathology represent personal and group conceptualizations, not merely biological reality, analysis of therapeutic transactions should focus on the interpretive strategy of the clinician. Thus, in a meaning-centered approach to understanding clinical practice, the cultural or meaningful character of symptoms and the clinical task of understanding and interpreting those symptoms are central issues.

In this paper we will briefly criticize an empiricist model for understanding the relationship between culture and symptoms. We will outline a meaning-centered framework for understanding clinical practice and a cultural model that may be employed by clinicians. Finally, we will describe experiences we have had teaching this model to primary care physicians in a Family Practice residency program.

THE EMPIRICIST MODEL OF THE RELATION OF
CULTURE AND SYMPTOMS

The following case was reported by a Family Practice resident in our Clinical Social Science Seminar. The resident is Chinese-American and was treating a Chinese refugee from Vietnam who complained of "heaviness of her chest." The case raises important questions about the analysis of the meaning of symptoms in clinical practice.

Case I

A 63-year old Chinese woman, a refugee from Vietnam who arrived in the United States in 1975, came to the clinic in April, 1978 complaining of "heaviness in her chest," shortness of breath, dizziness, and back ache. The patient spoke only Chinese and was accompanied by her married daughter, who acted as translator. The chest feelings were reported to be brought on by exertion and relieved by rest. The heaviness had been experienced for more than 10 years, and treatment by unknown medication while in Vietnam was reported to have given relief. The patient had no history of heart attack or high blood pressure. The resident ordered tests for heart disease, and results from a treadmill test reported documented angina: "strongly suggestive for ischemia," "Functional Class II."

Over the following eight months, the resident ordered a number of cardiac medications for the patient. Each led to side effects: short-acting nitroglycerin led to headaches, propanolol to shortness of breath and fatigue, and nitrolpaste to increased chest pain. None relieved the complaints of heaviness of the chest, and compliance was a problem. The only medication that the patient believed helped her was Donnatal®, a drug she had requested because of stomach discomfort and because a friend had used the drug. By January 1979, when the resident joined our Seminar, the patient was being tried on long-acting nitrates, and the resident was feeling thoroughly frustrated. The chart contains references to "angina under poor control," "patient not compliant," and "possible occult CHF."

Several sessions of the Seminar were devoted to cross-cultural studies of health care beliefs, ethnicity and health care, and the cultural patterning of depression. When the resident described the case, readings on depression in Chinese cultures were assigned (e.g., Tseng 1975; Kleinman 1977). These studies indicate that "somatization of psychiatric disorders" is very common among Chinese patients; i.e., somatic complaints are more legitimate than psychological or affective complaints, and the most common idiom for expressing and experiencing distress is somatic. Depression is commonly experienced as an illness of the heart. For example, Kleinman reports:

. . . in Mandarin a common word for depression is *men*. The character for this term is written with the radical which represents the heart (classically and still popularly believed to be the seat of the emotions) inside a radical representing a doorway. Most Chinese somatizers whom I have studied point to their chest when they use this term. They report a physical sensation of pressure on the chest or heart. But when they describe it by using *men* they mean both the physical sensation of something "pressing on" or "depressing into" their chest, as well as its psychological concomitants – e.g. sadness. But they focus on the former as the chief problem. (Kleinman 1977:6)

Following discussion of culture and depression, the resident recorded an interview with the patient on video tape, in which the patient's explanatory model and semantic illness network were elicited.

During the taped interview and a subsequent clinic visit, both in March 1979, the patient described her view of the illness and the experiences she associated with the feelings of heaviness on her chest. She said she has had these feelings for nearly 30 years. She believes they may have been caused by the heavy weights she used to carry across her shoulders when she was young (she demonstrated how the load, carried on a pole, used to weigh her down). She described a history of leaving her home in China and immigrating to Vietnam, then fleeing Vietnam in 1975, each time leaving family and home behind. She said that she still occasionally cries for a nephew who is still in Vietnam. She associated her shortness of breath (she breathes deeply or sighs often during the interviews) with events 30 years ago when she was beaten by her husband and could not breathe. The patient said she does not know how her heart works or what causes the pain. She hypothesized that the pain travels through her leg veins and reaches up into her heart. The patient has two married daughters living in Sacramento, but she maintains her own apartment. At the time of the interview, she was living with one daughter because she felt unable to work around the house.

Following discussion of this interview, the resident began to consider a diagnosis of depression. The patient's appetite is poor, although she continues to eat; she reports dryness of mouth; no change in sleep pattern is reported. In April, the chart notes that "the patient is feeling better. Still has heaviness in chest with activity but states she feels she is improving. Patient will be tried on protriptyline (an anti-depressant medication) since patient may actually be depressed and referring symptoms to heart in a manner that is culturally acceptable in the Orient." The resident introduced the medication to the woman by saying that she "had talked with some doctors who said the drug is especially good for heart problems in Oriental people." The patient was anxious to try the drug. However, in May the patient reported having stopped taking the drug because it exacerbated the dryness of her mouth. The medication was discontinued.

The resident reported feeling much easier about the case. "The major thing is that I've gotten over being frustrated with her." She has continued to prescribe long-acting nitrates, although it does not relieve the symptoms, and she believes the heaviness of chest to be a culturally appropriate expression of depression. She understands the patient's symptoms to have their meaning – in part – in their relationship to experiences and meanings associated by the patient with the symptom. For example, the chart notes from March include the following interpretation of the patient's shortness of breath: "She relates many activities with her SOB – sadness makes the heaviness worse; activity leads to SOB; swallowing sometimes leads to feeling of suffocation. She thinks having been beaten (at that time she could not get her breath) approximately 30 years ago may have led to her current condition." The resident's treatment goals are to continue to monitor the chest pain and to help the woman's family by enabling the patient to live at home. The resident reports that she remembers the videotaped interview as the most important thing she did to understand the woman and her illness.

In this case, focusing attention on the meaning of the patient's symptoms led the resident to a new interpretation of the case. She came increasingly to view the patient's illness as an image or symbol that condensed in a culturally appropriate idiom a series of personal tragedies. This interpretation led the resident to feel less pressure to eliminate the chest sensations and complaints. She stopped trying new cardiac medications and chose not to undertake further invasive diagnostic or therapeutic regimes, which her frustration might have led her to employ. Following discussions with the doctor about her personal history, the patient reported feeling better and was hopeful that she is improving.

The cultural approach to this case suggested two alternatives to the diagnosis of cardiac disease: a culturally patterned depression, or concurrent angina pectoris and depression resulting in chest sensations indistinguishable to the patient. Cardiac medications have failed to eliminate the complaints, and the patient's refusal to follow a course of anti-depressant medication made it impossible to confirm depression pharmacologically. It is possible that further diagnostic tests could differentiate between the two potential diagnoses. In addition to suggesting diagnostic alternatives, the cultural approach revealed the meaning complex that provides the semantic context of this patient's symptoms. Her complaints of heaviness of chest and shortness of breath are grounded in popular Chinese medical culture, in traditional views of the heart, and in modes of expressing distress that the patient shares with members of her subculture. Language of the heart provides the patient a socially appropriate idiom for articulating the losses and personal tragedies suffered in her life and for seeking attention and care.

This case raises important questions about the clinical importance of the meaning of symptoms. What is the relationship between a particular expression of distress, which is grounded in both personal and social contexts of meaning, and physiological disorder? How are patients' understandings of illness – the models used to explain a disorder, life problems associated with the illness, semantic illness networks — to be interpreted by the clinician? In this case, how is the complaint "my chest feels heavy" to be interpreted? Does the symptom reflect a cardiac disease? Does Chinese culture lead the patient to focus on one of the numerous symptoms of the depressive syndrome, to select that symptom as primary and disregard others? Does the set of symptoms represent a unique or culturally specific depressive illness? Do the complaints represent a culturally appropriate means of articulating personal or even intrapsychic suffering? Potential answers to such questions about the meaning and interpretation of symptoms are embedded in particular models of clinical practice.

The predominant theoretical framework in contemporary medicine for the clinical interpretation of symptoms is one that we may label "the empiricist model of clinical reasoning." This model assumes, simply, that symptoms — complaints of distress or behavioral aberrations — are to be interpreted as reflections or manifestations of disordered somatic (biochemical, neurophysiological, etc.) processes. Symptoms achieve their *meaning* in relationship to physiological states, which are interpreted as the referents of the symptoms. Complaints of intolerance of fatty foods reflect an obstruction of the hepatic duct that prevents digestive enzymes from reaching the small intestine; vegetative signs and dysphoric affect are manifestations of neurotransmitter abnormalities. Clinical reasoning, from this perspective, is unabashedly reductionistic. Somatic lesions or dysfunctions produce discomfort and behavioral changes, communicated in a patient's complaints. The critical clinical task of the physician is to "decode" a patient's discourse by relating symptoms to their biological referents in order to diagnose a disease entity. The process of clinical reasoning through which this decoding is achieved is illustrated most clearly by Alvan Feinstein's analysis of clinical judgment:

Each manifestation is attributed to a functional abnormality at a particular site in the body (or in the body as a whole). Each of these abnormalities is then attributed to an underlying abnormality, and the latter abnormality is ultimately ascribed to a particular diagnostic entity....

This sequential search for entities that are "immediate causes," each providing an explanation for its antecedent entity, is the intellectual characteristic that distinguishes diagnostic reasoning. (Feinstein 1973:220)

Diagnostic reasoning in modern medicine is a process of converting observed evidence into the names of diseases. The *evidence* consists of data obtained from examining a patient and substances derived from the patient; the *diseases* are conceptual medical entities that identify or explain abnormalities in the observed evidence. (Feinstein 1973:212)

While the thoughtful clinician would not claim that the "functional abnormality" is the only meaning of the "manifestation" or symptom, the primary interpretive strategy of diagnostic reasoning is to search for somatic referents of a patient's discourse.

What we have called the empiricist model of clinical reasoning is grounded epistemologically in what Harrison has called "the empiricist theory of language" (1972). This theory holds that meaning attaches to basic utterances in a language through a conventional association between a "language element" and a given "world element" (Harrison 1972:33; cf. B. Good 1977). The meaning of a statement — such as a patient's complaint or a proposition in a medical theory — depends first, then, upon "how the world is, as a matter of empirical fact, constituted" (Harrison 1972:33). Statements are meaningful if they accurately reflect empirical reality. Viewed in this framework, the ideal form of medical discourse is that which is "transparent" to biological reality, that which can be mapped onto an underlying reality in a one-to-one fashion. The "order of words" has meaning as it reflects and reveals the "order of things," and the two together constitute a two dimensional reality (see Foucault 1970; cf. White 1973).

In clinical practice, the mode of medical discourse or symptom expression often considered paradigmatic is that which clearly reveals pathological processes and disease entities. Every clinician recognizes, however, that complaints of many patients relate to somatic reality indirectly, obscuring disease processes for the diagnostician. Some patients express symptoms that have "no meaning": they reflect no somatic disorder. After ruling out all possible physiological meanings of a symptom, the clinician is forced to interpret symptoms as arising independently in the behavioral sphere or as having a psychological meaning. A second kind of skewing of the relationship between complaints and biological processes is represented by the cultural patterning of symptoms, the systematic "distortion" of symptoms resulting from the cultural "biases" of the patient. Because the patient's expression of symptoms may not accurately reveal somatic reality, the ideal of some in the biomedical community is a clinical practice that does not depend on a patient's discourse: ". . . the quest of modern clinical science is for precise pathognomonic tests that can accurately identify the presence of a disease, regardless of the associated symptoms" (Feinstein 1973:230).

The reductionism of biomedicine and the quest for a clinical science that is essentially independent of a patient's discourse have been sharply criticized (e.g., Eisenberg 1977; 1979; Engel 1977; Fabrega 1972; Kleinman 1978; Kleinman et al. 1978; and Klerman 1977). Some have argued that exclusive attention to the physiological is leading to the impoverishment of the caring function of medicine. Some have called for a fundamental reconceptualization of the relationship between the order of medical words and the order of medical things as the basis for a reformulation of biomedical theory and clinical reasoning in contemporary medicine. George Engel, for example, recently criticized the biomedical model for its failure to conceptualize adequately the "relationship between particular biochemical processes and the clinical data of illness" (Engel 1977:132).

It serves little to be able to specify a biochemical defect in schizophrenia if one does not know how to relate this to particular psychological and behavioral expressions of the disorder. The biomedical model gives insufficient heed to this requirement. Instead it encourages bypassing the patient's verbal account by placing greater reliance on technical procedures and laboratory measurements. In actuality the task is appreciably more complex than the biomedical model encourages one to believe. (Engel 1977:132)

Psychological, social and cultural factors strongly influence the way a particular biochemical condition will be experienced by an individual and manifested clinically. Bypassing verbal data to increase precision results in a basic failure to provide care, which has important implications for outcomes and patient satisfaction. Interpretation of patients' complaints as though they directly reflect biological processes ignores a growing body of evidence of cultural patterning of symptoms.

Several traditions of research indicate the complexity of the relationship between disease processes and clinical data. First, sociologists have demonstrated the validity of physicians' observations that patients of different ethnic or cultural backgrounds vary systematically in their clinical behavior. The classic studies in this tradition were carried out in Boston and New York in 1950's and 1960's, contrasting clinical behavior of Irish, Italian, Jewish and Old American or Yankee patients. Later studies, utilizing similar methods, were carried out with immigrants and ethnic groups in Australia (Pilowsky and Spence 1976; Minc 1963) and Israel (Antonovsky 1972). In his seminal studies in New York City, Zborowski (1952, 1969) showed that patients vary systematically in pain-related behavior – in their expression of pain, their complaints in various settings, their concerns about the meaning of pain, and their response to particular therapeutic strategies (cf. Fabrega 1976). Zola's studies in the outpatient clinics of Massachusetts General Hospital demonstrated a similar pattern in other aspects of clinical behavior. These studies, along with comparable studies by Mechanic (1963), Twaddle (1969) and Croog (1961), confirm hypotheses that clinical behavior varies systematically and suggest some of the dimensions of that variation. Groups vary in *the specificity of their medical complaints*; for example, first generation Italians tended to present diverse medical complaints, related to various organ systems, while Irish patients presented far fewer and more limited symptoms. Groups vary in their *style of medical complaining in various medical contexts*. For example, in clinical settings, Jewish and Italian patients alike were observed to openly and dramatically express their suffering, the Irish to deny symptoms, and Old American patients to suffer quietly and to try to view their pain as detached observers. The groups also vary *in the nature of their anxiety about the meaning of symptoms*. Protestants seemed most concerned about symptoms that are incapacitating (Twaddle 1969); Jews were most concerned about the potential implications of symptoms as indicating serious disease; and Italians were most concerned with pain itself. The research provided some indications that groups vary in their *focus on particular organ systems*. For example, Irish patients complained more of eye, ear, nose and throat symptoms than Italian patients in ambulatory care. And finally, the groups varied in their *response to therapeutic strategies*, such as reassurance or drug treatment of pain, depending on the meaning they attributed to their suffering.

Taken together with other research by medical sociologists, these studies show that the medical culture of patients and their families — their medical understandings, theories and values — affect their evaluation, experience and mode of expressing symptoms (Mechanic 1972), their pattern of care-seeking (Chrisman 1977; Lin et al. 1978; Mechanic 1978), and their evaluation of therapeutic treatment of their suffering. Given a certain disease or pain stimulant, culture affects the way an individual attends to the diverse sensations and transforms them into medical complaints. The most critical and problematic variables seem to be the meaning a symptom has for the patient and the idiom or language in which distress is experienced and communicated.

The sociological literature might be interpreted to imply that in different cultural or ethnic groups, the same disease will be represented by different symptoms. Given the same set of body sensations, members of different cultural groups will selectively attend to, complain about and seek professional help for some symptoms and not others. For example, university students are likely to consider tiredness as not only normal but normative, whereas a laborer or housewife may be more likely to consider tiredness a sign of ill health. The anthropological and cross-cultural psychiatric literature suggests that the relativity of human illness may be more profound than this, especially for psychiatric diseases. For example, studies of depression across societies show that guilt feelings, self-recrimination and depressive affect are absent in some societies (Marsella 1978). The existence of somatic symptoms associated with vegetative signs in such societies has led some theorists to proclaim depressive disease universal and invariant (Singer 1975). Others, however, have concluded that it makes little sense to apply a Western disease label to syndromes that are experienced and expressed so differently. Marsella, for example, argues that depression is a disorder associated with

cultures which tend to 'psychologize' experience. In these instances, experiential states become labeled and interpreted psychologically and this adds the components of depressed mood, guilt, self-depreciation, and suicidal ideation. At this level, the experience of depression assumes a meaning which is clearly different from that associated with purely somatic experience of the problem. (Marsella 1978:350) We must cease the labeling of individuals as depressed if they do not share common expressions and experiences of the problem. (Marsella 1978:351)

Whatever the biological substrata of disease, if disorders vary profoundly in their psychodynamics (e.g., Opler and Singer 1956; Levy 1973), their phenomenological and behavioral expression (e.g., Reynolds 1976; Carr 1978; Rin, Schooler and Caudill 1973), and their severity and duration (Waxler 1979), the assumption that cultural variation is essentially epiphenomenal is unwarranted and ethnocentric. This does not imply that psychiatric disease is not universal or that there are not commonalities across cultures, but it suggests fundamental difficulties with the "two-dimensional" model of the relationship of culture and disease. Such conceptual problems are not limited to exotic culture-bound syndromes, but are inherent in the study of the most common and difficult problems in primary care, such as hypochondriasis, somatization, the atypical and masked depressions, and chronic pain.

How can such research findings be translated into models that are applicable by the clinician to individual patients? One could incorporate cultural data into the basic empiricist paradigm. If the same disease is represented by different manifestations in various cultural groups, the social scientist might try to provide a "cultural code" for remapping symptoms onto appropriate disease entities. Heaviness of heart and somatic symptoms translate as depression among Chinese patients. Complaints of pain in many organ systems should not be interpreted as hypochondriacal among Italian patients. This approach faces serious problems. The research findings represent characteristics of groups — groups whose "distinctiveness" is "diminishing" generation by generation (Greenblum 1974) — and such data does not translate easily into clinical models. Medical students or residents can be taught some of the most common ethnomedical traditions, folk illnesses, and culturally specific symptom forms; but employed within the empiricist clinical framework, such data is applicable in only a few limited cases where culture seriously "distorts" symptoms. If the failure of clinicians to systematically attend to the cultural data present in *all* cases is to be overcome, if understanding the meaning that an illness or symptom has for each individual patient is to be made an explicit and relevant task of clinical care, a more basic reconceptualization of clinical practice is necessary.

TOWARD A MEANING-CENTERED APPROACH TO CLINICAL PRACTICE

... there is no societal reality, with all its concrete forces, that does not bring itself to representation in a consciousness that is linguistically articulated. Reality does not happen "behind the back" of language; it happens rather behind the backs of those who live in the subjective opinion that they have understood "the world" ... ; that is, reality happens precisely within language. (Gadamer 1976:35)

Recent work in the social sciences has provided the basis for what we might call a "meaning-centered approach to medical anthropology". The regular appearance of such terms as meaning, discourse, interpretation, translation, semantics, and the social construction of reality all indicate a new understanding of culture as configurations of meanings and discourse in terms of which human reality is constituted.[2] An interpretive social science involves conscious translation across meaning systems to arrive at understanding of the realities of others. A meaning-centered or interpretive medical anthropology approaches sickness not as a reflection or causal product of somatic processes but as a meaningful human reality. It views healing as transactions across meaning systems — popular, religious, folk, professional — that result in the construction of culturally specific illness realities and as therapeutic efforts to transform those realities. Critical research issues in medical anthropology, as in clinical medicine and psychosomatics, revolve around the relationship between meaningful and somatic aspects of sickness and healing. Those complex relationships can be analyzed appropriately, however, only if prior attention is given to conceptualizing and studying the meaningful experiential aspects of illness and healing. It is our contention that a meaning-centered understanding of health care and healing can provide an alternative to the empiricist understanding of clinical data, and that from such a perspective we can generate alternative models for clinical practice. We will briefly outline the theoretical background for such an approach, then describe a cultural model that may be employed by the clinician.

The development of a clinical approach that makes social and cultural aspects of a patient's life relevant to the clinician must, it seems to us, be based on a two-fold recognition that *human illness is fundamentally semantic or meaningful* and that *all clinical practice is inherently interpretive or "hermeneutic"*. First, while all disease has biological or psychological correlates or causes, sickness becomes a human experience only as it is apprehended, interpreted, evaluated and communicated — that is, as it enters the world of human meaning and discourse. Illness is constructed from popular medical culture, as the sufferer draws upon available theories and networks of meaning to interpret, reinterpret and communicate a particular experience. Illness, as a personal and social reality, and therapeutics directed toward treatment of that reality are inextricably bound to the medium of language and signification.

Illness realities are grounded in the conceptualizations of distinct and complex medical subcultures. For example, professional medicine includes the very different worlds of the cancer ward, the emergency room, the psychiatric hospital and the office of the rural family physician. Popular medical subcultures are even more diverse: traditional ethnic traditions of healing, often rooted in antiquity; Christian spiritualism and faith healing; the recent middleclass holistic health subculture, including health optimizers, natural foods groups, natural birthing movements, and new psychotherapies; and many other coherent medical subgroups in American society. Each medical subculture provides distinctive interpretations of human suffering and healing. Each provides explanatory models of illness, models of human physiology and personality, and forms of therapies, and each is grounded in a particular cosmology, epistemology and set of values. Clinicians routinely treat patients whose understanding and experience of illness are rooted in medical subcultures that have little in common with their own.

Any illness may be conceived as a coherent syndrome of meaning and experience that is linked to a society's deep semantic and value structure. The empiricist model understands a "syndrome" as "a concurrence or running together of constant patterns of abnormal signs and symptoms" that reflect a particular somatic dysfunction (Durham, quoted by Feinstein 1973:272). Symptoms are thus integrated or related to one another in a physico-functional manner. A meaning-centered approach views any illness as a concurrence or running together of configurations of meanings and experiences (B. Good 1977). Freud understood that a psychiatric symptom or dream symbol condenses a network of conscious and unconscious meanings, and that the most powerful symbols are those that are the most dense or "polysemic" and are linked to the most powerful affects. Similarly, an illness or a symptom condenses a network of meanings for the sufferer: personal trauma, life stresses, fears and expectations about the illness, social reactions of friends and authorities, and therapeutic experiences. The meaning of illness for an individual is grounded in – though not reducible to – the network of meanings an illness has in a particular culture: the metaphors associated with a disease, the ethnomedical theories, the basic values and conceptual forms, and the care patterns that shape the experience of the illness and the social reactions to the sufferer in a given society (B. Good 1977; Sontag 1977). In any episode of major illness, deep personal meanings are grounded in networks of signification and linked to basic values of a society or subculture. It is not our argument that disease is not biological or that meanings of illness and symptoms are independent of physiological conditions. An illness reality, however, is not a simple reflection of disease processes: the relationship between disease and culture is "three-dimensional" rather than two, and the integration of an illness syndrome is semantic or logico-meaningful.

Each illness reality in a society is constituted as a unique semantic network: it condenses a unique configuration of meanings. We would expect each illness – cancer, lower back pain, schizophrenia, *susto* in Mexico, spirit possession in Puerto Rico – to be associated with a typical set of personal stresses and social responses, to have specific links to basic social values of worth and well-being, and to provide a framework for individual episodes of illness. Two examples will illustrate. In American society, obesity or fatness is a cultural reality that condenses a specific configuration of meanings and experiences associated with large body size: the shame of being a fat (slow, ugly) kid in gym class; embarrassment in dating situations or when buying clothes; implications of low status or social class; repeated failure in attempts to lose weight and curb appetites; fat clinics and weight watchers; and social condemnation for lack of self control (MacKenzie 1979). Large body size has come to signify loss of self-control and lack of competence, the central virtues of the Protestant ethic. These meanings are condensed in the powerful image of obesity in American society. Such meanings cut across differences in theoretical frameworks and explanatory models of nutritionists, behavior modifiers, joggers, family physicians and the public. They invade discourse in a variety of contexts. And they link together social meanings and values with personal experiences and self-consciousness. Together they constitute a syndrome that is unique to American culture.

A second example is provided by our work in Iran. When Iranians experience the physical sensation of heart palpitations, often when they are upset or mildly depressed, they complain that their hearts are in distress and often seek relief from a physician. While notions of the heart as an organ of emotion are grounded in classical Islamic and Greek medicine, heart distress is given significance by a unique network of meanings in Iranian culture (B. Good 1977; M. Good 1980). The sensation of heart palpitations is treated as a symptom or an illness syndrome associated with several clusters of stresses and symbolized values in

Iranian culture: those associated with the issue of female sexuality, the status of women, and the religious pollution attributed to childbirth, menstruation and bleeding; those associated with grief, loss and old age; and the experiences of family conflict, anxiety and worry. This cultural configuration transforms a physical sensation into a form of experience; the symptom can only be interpreted within a personal and social context of meaning. For the individual sufferer, personal meaning is joined with social signification to form a unique illness reality.

For the physician as well as the anthropologist, the semantic structures of various illnesses have great importance. They provide the framework from which the interpretation of the symptoms of individual patients must begin. We have hardly begun to analyze the meaning of most illnesses in our society, despite their symbolic potency, or to investigate the implications of our discourse for therapeutic outcomes. Such research provides an important challenge to medical anthropology.

It follows from the recognition that all illness is an essentially meaningful phenomenon that all clinical practice is fundamentally interpretive or "hermeneutic."[3] The clinician's task is hermeneutic not only because he or she interprets a patient's condition, drawing upon a particular medical model, but also because the data interpreted – the patient's expression of illness symptoms – are themselves subjective and meaningful. The clinician is thus constantly engaged in translating across systems of meaning, in particular, translating between professional biomedical models and popular or folk models of illness.

In any clinical encounter the physician employs a particular medical model to identify certain data as relevant, to abstract from the complex totality of the sick patient, to interpret the abstracted data, and to construct a clinical reality that becomes the object of therapeutic endeavor. Any physician and any medical discipline has a repertoire of interpretive models – biochemical, immunological, viral, genetic, environmental, psychodynamic, family interactionist, pharmacological, and others. Each model has its own "structure of relevance" (Schutz 1970): it makes relevant certain data or certain aspects of reality ignored or left unanalyzed by other models. Each model employs particular "interpretive strategies" for constituting the meaning of the abstracted data, be they the patient's complaints or laboratory findings. And any clinical model posits certain pathological entities or conditions that become the focus of therapy. The utilization of interpretive models for the treatment of individual patients is a basic characteristic of all clinical practice, whether the clinician is an internist, psychiatrist, spiritualist healer, Chinese shaman or Iranian prayer writer.

An important part of the data interpreted by the clinician consists of reports by patients of their experiences of sickness. The patient's experience does not reflect simply underlying biochemical or psychophysiological processes. Consciousness of suffering is meaningful; all symptoms have personal significance and are inherently "culturally patterned." Thus the clinician is not merely engaged in the interpretation of objective data; all clinical practice involves the understanding and translation of subjective realities.

From a meaning-centered view of health care transactions, all clinical discourse involves *mutual* interpretations or translations across systems of meaning — across medical models and idioms, across perspectives, and across medical subcultures. The therapist interprets the intentions and the contexts of the patient's discourse in order to identify and construct a pathological entity. The patient interprets the therapist's discourse to construct new understandings of the illness. This mutual process of understanding and interpretation is a basic element in effective healing. Evidence suggests that whatever the pharmacological or physiological effect of "rational (biomedical) treatment" (Kety 1974), the therapist's ability to influence the patient's reality, to combat demoralization and construct new realities, is a powerful healing force (Frank 1974; Kleinman and Sung 1979). Clinical models are thus "models of" reality, mirroring or making sense of observed phenomena; at the same time they are "models for" reality, influencing perception and behavior, shaping the course of illness and the evaluation of medical outcomes, and producing the realities they posit (cf. Geertz 1973:93).

A meaning-centered analysis of clinical practice suggests both long-range and more modest goals for the social scientist in clinical settings. It is important that anthropologists and sociologists participate with medical researchers in the construction of "a new medical model," which expands the range of antecedent conditions believed to cause disease, which incorporates multifactorial views of causation, and which more profoundly conceptualizes the relationship between culture and disease (Klerman 1977; Engel 1977). However, an all-inclusive model that would mirror all aspects of sickness would not necessarily be clinically valuable, even were it theoretically possible. The more modest goal of the clinical social scientist should be to develop specific and limited clinical models to add to a clinician's repertoire. Such models should specify the data considered relevant, procedures for elicitation of that data, interpretive strategies for understanding the data, and the therapeutic uses of the model. The following paragraphs outline briefly a cultural hermeneutic model developed to be used by clinicians, contrasting it with biomedical models commonly employed in clinical practice.

A Cultural Hermeneutic Model of Clinical Practice

The cultural hermeneutic model provides the clinician with a model of a patient's illness as a syndrome of meaning. As a clinical model, its purpose is to enable the physician to elicit and analyze the meaning illness has for a patient and to consciously and successfully translate across medical subcultures. Unlike the biomedical model, which conceives disease as a biochemical or physiological abnormality, the cultural hermeneutic model conceives illness as a meaningful experience of an individual. Thus while the data made relevant by biomedical models are clinical data that reflect underlying physiological disorder, the primary data made relevant by the cultural model are those that yield special insight into the semantics of sickness. (See Figure 1 for an outline contrasting the biomedical and cultural hermeneutic models.)

Characteristics of the biomedical (empiricist) clinical model	Characteristics of the cultural (hermeneutic) clinical model
Pathological entity: Somatic or psychophysiological lesion or dysfunction.	Meaningful construct, illness reality of the sufferer.
Structure of relevance: Relevant data those that reveal somatic disorder.	Relevant data those that reveal meaning of illness.
Elicitation procedures: Review of systems, laboratory tests.	Evaluate explanatory models, decode semantic network.
Interpretive goal: Diagnosis and explanation (*Erklären*)	Understanding (*Verstehen*)
Interpretive strategy: Dialectically explore relationship between symptoms and somatic disorder	Dialectically explore relationship between symptoms (text) and semantic network (context).
Therapeutic goal: Intervene in somatic disease process.	To treat patient's experience: to bring to understanding hidden aspects of illness reality and to transform that reality.

Fig. 1. Comparison of the biomedical and cultural hermeneutic models of clinical practice.

The primary technique of elicitation of clinical data in the biomedical model is the review of systems, followed by lab work. Elicitation techniques in the hermeneutic model include investigation of a patient's explanatory model and the "decoding" of a patient's semantic illness network. First, the physician can elicit a patient's model of the onset, etiology, pathophysiology, course and appropriate treatment for an illness (see Kleinman et al. 1978 for a more detailed account). Explanatory models are often drawn from folk or professional therapeutic traditions or from popular medical subcultures. Quite often, however, individuals develop personal and highly idiosyncratic models of their illness. Second, the clinician can explore the semantic illness network of the patient. An illness or symptom, conceived as a syndrome of meaning, condenses a network of significant experiences and symbols that the clinician must elicit in order to understand the context of the patient's behavior. Focusing on those experiences that are potent and affect-laden for the patient, rather than those of particular biomedical significance, will help the physician understand the structure of the patient's reality. As such experiences are elicited, they are likely to be found to cluster together and be linked to important values of the patient's subculture or to powerful conscious or unconscious affects of the sufferer. Several such clusters of seemingly diverse phenomena may be condensed by a single illness or symptom, and these clusters related to each other through a network of cross-cutting meanings. Elicitation of the semantic illness network should focus both on the group conceptualizations and values and the deep personal meanings associated with the illness or symptom. No simple set of questions can be specified to elicit elements of the patient's semantic illness network. The following kinds of questions, however, may be useful: When this problem began, what other things were happening in your life? How do you think those are related to your problem? What previous experiences have you had with this illness? What problems in your life have been caused by your illness? What have you had to give up because of it? Do you know others who have had this condition? What problems did it cause for them? How serious do you think your illness will become in the future? What are the most difficult or important experiences that you associate with this problem? Are such experiences especially important for you, for your family (church, social group, ethnic group)? What do other people think about your having this problem? How do they react to you? How do you feel about their reactions? Responses to questions such as these may be interpreted by the clinician to construct the patient's semantic network, the interrelated cluster of meanings and experiences that provide the semantic context for the patient's illness. While analysis of the patient's semantic network may be useful in longer therapeutic sessions, it is important that the clinician integrate such questions into history-taking and routine clinical activities, rather than approach these issues only after tests reveal negative findings for a patient's symptoms.

According to the interpretive strategy of biomedical or pathological models, symptoms should be understood as reflecting underlying physiological or psycho-physiological processes and should be interpreted reductionistically to deduce disease processes. Ultimately, the interpretive task is diagnosis and explanation, the determination of a disease entity that provides a causal explanation of clinical phenomena. By contrast, the interpretive goal of the cultural hermeneutic model is *understanding*.[4] Symptoms are viewed as an expression of the sufferer's reality and as linked to associated stresses and experiences that constitute the personal meaning of the illness. The interpretive task is to understand the meaning of the symptoms and the illness for the sufferer. As in classical hermeneutics, this involves moving dialectically from the part (the "text", the symptom) to the whole (the "context", the illness network) and back again, to bring to under-standing the illness from the sufferer's perspective. The cultural model makes certain causal assumptions — that behavior is, at least in part, rationally moti-vated and that behaviors (symptom expression, noncompliance, etc.) result from beliefs and meanings — and may help "explain" seemingly strange behavior. The hermeneutic mode of "explanation" consists of making the behavior understandable by establishing its meaningful context. Explanation is meaningful rather than mechanistic in form.

The therapeutic goal of the biomedical model is to intervene in the disease process, based on an understanding of its causality. The therapeutic goal of the cultural model is to bring to understanding hidden aspects of the illness reality and to transform that reality, reformulating the patient's self-understanding. The cure of disease without a concomitant healing of illness — that is, a transformation of the patient's sense of ill health as a basic reality — has been a major failure of contemporary medicine (Eisenberg 1977, 1979). The cultural model focuses attention on the patient's experience as an outcome of treatment.

It should be obvious that what we have called the cultural hermeneutic model is not intended to replace the biomedical model. It is useful, however, for dealing with precisely those problems most poorly managed using the traditional pathology models. It provides a valuable clinical approach, first, for determining what issues are of most concern to the patient, what lies behind a patient's seeking help at a particular time, why an illness crisis arises when it does, what problems are associated with an illness for a patient. Second, the model provides a method for "patient education," now understood as translation across models, and for exploring problems of "compliance," i.e., for understanding the rationality of a patient's behavior. Third, the model provides an approach to negotiation of therapeutic alliances and to cognitive aspects of healing.

In the final section of this paper we describe our experience using this model in a teaching setting.

EXPERIENCES WITH THE CULTURAL HERMENEUTIC MODEL: CASES FROM A RESIDENCY TRAINING PROGRAM

The clinical cases discussed below were originally presented in a clinical social science seminar the authors teach for Family Practice residents three hours per week for rotations of three months. The seminar's focus is on the social and cultural aspects of illness encountered in an urban primary care clinic that serves diverse ethnic and social class populations. The seminar — a kind of "cultural Balint group"[5] — combines clinical case discussions with analysis, didactic readings and lectures. It provides the context for teaching, consultation and research — for developing new clinical models and evaluating their efficacy in managing routine as well as particularly difficult clinical cases.

The two basic premises of the seminar are (1) that the medical model is limited in its effectiveness for managing the vast majority of problems encountered in primary care practices (Good et al. 1979), and (2) that translation between popular and professional medical subcultures is a major function of the family physician. Throughout the seminar (and in a concurrent group process seminar conducted by a clinical psychologist), residents are encouraged to integrate alternative models, which emphasize psychosocial and cultural aspects of illness and care, with the medical model in their day-to-day clinical practice. The purpose of this effort is to develop residents' awareness of non-somatic factors in the illness experience and thus to increase their consideration of new types of data that are frequently not elicited or are dismissed as irrelevant in clinical practice.

Several clinical techniques are taught to the residents to increase their ability to elicit and analyze the meaning illness has for a patient. While some didactic training is given in the content of popular or ethnic medical traditions, the primary model of teaching is "process" oriented. During a meeting of the seminar, residents are introduced to a clinical skill and may role-play a clinical encounter. They are then asked to use the technique with patients during the following week, to video-tape an interview, and to bring back accounts or video-tapes to the seminar for discussion. Learning is most successful when a particular clinical technique helps a resident solve a problem with a patient. The most difficult aspect of teaching is to bring residents to break established clinical patterns and actually try out alternative modes of elicitation, clinical judgment or therapeutics.

Residents are first taught to distinguish "disease" and "illness", to diagnose and record illness problems (e.g., family problems secondary to physical or psychosocial impairment of a member, acute life crises, chronic maladaptive behavior patterns, abuse of sick role, conflicts in negotiating illness labels, etc.), and to develop treatment plans for managing such problems (Kleinman et al. 1978; Kleinman 1979). Second, residents are encouraged to elicit "patient requests" (requests to have a feared condition ruled out, troubling symptoms explained, a specific medication or test given, an illness legitimized, or a referral made) and "negotiate" a satisfactory response to such requests (Lazare et al. 1975). Third, residents are taught to elicit the "explanatory models" of patients and their families, analyze conflicts between biomedical and popular models, and negotiate acceptable alternatives if a patient's model is producing maladaptive behavior (Kleinman et al. 1978). Fourth, residents are taught to elicit and "decode" patients' semantic networks, to uncover the personal and evaluative meanings that provide the context for the patient's experience (Good 1977). Through utilization of each of these clinical tools, residents are taught to become conscious of their role as *translators across medical subcultures*. Although general knowledge of the range of alternative medical traditions is useful, the physician need not have explicit and detailed information about a patient's medical subculture in order to use the cultural hermeneutic approach in clinical practice. Residents are encouraged to integrate a few questions from this approach into routine clinical practice, to make fuller use of the approach for cases in which cultural and psychological factors seem prominent, and to ask for a cultural consult for particularly puzzling cases.

The following cases were presented in the seminar and illustrate issues discussed in this paper.

Case II

Mr. T. is a 28 year old black male, employed in the maintenance department of a large firm, who came to the clinic several times for treatment of a lower back injury sustained at work. When first seen at the clinic, he was diagnosed as having paravertebral lumbar muscle spasm/strain, treated in the office with Fluori-Methane Spray and Stretch®, prescribed hot baths, Williams exercises, and anti-spasmodic medication, and educated in proper lifting habits.

A short time later he reinjured his back at work. He blamed his foreman for treating him as a malingerer and not assigning him lighter work until his back healed. He was sent to the company doctor and then visited the clinic again, each time complaining of continued back pains and seeking a medical order to reduce his work load. Mr. T.'s physician, a resident in our seminar, feared his problem would become chronic and asked us to do a consultation.

In our interview with Mr. T., he revealed a very clear explanatory model of his back problem. He believed that when he was first injured, a muscle in his lower back had been stretched — "like a rubber band that is stretched too far and loses its elasticity". Healing would occur, he believed, when the muscle was allowed to rest and regain its former strength and elasticity. The physician had ordered him to do various stretching exercises, but he admitted doing very few of them. "I don't understand it. The doctor says I should be doing stretches, but it is that stretching that caused the problem and that's what I am trying to avoid."

When asked what he believed might be the underlying cause of his back problem, Mr. T. said that he had been having some difficulties in his life that he thought might be related. He was having financial problems, his mother was ill, and for the past six weeks he had been having difficulties with his girlfriend. These indirectly caused his back pain, he believed, by preventing him from eating and sleeping well and generally weakening or "zupping" his physical condition.

Immediately following the consultation, the physician (who had not seen the interview) met with Mr. T. He briefly discussed the progress of his back pain, suggested that he continue with the stretching exercises, and prepared to give him a "spray and stretch" treatment to relax the muscle spasm. Mr. T. then offered the physician his model of why stretching should be avoided. The physician countered with a clear model of a muscle spasm. "It is like a charlie-horse. What do you do for a charlie-horse? You slowly stretch it out. You should do the stretching exercises only to the point of pain to stretch out the cramped muscle." Mr. T. was dubious but agreed to try.

The physician then asked rhetorically, "Is there anything else?", expecting that the interview was concluded. Mr. T., having rehearsed his problems for us, briefly outlined his life difficulties and asked if they might be related. The physician went through his problems with care. The financial problems were manageable, they agreed. The doctor assured him his mother's medical problems were not too severe. They then explored together the problems he was having with his girl friend. The physician agreed that these difficulties could be prolonging the back pains, suggesting: "Your body may be trying to tell you something." He supported the patient's inclination to break off the difficult relationship and urged him to come to some decision before he returned in two weeks.

Two weeks later Mr. T. missed his scheduled appointment. The physician feared the illness was unresolved and that the patient might be seeking care elsewhere. A few days later, however, he met the patient by accident. Mr. T. assured the doctor that his back was much improved, though not totally free of pain, and was no longer bothering him significantly. He also reported with relief that he had resolved his problem with his girlfriend.

The cultural model clarifies several aspects of this case. First, the illness reality as perceived by Mr. T. was a back pain caused by a stretched muscle. He interpreted his pain in these terms, noting that whenever he bent forward or sideways,

directions that stretched his back, it caused him pain. And he acted on the
basis of that perception, refusing to carry out the stretching exercises ordered
by the physician because they seemed irrational in terms of his explanatory
model. The physician was treating a quite different reality (a muscle spasm). He
assumed that the patient understood the problem as he did, and that failure to
comply with the medical regime indicated resistance to treatment. Even when
Mr. T. described his perception clearly, prompted by his interview with us, the
physician rejected the patient's model and again — even more clearly — stated
his own. Because of the conflict between explanatory models, the patient remained unpersuaded and unwilling to comply with the treatment regime.

Second, the patient understood the meaning of his back pain in terms of a
network of associated stressful experiences. The patient's personal semantic
illness network was embedded in a broader set of meanings associated with back
pain in American medicine (see Figure 2). For patients and physicians alike,

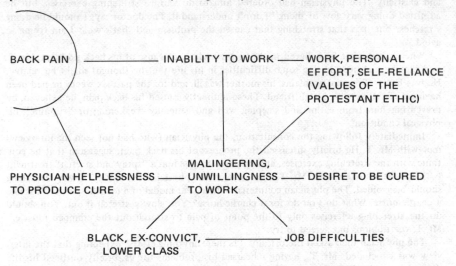

Fig. 2.   Partial semantic network of back pain in American medicine.

lower back pain is often frustrating and difficult to manage. The patient is often
partially incapacitated and unable to work; and because the cause of the pain is
often difficult to document and the physician helpless to produce a cure, the
back pain patient is often suspected of malingering and hypochondriasis. In a
society in which work, self-reliance, will power and personal effort are central
values associated with the Protestant ethic (Hsu 1972), an inability to work
because of pain, especially pain of undocumented origin, evokes mistrust, anger
and negative sanctions. This is even more likely if the patient is lower class,
black, or an ex-convict. This semantic network, specific to back pain in American
society, provided the context for social responses to Mr. T. and invaded the
clinical transactions between him and the therapists. Mr. T. came to his present

job nearly a year ago while on probation. His supervisor was unhappy with his appointment and tried to have him fired. Mr. T. feared that loss of his job might jeopardize his parole. In this context, his symptom — "I hurt my back and I cannot bend or lift" — would certainly reopen this conflict with his supervisor. While Mr. T. could request a lightened work load because of the job-related injury, the foreman could use this as an example of poor work and threaten Mr. T.'s tenuous position. Mr. T, sought to legitimize his condition by consulting a physician. When the doctor hesitated to "reward" his back pain and Mr. T., in response, sought further consultations, the physician began to suspect he was malingering and trying to manipulate the medical system. It was at this juncture that a consultation was requested.

Mr. T. also experienced his back pain as directly associated with problems he was having in his primary relationships — with his mother and his girlfriend. These problems, he believed, led to loss of sleep and appetite and a general loss of energy. His mother's ill health reminded him that she might die, and he hinted at unfinished business with her ("she always told me I had a black heart, and that was before black was beautiful . . ."). He felt conflicted about his relationship with his girlfriend — angry about her unacceptable behavior, guilty about the way he began the relationship, anxious to end the relationship but not to hurt her. In these two relationships, as in his problems at work, Mr. T. hinted that he was unable to express his affects or had to control them with great care.

For Mr. T., all these problems were a significant part of the meaning of his back problem. His illness experience was organized along a network of everyday meanings and interactions that linked his sickness with the basic stresses that were part of his life. The physician's most significant treatment was to bring hidden aspects of that network to understanding and to support Mr. T. in his decision to make significant changes in his life. "Decoding" the meaning of the symptom led not to its physiological correlate but to its social and meaningful grounding. This case suggests not only that a physician needs to elicit the web of personal, family and cultural meanings in terms of which illness is evaluated and experienced. It also suggests that teaching patients to confront their own networks of illness meanings is a basic clinical task. For Mr. T., the consultation and the physician's treatment brought to consciousness a part of the personal and semantic context in which the symptom was grounded. Unlike the stretching exercises, understanding these issues and working out changes in a significant relationship led to healing for the patient.

The resident made mistakes in this case, in particular in failing to recognize the patient's explanatory model. However, he successfully elicited and treated the problem most critical to the patient and was rewarded with a successful outcome. In the seminar, the tape of this interview has been used to demonstrate the problems resulting from discrepant explanatory models, the semantic network that provides the symptom with meaning, and the therapeutic value of eliciting and treating the patient's subjective illness reality.

The next case was presented to the seminar for discussion by one of the Family Practice residents. The case illustrated for the seminar the need for the physician to translate among the biomedical model, a folk illness model drawn from popular Mexican-American culture, and a popularized biomedical model. At the same time, it illustrated that folk illnesses, just as biomedical diseases, may condense meanings and experiences for the patient that are hidden from the physician.

Case III

While on call the previous evening, the resident received an emergency page from the hospital operator, who reported that Mrs. A. had called for a physician, convinced that it meant "life or death for my baby." The resident returned Mrs. A.'s call and found her hysterically exclaiming, "my baby is going to die." She responded to the resident's questions, saying that the "soft spot" on top of her two month old child's skull had collapsed and become depressed. The baby had been cranky and spitting up when a friend (a traditional Mexican woman), who was visiting Mrs. A., noticed the depressed fontanel and warned Mrs. A. that the collapse of the soft spot was an omen of impending death. Mrs. A. interpreted this to mean that "there is an abnormal connection between the brain and the skull" and that "the brain will be contaminated." On further inquiry, the resident discovered that the baby was being treated at that moment by Mrs. A.'s friend for "fallen fontanel". The friend was pressing upward on the baby's soft palate, and was rubbing alcohol on the palate and on the top of the infant's skull, to force the fontanel back into position.

After inquiring about the child's vital signs and hearing no cause for alarm, the resident attempted to calm Mrs. A.'s fears, to explain to her that her friend's belief "isn't what people believe today." However, Mrs. A. insisted on bringing the child to the Emergency Room for examination, and the physician agreed to meet her immediately.

When the resident met Mrs. A., her friend, and her child, he found that Mrs. A. was much calmer, explaining that her friend's treatment "had worked for the moment". The infant was observed to be quiet and content, but to have a striking assymetry of the frontal skull. Mrs. A. was a young woman in her middle twenties, the daughter of Mexican parents. She had two other healthy children, ages seven and eight. Her third child, the identified patient, was born with frontal skull asymetry and with bilateral hernias, which were surgically corrected. Mrs. A. told the resident, "I am scared my baby is going to die. I am afraid my baby will have brain damage. There is too much going on with my baby." She asked if her child would be admitted to the hospital and requested the resident examine the child's palate. The resident assumed that Mrs. A. wanted the palate checked for damage that might have occurred from the traditional cure.

The resident's response to Mrs. A. was to examine the child and attempt to negotiate an acceptable interpretation of the symptoms. Upon physical examination of the infant, the resident found nothing to warrant medical treatment and no evidence of a depressed fontanel. In attempting to negotiate the meaning of the symptom with Mrs. A., the resident explained that doctors also appreciate that the state of an infant's fontanel is a significant sign; if depressed, it may indicate dehydration, or if bulging, may indicate meningitis. Mrs. A. responded that her friend told her that "doctors don't understand what is going on (with fallen fontanel) and babies have been sent home to die because doctors thought nothing was wrong." The resident attempted to reassure Mrs. A. that there was no evidence that her baby was in crisis or subject to impending brain damage. He scheduled her for a clinic visit the following week and sent her home. He felt, however, that he had been less than successful in negotiating an acceptable model of the meaning of the symptom.

In the seminar discussion it became clear that Mrs. A.'s friend had diagnosed the child using a traditional Mexican-American illness category, *caida de la mollera* ("fallen fontanel"). According to Rubel,

Infants are conceived of by the Spanish-speaking population as possessed of a fragile skull formation. The skull includes a section which in this immature stage easily slips or is dislodged from its normal position. The *mollera* (fontanel) is that part of the skull pictured as sitting at the very top of the head. It is normally sustained in proper position by the counter-poised pressure of the upper palate. A blow upon the youngster's head ... is believed to dislodge the fontanel, causing it to sink. The sinking of the dislodged fontanel forces the upper palate to depress, in turn blocking the oral passage. (1960:797)

Mrs. A.'s friend had diagnosed the condition and used a traditional technique for treating it.

Mrs. A. is culturally less traditional than her friend and knew less about the illness. She believed her friend, however, and was terrified for her baby. The resident had elicited her model, taken her concerns seriously, and had tried to negotiate a common model. The prediction that physicians would not understand this illness made it difficult to negotiate a reality that would reassure the mother.

We asked the seminar to further consider the meaning of the illness crisis for the mother. What experiences, what fears and concerns, what meanings were condensed by this illness? Why had the illness been diagnosed *at this particular time*? Why had the crisis arisen now? The Family Nurse Practitioner who usually treats the family was asked to join the seminar to give additional background on this case.

The FNP noted that the child's skull asymmetry was attributed to positioning during pregnancy, although Mrs. A. had been concerned that a pelvic fracture she suffered in an accident might have been related to the deformity. Mrs. A.'s pregnancy was otherwise uneventful. At the delivery, the physician assumed the asymmetry was temporary and would eventually correct itself. The bilateral hernia surgery was successful, and the child was "developing beautifully, normally," according to the FNP. The FNP characterized Mrs. A. as "anglocized", as not a traditional Chicana.

The FNP reported that Mrs. A. had called her the morning after her visit to the Emergency Room to express her concerns that her child might suffer brain damage. Mrs. A. recounted that in consultations with pediatric specialists a week earlier regarding the child's skull asymmetry, she was told that "if the suture line of the skull closed early it would not allow for normal brain growth". She feared that the collapse of the fontanel implied her child was in crisis and subject to immediate brain damage. She also told the FNP that her husband was away on a business trip. It was evident that the infant's skull asymmetry and fears about brain damage provided the context for the current crisis.

In response to questions raised in the seminar's discussion of this case, the FNP scheduled a visit for the family. From this visit, it was learned that Mrs. A., who had not had an infant for seven years, was anxious about her mothering abilities. She reported she had been overly protective and a worrier with her first two children as well. Given the difficulties Mrs. A. had with this infant and given the absence of her husband's support, her fears were readily aroused by her friend's diagnosis. In addition, Mr. A., a Chicano, who accompanied his wife on this visit, told the FNP that he too believed that a fallen fontanel would lead to brain damage. He felt his child had a slight depression of the fontanel. With this knowledge, the FNP began to instruct the parents on the anatomy of the skull, to discuss their concerns about potential brain damage, and to clarify what the pediatric specialists meant by "premature closing of the sutures". Additional sessions were scheduled for Mr. and Mrs. A.

Several important points were illustrated by this case. First, the meaning attributed to an illness symptom is structured by the complex interaction of various cultural systems within which an individual participates. In the case of Mrs. A., it was not possible for the resident to understand her hysterical reaction and her fears that her infant was in a life-threatening crisis without unpacking the meanings she attributed to the child's symptoms. Elicitation of these meanings required not only knowledge of the infant's medical history but also an understanding of the way in which Mrs. A. interpreted that history. The resident needed to recognize that Mrs. A.'s explanatory model integrated a traditional folk model with her own understanding of the pediatric specialists' model, and these led her to interpret the child's symptoms as indications of a life-threatening condition.

Second, the case illustrates that understanding and responding to symptoms requires more than a simple translation between a folk or popular illness model and a biomedical model. The resident found he was unsuccessful in his attempts to find equivalents between Mrs. A.'s Mexican folk illness model and his own biomedical model. Such problems of translation may be especially acute for those folk illnesses to which children are susceptible. In many societies, childhood illness may be attributed to such causes as fright, evil eye, fallen fontanel or witchcraft. While anthropological analyses, using biomedicine as the comparative base, have often focused on what diseases or symptoms lead to the diagnosis of a folk illness, attention should be directed to aspects of the social context and to the mother and family members who make the diagnosis. Folk illnesses provide frameworks for interpreting and condensing concerns that may be rooted in the mother's own life or in family dynamics. Treatment of a folk illness requires not only that the explicit explanatory model be understood, but that the associated network of meanings be decoded and treated. In this case the symptom fallen fontanel stimulated a crisis, because it condensed a network of fears and anxieties aroused by the child's deformity, previous surgeries, and consultation with medical specialists, coupled with the mother's anxiety about her mothering abilities and the absence of her husband.

Although the resident felt his initial success in managing this crisis had been limited, analysis of the case was useful both in teaching and in developing a treatment plan for the family. The resident began to develop an understanding of the complexities of the case far beyond that of the family's regular physicians and specialists. He assisted the clinic's future management of the case with a cultural consultation to the Family Nurse Practitioner involved in Mrs. and Mr. A.'s care. The FNP responded with a series of consultations with the family in which she acted as a cultural translator, eliciting their concerns and providing patient education. As a result, an episode that would have remained baffling to the resident was made understandable, and the care providers began to address the issues of most concern to the family.

The final case was presented in the seminar by a second year Family Practice resident. He was very concerned about the weight of a five month old patient. He was baffled by the apparent resistance of the child's parents to his suggestions that they increase the child's solid food intake. A video-taped explanatory model interview (of 45 minutes) helped both the resident and the parents to clarify issues related to the child's growth and feeding.

Case IV

The resident began to care for this family shortly after the infants' birth. At six weeks, the infant was in the fiftieth percentile for height and weight. At four months, the child's weight dropped below the tenth percentile, and at six months, below the fifth percentile. The explanatory model interview was conducted during this month.

Family social history revealed that Mrs. J., the child's mother (age 37), had suffered numerous losses and difficulties in her life. As a child her mother had died; as a teenager, her first fiance had drowned. She left home at 17 because her father "destroyed her animals," sold her belongings, was "unloving", and subjected her to physical and verbal abuse, including attempts at sexual abuse. Her first marriage ended in divorce and was followed by a miscarriage when she was six months pregnant. Her second marriage was to Mr. J., the infant's father (age 40), who was currently unemployed. Both Mr. and Mrs. J. were rather obese. The couple appeared to have a good relationship, to be quite happy in spite of some difficulties adjusting to the change in their relationship brought on by their new baby. Both doted on the child. In previous visits, they told the resident that they wanted their baby to eat only natural foods and breast milk. The couple were not vegetarians. Mr. J. consulted La Leche League for assistance in coping with difficulties of breast-feeding.

During the explanatory model interview, the resident attempted to uncover the causes of the infant's low weight gain and the parents' perception of the problem. As the resident explored the parents' beliefs about feeding, he found they were concerned about "crib death" and breast-feeding.

The first point both parents made to the resident was that their child was "gaining a lot" and "doing great ... breast-feeding on demand and eating some solids twice a day". The defensive response was in reaction to the resident's expression of concern during the previous visit and his advice that solids be included in the baby's diet. As the interview progressed Mrs. J. commented, "I try not to feed her when she's going down, and if I do breast-feed her, I keep her awake for awhile because in crib death, one woman's baby died after feeding." Mrs. J. also noted that she was having some difficulties nursing, that her milk would not always "drop down", and that she became increasingly anxious when this happened and her baby could not nurse. "It hurts my feelings when I don't know how to make my milk come down." Mr. J. observed that "when [Mrs. J.] can't nurse, the baby's frustrated because she can't eat, [my wife] is frustrated because the baby isn't nursing, ... it's a vicious circle."

Several times during the interview, both parents expressed concerns about crib death and described various people whose babies had died of SIDS. Conversations with such people had occurred once during Mrs. J.'s pregnancy and several times in the past three months. When the resident inquired what each parent thought caused crib death, both responded with detailed explanations. Mr. J. commented, "When a baby has eaten and is really full, they should be contented and happy and they are. But I don't think that their little bodies can handle sleeping too. The digesting, the heart beating, the breathing – I don't think they are geared to handle it. I think that's a contributing factor in crib death, putting them down after eating. They just forget to breathe. . . they just forget to function. It's not even good for an adult to eat and lay down. If you have a whole load of food you're trying to digest and you're laying there, your heart is going BOOM! BOOM! You think you're relaxed but not really. You can't handle it . . . your body just shakes all over. Our hearts are bigger and it's just a shock to our system. It's a weird sensation."

Mrs. J. felt that by keeping the baby next to her own body her breathing would provide enough constant stimulation "to remind the baby to breathe". She noted it was almost impossible "to keep the baby awake for a long while after nursing." The parents felt a good solution to this problem was to keep the infant in bed with them in order to provide the outside stimulation necessary. [Although there appeared to be some tension between the parents over this practice, they continued to have the child share their bed up through the fourteenth month.]

Both Mr. and Mrs. J. told the resident that they felt breast-fed babies are less likely to die from crib death than formula-fed babies. Mrs. J. commented that the majority of crib death babies were not breast-fed and both parents told the resident that they would like to see research on the relationship between crib death and kind of feeding (formula versus breast-feeding).

Following the explanatory model interview and the seminar case conference, the resident outlined a program of dealing with Mr. and Mrs. J.'s concerns. It included patient education on SIDS, support for Mrs. J.'s efforts to breast-feed and additional information on nutrition and child development to encourage the parents to increase solid food in the child's diet. The interview and case conference clarified for the resident the meaning of feeding for this family. It also raised issues concerning the relationships among the couple, the infant and the resident.

The baby's weight gain began to follow an upward curve in the seventh month (one month following the taped interview), although the child's development continued to concern the resident. By the ninth month the weight was again about the fifth percentile, and at eleven months the child appeared developmentally normal, active, and "doing very well."

A second video-taped interview at this time indicated that the parents were no longer concerned about "crib death", because as Mrs. J. commented, the baby ". . . is old enough now, is not lethargic – she breathes very deeply." Food solids had been increased in the child's diet, although caloric intake continued to be a problem. The child was breast-fed on demand and was given multiple vitamins and food supplements, which the parents felt provided adequate nourishment for the child, even though they "filled the baby up" and reduced her desire to eat. The resident, again working with this knowledge of the parents' model, noted that vitamins do not have the calories necessary for growth and encouraged the parents to give the child solid food prior to nursing or feeding the baby supplements.

In our understanding of this case, the parents' reluctance to increase solid foods in their baby's diet was grounded in a network of meanings that had quite practical consequences for child-rearing. Both parents held strong beliefs that feeding an infant solid food may produce crib death, because babies are too small to handle all life functions and still digest heavy food. They both believed breast milk to be more easily digested than formula and thus less likely to cause crib death. This explanatory model made sense of the family's seemingly irrational behavior, but understanding of this case at a cultural or cognitive level is clearly too superficial. The parents' model of the baby's vulnerability and of the threats associated with nourishment clearly condensed a web of affects and psychodynamic meanings that need to be explored. The losses suffered by Mrs. J. in her childhood and the birth of her first child at age 37 led Mrs. J. to perceive the child as particularly vulnerable. As she once told the resident, "I lost everything when I was young. *Nothing* is going to make me lose this baby." Concern about the baby suddenly dying was based in deep-seated concerns of the mother over issues of loss. These concerns were indicated behaviorally by the mother's unwillingness to let the child ever leave her sight. In addition, Mrs. J. felt her success as a mother was defined in part by her ability to breast-feed. While her anxiety may have been partial cause for the failure of the let-down reflex and thus problems of milk production, it seems likely that her concern with breast-feeding and her resistance to alternative foods are linked to deep-seated personal affects. The parents' model also suggests issues of family dynamics. Remarks by both parents during the interview alluded to conflict over the amount of time Mrs. J. lavishes on the child. And while both parents defended their decision to have the baby sleep between them in their bed, Mr. J. went on to comment about his wife's belief that the child should not see him unclothed. The parents' model of feeding patterns and of SIDS and its threat to their child condensed a complex and multi-leveled web of meanings. The models, supported by a popular birthing and breast-feeding subculture, cannot be understood as a simple reflection of a psychodynamic structure. On the other hand, understanding of this family's discourse and their explanatory model requires exploration of the personal, affective, family and cultural meanings that are condensed and juxtaposed in their image of SIDS and breast-feeding. We would expect that in the future, the network of affects and meanings currently associated with problems of feeding will be condensed by new problems with the child and new models for understanding those problems.

The explanatory model interview and its discussion in the seminar was seen by the resident as a turning point in his understanding of the family. Behavior that had seemed quite irrational suddenly seemed reasonable. Knowledge of the parents' reality enabled him to provide information the parents wanted and to negotiate feeding issues, instead of feeling helpless to coerce a change in feeding. When presenting the case at a residents' conference, the resident expressed his belief that the infant's resumption of a more normal growth pattern dated from the explanatory model interview.

CONCLUSION

The implications of our work with residents is clear. Symptoms do not reflect somatic abnormalities in any simple way, and the relationship among symptoms does not mirror a set of mechanistic or functional physiological relationships. Symptoms are irreducibly meaningful. Illness and symptoms are experienced as realities and are thus integrated, logically and meaningfully.

Reconceptualization of the relationship between "biochemical processes and the clinical data of illness," as Engel suggests is necessary, must begin therefore with an appropriate analysis of illness as a meaning structure. We have suggested that anthropology and the interpretive social sciences provide tools for semantic and hermeneutic analyses of illness realities and therapeutic transactions.

Clinical practice often proceeds by treating symptoms "as if" they directly reflect somatic states, leaving other forms of interpretation to the residual "art" of medicine. Such an approach has serious consequences. Recent consumer critiques of medicine make it clear that one major cost of such scientific assumptions in medicine is a loss of humanistic patient care. When symptoms are treated as biological indicators rather than meaningful realities, when "disease" is treated to the exclusion of the personal experience of suffering, the physician loses a very fundamental and primitive healing function. Such problems are inherent in the interpretive strategy of empiricist clinical models and are grounded in the epistemology of contemporary medicine.

Philosophical and theoretical reformulation of medical theory is necessary but not sufficient. Such reconceptualization needs to be translated systematically into new clinical models and forms of training. The "cultural hermeneutic" model and associated clinical tools provide one approach to meeting this need. It provides realistic techniques for focusing the clinician's attention on understanding and translating illness realities, on decoding a patient's symptoms by seeking their grounding in their meaningful context rather than searching exclusively for their empirical or somatic referents. In this way it places the cultural or meaningful patterning of symptoms at the very heart of the clinical enterprise.

NOTES

1. The cases described in this paper were presented in the Clinical Social Sciences Seminar taught by the authors in the residency program, Department of Family Practice, University of California Davis Medical Center, Sacramento, California. The authors wish to thank the participants in that Seminar, in particular Pat Gee, Phil Brosterhous, John Burroughs, and Charles Sutter. The authors were supported in part by NIMH-Psychiatry Education Branch, Grant No. MH 14022.
2. A turn toward meaning and interpretation as a basic paradigm in the social sciences is illustrated by the following: Brown and Lyman 1978; Beidelman 1971; Berger and Luckmann 1966; Crick 1976; Douglas 1975; Fischer 1977; Gadamer 1976; Geertz 1973; Hanson 1975; Leach 1978; Rabinow and Sullivan 1979.
3. The "hermeneutic" or "interpretation theory" approach to studying social reality has been made accessible through publication of Ricoeur (1976) and the introductory collection edited by Rabinow and Sullivan (1979).

   I use the term "hermeneutics" in this paper to refer to the process of translating across diverse sets of meanings, which is inherent in all clinical transactions. This process, as Ricoeur (1976) argues, is analogous in important ways to textual interpretation, the subject of classical hermeneutics. As Taylor (in Rabinow and Sullivan 1979:25) indicates, both seek to make a coherent interpretation from incomplete or confusing texts or statements:

   > Interpretation, in the sense relevant to hermeneutics, is an attempt to make clear, to make sense of . . . a text, or a text analogue, which in some ways is confused, incomplete, cloudy, seemingly contradictory — in one way or another unclear. The interpretation aims to bring to light an underlying coherence or sense.

This means that any science which can be called "hermeneutical," even in an extended sense, must be dealing with one or another of the confusingly interrelated forms of meaning.

And both construct interpretations by moving dialectically from the meaning of the text to the text's larger context, and back to the text itself, with ever increasingly rich interpretations.

4. In the Neo-Kantian tradition, "understanding" (*verstehen*) was contrasted as the goal of the human sciences with "explanation" (*erklären*), the goal of the natural sciences.

5. During the 1950's, Dr. Michael Balint, a psychiatrist, led seminars for general practitioners who met to discuss the psychodynamic dimensions of their most difficult patients, their own psychological investment in these patients, and the effects of these on the therapeutic transactions (Balint 1957). These groups have provided an important model for teaching physicians to treat the psychosocial problems of their patients.

REFERENCES

Antonovsky, Aaron
    1972 A Model to Explain Visits to the Doctor: With Specific Reference to the Case of Israel. J. of Health and Social Behavior 13:446—454.
Balint, M.
    1957 The Doctor, His Patient, and the Illness. New York: International University Press.
Brown, Richard H. and S. M. Lyman
    1978 Structure, Consciousness, and History. New York: Cambridge Univ. Press.
Burr, Bill D., Byron J. Good, and Mary-Jo DelVecchio Good
    1978 The Impact of Illness on the Family. *In* Robert Taylor, ed. Family Medicine: Principles and Practice. Pp. 221—233. New York: Springer-Verlag.
Beidelman, T. O., ed.
    1971 The Translation of Culture. London: Tavistock Publications.
Berger, Peter L. and Thomas Luckmann
    1966 The Social Construction of Reality. New York: Doubleday & Co. Inc.
Carr, John E.
    1978 Ethno-Behaviorism and the Culture-Bound Syndromes: The Case of *Amok*. Culture, Medicine and Psychiatry 2:269—293.
Chrisman, Noel
    1977 The Health Seeking Process: An Approach to the Natural History of Illness. Culture, Medicine and Psychiatry 1:351—377.
Crick, Malcolm
    1976 Explorations in Language and Meaning: Towards a Semantic Anthropology. New York: Halsted Press, John Wiley & Sons.
Croog, Sydney
    1961 Ethnic Origins, Educational Level, and Responses to a Health Questionnaire. Human Organization 20:65—69.
Douglas, Mary
    1975 Implicit Meanings. Boston: Routledge & Kegan Paul.
Eisenberg, Leon
    1977 Disease and Illness. Distinctions Between Professional and Popular Ideas of Sickness. Culture, Medicine and Psychiatry 1:9—23.
    1979 Interfaces Between Medicine and Psychiatry. Comprehensive Psychiatry 20:1—14.
Engel, George L.
    1977 The Need for a New Medical Model: A Challenge for Biomedicine. Science 196: 129—196.

Erikson, Erik H.
  1964 Insight and Responsibility. New York: W. W. Norton & Co.
Fabrega, Horacio
  1972 Concepts of Disease: Logical Features and Social Implications. Perspectives in
         Biology and Medicine 15:583–616.
  1976 Language and Cultural Influences in the Description of Pain. British Journal of
         Medical Psychology 49:349–471.
Feinstein, Alvan R.
  1973 An Analysis of Diagnostic Reasoning, Parts I and II. Yale J. of Biology and Medi-
         cine 46:212–232, 264–283.
Fischer, Michael M. J.
  1977 Interpretive Anthropology. Reviews in Anthropology 4:391–403.
Foucault, Michel
  1970 The Order of Things. New York: Vintage Books.
Frank, Jerome
  1974 Persuasion and Healing: A Comparative Study of Psychotherapy. New York:
         Schocken Books.
Gadamer, Hans-Georg
  1976 Philosophical Hermeneutics. Tr. and ed. by D. Linge. Berkeley: University of
         California Press.
Geertz, Clifford
  1973 The Interpretation of Cultures. New York: Basic Books, Inc.
Good, Byron J.
  1976 The Discourse of Medicine: Medical Systems and Communication in Iran. Unpubl.
         Ms., presented at American Anthropological Association Annual Meetings.
  1977 The Heart of What's the Matter: The Semantics of Illness in Iran. Culture, Medi-
         cine and Psychiatry 1:25–58.
Good, Byron, David Hayes-Bautista, and Mary-Jo DelVecchio Good
  1979 New Constituencies, New Expectations: Towards a Redefinition of Health Care
         for the State of California. Manuscript commissioned by the California Policy
         Seminar, University of California, Berkeley.
Good, Byron J. and Mary-Jo DelVecchio Good
  1979 The Semantics of Medical Discourse. Forthcoming in Yearbook in the Sociology
         of the Sciences: Anthropological Perspectives in the Sciences. Everett Mendelsohn,
         Editor.
Good, Mary-Jo DelVecchio
  1980 Of Blood and Babies: The Relationship of Popular Islamic Physiology to Fertility.
         Social Sciences and Medicine 14B:147–156.
Greenblum, Joseph
  1974 Medical and Health Orientations of American Jews: A Case of Diminishing Dis-
         tinctiveness. Social Science and Medicine 8:127–134.
Hanson, F. Allan
  1975 Meaning in Culture. Boston: Routledge & Kegan Paul.
Harrison, Bernard
  1972 Meaning and Structure: An Essay in the Philosophy of Language. New York:
         Harper and Row.
Hsu, F. L. K.
  1972 American Core Values and National Character. In Psychological Anthropology.
         F. L. K. Hsu, Editor. San Francisco: Schenkman.
Kety, Seymour
  1974 From Rationalization to Reason. American J. of Psychiatry 131:957–963.

Kleinman, Arthur
    1977 Depression, Somatization and the "New Cross-Cultural Psychiatry." Social
        Science and Medicine 2:3–10.
    1978 Clinical Relevance of Anthropological and Cross-Cultural Research: Concepts
        and Strategies. American J. of Psychiatry 135:427–431.
    1979 Recognition and Management of Illness Problems: Therapeutic Recommendations
        from Clinical Social Science. Mass. Gen. Hospital Review for Physicians: Psy-
        chiatric Medicine Update. New York: Elsevier. Pp. 23–31.
Kleinman, Arthur, Leon Eisenberg, and Byron Good
    1978 Culture, Illness and Care: Clinical Lessions from Anthropologic and Cross-Cultural
        Research. Annals of Internal Medicine 88: 251–258.
Kleinman, Arthur and Everett Mendelsohn
    1978 Systems of Medical Knowledge: A Comparative Approach. J. of Medicine and
        Philosophy 3:314–330.
Kleinman, Arthur and L. H. Sung
    1979 Why Do Indigenous Practitioners Successfully Heal? Social Science and Medicine
        13:7–26.
Klerman, Gerald
    1977 Mental Illness, the Medical Model, and Psychiatry. J. of Medicine and Philosophy
        2:220–243.
Lazare, Aron, S. Eisenthal, and L. Wasserman
    1975 The Customer Approach to Patienthood: Attending to Patient Requests in a
        Walk-In Clinic. Arch. Gen. Psychiatry 32:553–555.
Leach, Edmund
    1978 Culture and Reality. Psychological Medicine 8:555–564.
Levy, Robert I.
    1973 Tahitians: Mind and Experience in the Society Islands. Chicago: University of
        Chicago Press.
Lin, Tsung-Yi, Kenneth Tardiff, George Donetz and Walter Goresky
    1978 Ethnicity and Patterns of Help-Seeking. Culture, Medicine and Psychiatry 2:3–13.
MacKenzie, Margaret
    1979 Fear of Fat. Book-length manuscript.
Maduro, Renaldo
    1975 Voodoo Possession in San Francisco: Notes on Therapeutic Aspects of Regression.
        Ethos 3:425–447.
Marsella, Anthony J.
    1978 Thoughts on Cross-Cultural Studies on the Epidemiology of Depression. Culture,
        Medicine and Psychiatry 2:343–357.
Mechanic, David
    1963 Religion, Religiosity and Illness Behavior: The Special Case of the Jews. Human
        Organization 22:202–208.
    1972 Social Psychologic Factors Affecting the Presentation of Bodily Complaints. New
        England J. of Medicine 286:1132–1139.
    1978 Effects of Psychological Distress on Perceptions of Physical Health and Use of
        Medical and Psychiatric Facilities. Journal of Human Stress 1978 (Dec.):26–32.
Minc, S.
    1963 Of New Australian Patients, Their Medical Lore and Major Anxieties. Medical J.
        of Australia I – (50th Yr):681–687.
Opler, Marvin and J. L. Singer
    1956 Ethnic Differences in Behavior and Psychopathology: Italian and Irish. Interna-
        tional J. of Social Psychiatry 2:11–23.

Pilowsky, I. and N. D. Spence
    1976 Pain and Illness Behavior: A Comparative Study. J. of Psychosomatic Research
          20:131–134.
Rabinow, Paul and W. M. Sullivan, eds.
    1979 Interpretive Social Science. Berkeley: University of California Press.
Reynolds, David K.
    1976 Morita Psychotherapy. Berkeley: University of California Press.
Ricoeur, Paul
    1976 Interpretation Theory: Discourse and the Surplus of Meaning. Fort Worth, Texas:
          Texas Christian University Press.
Rin, Hsien, C. Schooler and W. Caudill
    1973 Culture, Social Structure and Psychopathology in Taiwan and Japan. J. of Nervous
          and Mental Disease 157:296–312.
Rubel, Arthur J.
    1960 Concepts of Disease in Mexican American Culture. Am. Anthropologist 62:795–
          814.
Schutz, Alfred
    1970 Reflections on the Problem of Relevance. Richard M. Zaner, ed. New Haven: Yale
          University Press.
Singer, K.
    1975 Depressive Disorders from a Transcultural Perspective. Social Science and Medi-
          cine, 9:289–301.
Sontag, Susan
    1977 Illness as Metaphor. New York: Farras, Straus and Giroux.
Tseng, Wen-Shing
    1975 The Nature of Somatic Complaints Among Psychiatric Patients: The Chinese
          Case. Comprehensive Psychiatry 16:237–245.
Twaddle, Andrew C.
    1969 Health Decisions and Sick Role Variations: An Exploration. J. of Health and
          Social Behavior 10:105–114.
Waxler, Nancy
    1979 Is Outcome for Schizophrenia Better in Nonindustrial Societies: The Case of Sri
          Lanka. J. of Nervous and Mental Disease 167:144–158.
White, Hayden
    1973 Foucault Decoded: Notes from Underground. History and Theory, 12(1):23–54.
Zborowski, Mark
    1952 Cultural Components in Responses to Pain. J. of Social Issues 8:16–30.
    1969 People in Pain. San Francisco: Jossey-Bass.
Zola, Irving K.
    1966 Culture and Symptoms: An Analysis of Patients' Presenting Complaints. American
          Sociological Review 31:615–630.

9. A CULTURAL PRESCRIPTION FOR MEDICOCENTRISM

Contemporary American medicine is beset by conflicting expectations. There is a disparity between what the patient's expectations are of the doctor's role, the doctor's own view of the physician role, the medical student's of their faculty, and the resident's view of responding to responsibility.

"Physicians and other providers are not naturally motivated to ask questions and state problems from the patient's point of view. They continually see things in terms of the way they were trained and the speciality they entered" (Lawrence Weed 1978).

OVERVIEW

Applied anthropologists in clinical settings are involved in a crusade for a pluralistic world view. Anthropologists, by training, have a belief structure opposed to ethnocentrism and its professional offspring, medicocentrism. Medicocentrism is a world view that filters experience through medical filters in which the medical view is reality (cf. Kleinman 1978; and Green et al. 1977). Anthropologists as culturally oriented people perceive clinical encounters as examples of world view conflicts: to the patient, uncertainty about the course of his or her problem is part of the illness; to the physician, organic pathology (disease) is most valuable. The physician searches for objectified symptoms of disease in a medical territory where environmental design reinforces disease as the central object. The patient experiences discomfort, "my illness," and not a biomedical term, a disease (cf. Bryan 1979; Kleinman 1978). Thus, the anthropologist tries to understand the patient's perception of clinical reality, while the physician tries to fit patient experiences into objectified symptoms so that the transformation allows him/her to make appropriate clinical decisions in the biomedical realm.

The anthropologist's paradigm arranges the world in a pluralistic context: a myriad of explanations for misfortune, discomfort and illness. The physician's paradigm is reductionistic, as s/he tries to fit a bewildering array of messages, signs and symptoms into critical information that fits his/her biologistic problem-solving expertise.

The crusade ensues because anthropologists, in the clinical setting, try to sort patient meanings of illness into wider social contexts, and the physician tries to sort illness into narrower contexts. Pluralism confronts reductionism, relativism confronts medicocentrism.

A pluralistically oriented world view presupposes many world views, many

197

L. Eisenberg and A. Kleinman (eds.), The Relevance of Social Science for Medicine, 197–222.

paths to experience, and many communication models that distort experiential input. Such a view is necessarily at odds with a prevailing physician world view that separates the body from the mind and biology from social behavior. Engel (1977) articulates this biomedical model as embracing both reductionism and the mind-body dualism.

Anthropologists see culture as a distinctive achievement of human groups, a pattern that serves to embody ideas and values that generate behavior in those groups.[1] Cultural patterns set acceptable templates that generate behavioral action and condition responses to other's actions. Culture not only orders behavior but orders the categories through which biologic changes become manifest (Fabrega 1974). Thus, anthropologists presuppose that disease cannot be perceived *apart* from a cultural context. Evolutionary constraints operate within a cultural conditioning system and not alone. The presupposition of culture as part of disease, in any universalistic definition, including its illness component, sets anthropologists apart from physicians. In attempting to free physicians from medicocentrism (a culture-bound model), anthropologists wish to convince physicians of the essential value of options, pluralistic ideas and practices, and understanding behavior and meaning in the cultural context. This is the underlying motivation of anthropologists in the clinical setting.

The following will illustrate how cultural awareness can be introduced into the orthodox medical setting so that physicians can enhance their problem-solving skills with the valuable tool of cultural sensitivity. It is assumed that cultural awareness will be useful in identifying the meaning of illness to a patient. And if the meaning of illness (viz. pp. 212–217) is known, then communication and treatment plans will be more congruent between patient and provider. Each should then feel more understanding, more actively involved in the therapeutic process, and the caring relationship will be self-evident.

INTRODUCTION

This article will attempt to generalize from my experience in clinical settings, both ambulatory and hospital, in order to sensitize health providers towards the crucial role that cultural factors play in the definition of illness. I will attempt to set out practical strategies that allow the health provider to understand why patient's behavior during an illness is not predictable from provider expectations, and why patient responses to standardized treatments often run contrary to the provider's clinical expectations.

Where appropriate I will include clinical illustrations derived from actual experiences in the United States. Attempts to confront the biomedical *belief* that some medical disease can be cured, controlled and categorized without regard to social, psychological and cultural factors are fraught with frustration. (Clinical anthropology is not easy.) Abnormalities in biological phenomena may explain some variance in disease but never explain the considerable variance in the experience of illness.

Presently there is a tremendous public demand for "whole-person care" incorporating patient expectations for coordination, communication and cultural sensitivity. If physicians assume such obligations then their jurisdiction will be even more enhanced. If they continue to limit their professional focus to clinical detail and subsequent medical management then they will inexorably be moving to technician status (Carlton 1979:4, 6). If anthropologists, as medical critics, demand that physicians practice wholistic medicine, shouldn't they be confident that their field has substantive material for educating physicians? Shouldn't they also be prepared to defend the priority of their material over some other discipline that then has diminished time in medical training? Additionally, what anthropologist is willing to offer him or herself as a clinical consultant? (I have offered myself as one example with the resulting loss of prestige within main-stream anthropology and "outsider" status among physicians. An occupational hazard in dealing with practical issues is the confering of second class citizenship by anthropologists who consider applied anthropology impure.)

The legal consequences of decisions made on cultural consultant's advice are unknown to me. At least two issues must be considered: what role does the anthropologist take in regard to "final responsibility" for treatment outcomes, and how do anthropologists get malpractice insurance? These complex questions must be addressed if clinical practice is to be culturally sound. (I have skirted these problems by always functioning as a co-clinician.)

I believe that cultural intervention strategies, both to sensitize clinicians to the cultural domain and to improve therapeutic efforts, must include examples from the patient's and the provider's cultural framework.

The preceding discussion presupposes certain premises. It may be useful to reiterate these premises. Providers and patients filter world experiences through many screens including the social and cultural. Communication between two participants may be enhanced or diminished when they share or diverge in their use of cultural filters. I assume that when they recognize or share their cultural filters their resultant interaction is more congruent and more effective (cf. Bandler and Grinder 1975, Volumes I and II for an intensive analysis of such filters). I also assume that established and presumed culturally sensitizing experiences, such as working in an inner-city clinic or another culture, are not sufficient but what is required is a refinement of the clinical experience at every opportunity. Cultural perspectives will extend and refine clinical teaching.

THE CULTURE OF THE PATIENT

Anthropologists when presented with problems that require anthropological application use certain principles as rules to guide their behavior (the substance of which makes up the discipline of applied anthropology). These principles are retested in every case and when found deficient, modifications of the principles are developed. I will not recapitulate anthropological rules that have been proven useful (see the bibliography in Eddy and Partridge 1978 for a review), but will describe the themes that enable one to systematically analyze the patient's cultural context.

Each patient presents in the clinical setting with a formed culture including elements at the reference level (rules to guide behavior) and activities that are the behavior. These two characteristics are often described as symbolic and behavioral. Events occur that are guided by symbolic rules. The anthropologist tries to distinguish the two domains by observing, describing, recording, cumulating the data into patterns, and cross-checking these productions by observable future behavior.

Individuals come to a novel setting with a rule-guide for how to behave that is derived from their culture, but they also learn the rules of the new setting. Patients come to the clinical setting with illness behavioral rules that sometimes conflict dramatically with the provider's professional cultural rules. Individuals come to the clinical setting with a support structure that enables them to interact predictably with others, and if they are temporarily disabled there are specific rules on how to reenter the home world. Clinicians can evaluate the culture of the patient by attention to these principles.

Patients as culture bearers have rules for categorizing all things derived from their linguistic world and also from the values that they apply to things. Thus, food and medicines are cultural categories. An exercise that helps one understand the notion of cultural categories would be either of the following: (1) ask yourself what it is that makes breakfast separate from other concepts (does everyone you know define breakfast the same way?); (2) ask yourself what it is that makes drugs separate from other concepts (does everyone you know define drugs the same way?). The way people structure categories of the world implies their restrictive choice(s) for behaving in the world. Clinicians define certain concepts as "essential" in taking a good history (including deriving data about some of the following questions, point of onset, mode of progression, duration, periodicity, location, intensity, character, precipitating factors, relief factors, aggravating factors, associated signs and symptoms, family history, and age of onset). Patients define certain other information as "essential" in giving a history, responding to historical questions, and being a good historian. Cultural rules define what is good in this situation.

Thus, the anthropologist in approaching the clinical situation would automatically be looking for rule-guided behavior, and the rules that guide the behavior. These rules would usually include a listing of the concepts that are associated with a clinical encounter: illness, sick role, causal attributes of illness and rehabilitation, healer and healing attributes, body images (in wellness and sickness), vitalization of the body (including respiration, digestion, defecation, etc.), culturally shared symptom awareness (observation of like illnesses), results of treatment, and social support networks.

A method for assessing these variables by the clinican is presented in a later section of this paper: the Cultural Status Exam (pp. 206ff.). The use of this procedure does not produce an expert on the culture of the patient, but it does refine the clinical examination so that cultural factors are systematically collected and usable in patient care.

Some Cultural Prescriptions

Premise: every facet of the clinical encounter is pervaded by cultural charges. For example, a psychiatrist asked me why he had such difficulty with his patients keeping their appointments. My response was, "Are they working or unemployed, unionized or not, and do they keep appointments in their informal lives?" It turned out that these patients were referred to his mental health clinic by a company nurse, they were not given released time for this effort, were not covered in their contracts for mental health visits, and were primarily migrant workers. Appointment keeping was not valued in their personal lives, and their peers praised non-absenteeism on the job. They also did not talk about personal matters with other males, particularly higher status males; when they did talk it was to females. They valued present time discussions and not past time matters.

The psychiatrist had considered these patients as nonreflective, nontalkative, and resistant to therapy. If he had looked at their cultural "talk lives" he would have discovered that one glass of beer, after work, and the presence of a woman made them very talkative and more introspective.

Cultural prescription: If your values for a "good" patient include insight, fluid discussion, and time bound personal sessions, examine what your patient's values include in these spheres. When, where, to whom, and in what setting do they evidence "your" values? Do they share a different set of expectations about the appropriate place and person for a talk time? My reflection of these issues to this therapist helped him to plan his office and workday differently. He rearranged his office so that many sessions took place in a den-type setting with his support staff present. He rearranged office hours so that he could meet with some of his clients in local bars. By meeting later he also had more mornings free for some of his own family needs. Reflecting on these changes, he shared with me a cultural lesson: "My definition of the optimal therapeutic stage has been drastically altered, I think I am more humble because of this, and more successful." (Alas, I failed to systematically validate his perception or collect appropriate follow-through data on his "accomplishments.")

Premise: Patients are not always actively involved in their recovery. A mechanic was in the intensive care unit of a university hospital. He was on a respirator for two weeks, and had serious internal bleeding compounding his primary problem of myasthenia gravis of sudden onset. His treatment team agreed that if his bleeding did not stop he was probably not going to survive. One of the residents working with him knew that he was my personal mechanic and asked me to help. I asked his nurses and his doctors what level of involvement they could discern from the patient. They all agreed that he was completely passive both physically (compounded by nasogastric tubes, respirator, assorted I.V. attachments, and he could not speak) and psychologically.

Cultural prescription: I spent several hours interviewing his wife and I also watched him, then I designed a system of tapping letters so he could communicate. Next I asked him to concentrate on various organ systems that were malfunctioning. I gave him image exercises for every twenty minutes, starting with reduced bleeding time, and within a few days working up to the beginning of voluntary breathing. From interviewing his wife I reasoned that he perceived the medical setting as a mechanic would, "a spare parts place." Thus he had resolved to wait for the appropriate part, which was his "active" involvement in the repair job. His bleeding stopped and he began to be less dependent on the respirator and was eventually weaned. I have no control to verify whether he would have improved without my involvement but I took for a given that his personal world view of disablement used the image of a passive machine. I was cued to this by the unanimous view of his treatment team that he was seemingly uninvolved in his case.

In another case, a 45 year-old, religiously committed Black southern female was diagnosed as cancer phobic, morbid and depressed. In the last six months she had lost her father, who was very close to her. She had also learned from several sources that her husband had had intercourse with her mother. She was convinced that she was dying of stomach cancer, and she also maintained that no one in her family would befriend her as her mother had alienated everyone from her. The resident was beginning to build a bond with her but would be finishing his rotation on her service in a few days. The team was unsure of what to do.

Cultural Prescription: I questioned her about religious images, about the polluting effect of incest (in her definition), and how close she had been to her father. I then suggested a plan that would have her oldest daughter (who her father had estranged from her) kneel with her when she prayed and, during prayer, talk to her father. I hoped by this method to build a bond for her with her daughter, to cancel the grandmother's influence, via the shared religious emotion, and to create a friendship option for her that was not tied to the vagaries of a resident's schedule (who would also not be available when she left the hospital).

In another case, several residents asked me how they could obtain better historical information from certain patients that they had in the clinic. Cultural prescription: I did some homework on the patients' background and discovered that they were from a small religious group that viewed healers as communication mediums to the other world. They were acting in accordance with their cultural expectations of the healer/patient situation: they should be mute and wait for the healer to receive instructions from the divine spirit. They were not retarded, nor resistant as the residents jokingly claimed, but perceived the healer from a different reality. They were high non-compliance risks because the residents "naturally" asked them to take their medications individually, rather than in a social setting with the assistance of significant others, which is how they usually followed their healer's advice.

TEACHING RESIDENTS TO BE CULTURALLY AWARE

For the last six years I have been in various settings where my covert agenda has been to overcome medicocentrism. Underlying this work are two basic presuppositions to my approach: (1) the most appropriate setting in which to attempt physician behavioral change is the clinical setting, and (2) cultural awareness is based upon understanding your own cultural biases. From these premises flow my cultural intervention plans: model cultural sensitivity in the clinical context, and use humor and scientific curiosity to allow the residents to ask about their culture (both the physician-specific and the American culture).

Certain behaviors would then seem to be counterproductive. For example, the social scientist should not fantasize an ideal setting where all student-physicians attend lectures or seminars in cultural or social science. Lectures are remembered as rituals of sit-down, one-way communication that prepared the medical student for examinations, were forgotten quickly and were usually seen as irrelevant to clinical decision-making.

Anthropological anecdotes on exotic cultural differences and customs should be saved for teaching anthropologists. If anthropology is relevant and liberates us from ethnocentric professional and personal constraints, then bring it home to the social world of the student. Therefore, the anthropologist's expertise should be on cultural values and behaviors in local populations, all the hybrid ethnic Americans that become patients in American settings. Anthropology is liberating because it can expand one's vision and preadapt the anthropologically aware person to accept many options in problem solving.

When a physician is designing a treatment plan s/he should be aware of the circadian cultural rhythms of patients. For example, what are their food habits and customs? If they drink wine with meals suggest that they take their medicine with wine — not with water. If alcohol is contraindicated with their medicines, one can ask, "what alcohol-like substances can be substituted" (sparkling sodas, grapejuice, etc.)? If the patient population has food categories that relate to health and illness behavior find out what they are. For example, many Hispanic-American, and Asian-Americans have hot-cold and other balance classifications associated with foods, beverages, bathing and medications (see, Harwood 1971, for details). The physician should find out the specifics of the categories and which substances neutralize which others. It is also useful to find out the categorization of spices and salt-rich substances. Is water or milk taboo, or not a beverage, as in many parts of France? This may influence physicians' recommendations, or the kind of expanded history they want to take. Some groups do not categorize either water or soft drinks as a food. If diet is an important part of a prescription what are the social, ritual, and emotionally powerful associations those patients have with their dietary regimen? When doctors prescribe, it is useful to remember they are often trying to change deeply valued, internalized patterns.

If patients' lifestyles prevent routine eating, how can they take pills on a routine schedule? How routine should the pill be taken, and what outcome measures occur when optimal medication schedules are suboptimal? (For a superb review of sociocultural factors in compliance see Sackett and Haynes, 1976.) What behaviors do they indulge in routinely? It is best to assume there is no routine; discover what it is.

An easy way to learn that three and four times-a-day drug routines are difficult to comply with can be gained by keeping a record of interns' meal times. Simple reflection on this bizarre pattern may help the resident empathize with other's priorities.

A way to learn about other life value priorities is to ask a physician to conduct a conference on physicians' counterproductive lifestyles, or on the medical treatment of a physician's family. Even among the culture-bearers of health, congruence between ideal and practice does not occur.

The Provider Problem List

Another device that I have found useful in sensitizing clinicians to other explanatory models and other views of reality is a list of their professional and personal problems.

Increasingly, professional and personal attention has been directed to the signs of stress-related problems among physicians. High rates have been reported including rates of suicide, drug addiction, alcoholism, depression and other emotional problems. Suicide rates, for example, may be as high as eight times the rate for the general population (Medical Tribune 1967). As Mawardi notes,

"No one . . . will forget the statement that the United States loses the equivalent of graduates from seven entire medical schools (approximately 700 physicians) per year due to suicide, drug addiction, and alcoholism" (Mawardi 1979:1485).

Physicians who write about physician patients often note that when physicians are patients they act as if they believe in a magical protection ascribed to their role. They are then devastated when they become ill, often overwhelmed and helpless. They lose their control, their power and their magic in such situations and resort with too early return to work.

In my own work with residents several specific problem areas are uniformly mentioned: long hours, night call, sleep loss, sexual and social deprivation, professional and personal responsibility conflicts and lack of time for self. Young physicians seem to labor under the image that a time will come when s/he can do what s/he wants but that time never seems to come (cf. Donnelly 1979 for an entire thesis on intern stress.)

A common problem among interns is that they feel a tremendous conflict between going home and staying in the hospital. They seem always to feel a conflict about where they are supposed to be. So, in conducting cultural rounds I would usually take a few minutes individually, or in a group if there was previous evidence of support, to create a problem list on them. In this case Problem Number 1 would be titled *Dual Homes*. We would then spend a few moments more clearly spelling out the specifics of the problem, how common it was, and then formulating a plan for further information, or a design for problem resolution. Then we would return to patient problems and see if we couldn't find a parallel conflict among any of their patients, briefly review the plans for resolution and see if any of those plans were relevant to the resident.

What do we accomplish in this manner? First, we allow the physician to disclose his or her own problems, particularly in the psychosocial domain. I assume that self-disclosing behavior enhances empathic communication for most interpersonal situations (cf. Gazda 1975). Secondly, we allow the resident to admit that patient problems are not always so far removed from doctor's reality, and that resolution strategies are generic to all personal problems, not just patients.

I use the problem list concept because it is part of the everyday vocabulary of the physician and is thus not an alien concept such as "identity redefinition skills" or psychoanalysis (cf. Pfifferling 1977). By taking a few minutes at the end of each rounding period, or once a week, we symbolically tell the resident that their health and personhood is important and that they are human too. We admit that the residency experience is difficult and that attention to their personal feelings and difficulties is appropriate. The Provider Problem List allows regular ventilation of patient/hospital/education-related stresses, *and* poses a way of identifying and beginning to resolve these burdensome issues.

Problem lists could include cognitive areas such as inadequate nutritional data, destressing strategies, cultural ignorance (with specific examples), or role expectations of other health workers. The list could also include emotional or feeling tone problems of the residents such as fatigue, anger, hostility, overobjectifying, etc. Or it could include logistic or interpersonal problems such as unavailability of technical, record or procedural items and uncooperative nurses, patients, peers, attendings etc.

How does the problem list concept work to increase cultural sensitivity? It allows the providers to consider their medical decision-making strategies as appropriate to their own problems. They must define their problem, decide on further necessary data, plan to implement problem clarification or resolution, and develop a feedback mechanism: the revised problem list with relevant progress notes. They relate their progress notes to their personal data (subjective) and to objective data. They become *distanced* as insider-outsiders in resolving their own problems. By taking on this strategy they become more capable of "objectively" viewing their realm with all its rituals and magical thinking. Becoming more anthropologically aware of their own place in the initiation ritual of adult medical socialization (i.e., housestaff training) and intervening in the discomforting aspects of their training help them to see anthropology as relevant. By jointly problem solving with the anthropologist and/or their peers, they discover the hidden resource of increasing their options in problem solving when they deal with someone from another, alien field: anthropology.

By jointly problem solving, with both the anthropologist and their peers, they discover one of my hidden agendas: increasing their problem-solving options by sharing impasse situations with unexpected others. The anthropologist can, in turn, incorporate not only anthropological insights but mobilize patient resources. Patient activation can reduce societal and professional pressures to maintain physician overdominance. As Weed has written,

For many aspects of management, a physician's partially-recalled knowledge cannot possibly compete with a patient's *organized* (my italics) knowledge of himself. Our job is to give the patient the tools and responsibility to organize the knowledge and slowly learn to integrate it (1978:XVI).

How well does the Provider Problem List work? Unfortunately, these ideas have not been validated against specific outcome criteria. Several reasons seem to explain this problem. Chiefly, there seems to be no funding for this kind of research. Also, medical staffs do not perceive the anthropologist as an appropriate clinical consultant and social science faculty prefer to ply their trade in the lecture hall rather than in the clinical setting. From the subjective responses I have received from medical students and residents, however, these innovations have been extremely useful and enriching. But testimonials are only a beginning, and it is to be hoped that clinical social scientists and clinicians will replicate such attempts and analyze their outcomes.

The Cultural Status Exam

I have used a few concepts to try to sensitize clinicians to culturally significant parameters. They revolve around the patients' models of clinical relevance. Lay persons have explanatory models for the cause, temporal onset, underlying biological involvement, the process of the illness and its role transformations, and appropriate treatment. They have models generating healthful and unhealthy lifestyles, and for locating their place in an esteemed network (identity, self-worth, and energy allocated to "health" issues). By and large these models are given poor credence or disdained by physicians. Each partner in the clinical transaction has a folk model of reality and often they are incongruent; rarely are the differences negotiated.

If the physician is aware of the patient's explanatory model including the perception of the healer role, and the system of which it is part, historical information will be more easily elicited, satisfaction will be enhanced, compliance will be higher, and hidden agendas will not surface at inappropriate times (Wallston and Wallston 1978; Somers 1976; Roter 1977; Fink 1976; Becker 1976).

The following set of questioning frames should enable the provider to elicit information that approaches patient perceptions of clinical reality. I have found these questions to be helpful in teaching residents and medical students to "hear" the patient's reality. It has also been my impression that when these questions are appropriately tailored (i.e., tuned to the local set and the setting of the patient) the provider is judged to be genuine, empathetic and warm.

CULTURAL STATUS EXAM

I. How would you describe the problem that has brought you to me?
  (a) Is there anyone else with you that I can talk to about your problem? (If yes, to significant other: Can you describe X's problem?)
  (b) Has anyone else in your family/friend network helped you with this problem?

II. How long have you had this (these) problem(s)?
  (a) Does anyone else have this problem that you know? If yes, describe them, how old they are, and their different manifestations.

III. What do you think is wrong, out of balance, or causing your problem?
  (a) Who else do you know who has, or gets this kind of problem?
  (b) Who, or what kind of people don't get this problem?

IV. Why has this problem happened to you, and why now?
  (a) Why has it happened to (the involved part)?
  (b) Why did you get sick and not someone else?

V. What do you think will help to clear up your problem?
  (a) If they suggest specific tests, procedures, or drugs, ask them to further define what they are and how they will help.

VI. Apart from me, who else do you think can help get you better?
  (a) Are there things that make you feel better, or give you relief, that doctors don't know about?

Each of the question frames in the Cultural Status Exam (I also refer to it as the Cultural Rule Out) is designed to elicit material in culturally significant dimensions, and each set of dimensions can easily lead to many other branching questions.

Question (I) attempts to force the provider to allow patients to carefully define the problem from their perspective. The provider should not interject any "clarifying" remarks during this period. Before proceeding to further questions I feel it is valuable to ask if there are other persons who have valuable information. If the response is affirmative I solicit the other's information — either then, with patient permission, or at the end of my interview. Inconsistencies in others' opinions of the patient's problem can be a goldmine that is usually untapped. Often the elicitation of this information with the patient present produces dramatic rapport. During this information gathering stage it is also useful to solicit self-care activities which often are a clue to social support structures or persons.

Question (II) attempts to force the provider to hear the patient's interpretation of *time*, and the perceived severity of the problem. Delay, recentness, and suddenness of problem all contribute to eliciting the patient's time perspective. If you know what view of time your patient has (e.g., concern with past and unresolved guilt; concern with present and immediacy of focus; concern with future and impact on life goals) you can often predict compliance potential, rehabilitation effect, and patient's need for intensive professional support. This question often leads one into folk epidemiology, e.g., who else has these symptoms, and how are they distributed among valued others. By collecting folk epidemiological material expected life cycle concomitants can be elicited (cf. Pfifferling 1975). Useful background data on the value of eliciting time categories in the medical context are found in Zborowski (1969), Spiegel (1959, 1976).

Question (III) continues in the folk etiology vein; it allows patients to participate in the etiologic search, and to inform you of their model of misfortune. By identifying their causal perspective physicians can often translate their putative agent into their patient's model. For example, if a patient has a yeast infection (moniliasis), and perceives illness as bodily imbalance, then one can instruct her on how to correct the vaginal "imbalance" caused by Candida.

Question (IV) focuses on the individual's perception of his/her place in a valued (or disvalued) network. It is my impression that most patients have causal explanations for generic categories of illness, and also specific explanations for individual manifestations of illness. By collecting this data one can discriminate between social and individual disruptions. Usually this focus allows the physician to anchor the interview specifically and comfortably prepares the patient for a physical examination. By asking, "Why has it happened to you and not to someone else?" the doctor cross-checks earlier etiologic and psychologic data. If someone has suppressed their reasoning earlier in the interview you should now have established sufficient rapport to elicit an honest response.

Question (V) attempts to allow the patient to spell out his/her treatment objectives. I have found that most patients have a treatment agenda before they walk into your office. It has been my impression that if you do not allow these plans to surface, and discuss them, many people will implement them anyway. They may be detrimental or helpful. I consider the release of these agendas preventive medicine for provider frustration.

Question (VI) attempts to assure patients that doctors are trying to help them and are interested in doing anything they can to resolve their patients' problems (within their ethical framework). Doctors are also trying to incorporate their patients' healing network into their armamentarium. By *not* knowing who they are using as healers, external to the allopathic system, doctors deny their patients' resort system, and reinforce medicocentrism. Often, contacts with these other healers produces vital information that would not be attained in any other way. By eliciting the patient's perceived treatment activities — external to biomedical prescriptions — one may gain vital information that could cause treatments to fail or be dangerous. For example, if doctors are trying to maintain a controlled electrolyte, blood sugar, or carbohydrate balance, shouldn't they know their patients' herbal beverage intake, etc.? It seems logical that the more doctors maintain their humility the less they will be expected to perform superhuman feats; an unnecessary and potentially dangerous burden that can be removed.

The preceding questions have been useful to me, and to my students, but they must be systematically researched, and the results reported. I would expect that such a study would validate which questions reveal vital information, how often, and for which classes of patients. For the interested reader there is a more complete list of questions available. I hope that this essay will stimulate both validation of this domain and the sharing of these questioning frames.

CULTURAL PREMISES OF THE PHYSICIAN'S WORLD

Just as patients define clinical reality different than physicians and other patient groups, so do physicians have many different clinical realities. However, physicians are socialized through a common experience, medical education, and share more cultural rules than do their patients. The following discussion is an initial formulation of American physician's cultural premises. It is intended to foster self-reflection among physicians and to offer an inside glimpse on the physician mentality for patients.

Physicians are socialized to value certain kinds of activities, processes and behavior as basic to their definition of the clinical encounter. These defining premises generate a world view of what they ought to see, do and regard as important. As Carlton has written,

When we look at how physicians solve problems in the medical setting we find that they invoke a particular mode of thinking and argument that is universally shared by university-trained physicians (1979:66).

Carlton calls this mode of thinking "The Clinical Perspective."

Physician to physician discussions center around interesting patient-relevant problems. *Interesting* problems are those that involve diseases that, if identified accurately, will segregate the clinician from his or her peers by virtue of clinical acuity, reinforcing competition as a value. Careful biomedical description of biological parameters within a particular case enhances peer esteem and raises individual stature in the hierarchy.

The delineation of the patient's problem(s) should be by the clinician and not by a nonphysician. Synthesis and articulation of a diagnostic end-result are behaviors reserved for physicians and when others, such as nurses, are perceived to usurp such a role they get into hot water.

Activities that allow the physician to display sensory acuity (fine motor, auditory, visual or quantitative skills) or mnemonic expertise are more valued — and more rewarded — than communication facility (e.g., teaching patients).

Desirable medical settings involve environmental designs that orient around the habits and needs of the providers. One has only to look at the location of new medical offices to validate this point; they are located near hospitals and away from the hub of the local population's social activity. Physicians that ply their trade alone or alone among nurse-clinicians, for example, are marginalized by their peers. Prestige and rewards accrue to those that are acknowledged leaders in special areas, specialists, rather than generalists.

Medicine's social architecture is composed of specialists, credentialists, and information explosionists with the physician as the central, and dominant actor.

Credentials are charters for clinical behavior and those with lesser or no formal credentials are not considered to possess clinical skills or knowledge. Feats of memory are important ritual displays for upward mobility and key signs that you are in a medical arena.

Decisions should be made around single cases, based on cumulative descriptions of single cases. It is expected that the scientific accumulation of single-case phenomena will lead to scientific medicine. Identifiable biologic aberrations in a single case should lead to the appropriate path for clinical solutions.

I have summarized these premises in Figure 1. Evaluation of quality medical education and care should be based on the establishment of the optimal criteria of process behavior and the audit of physicians displaying that style of process management. Outcomes of clinical behavior are derived from observations of process records, those activities that are recorded in the immediate presence of the clinical observer. Biological processes that are subject to modification by physician intervention, and can be observed or quantified, are to be used to determine the decision-making skill of the physician-in-training.

CURRENT CULTURAL PREMISES
IN ORTHODOX MEDICINE

Physician-Centered

Specialist-Dominated

Credential-Oriented

Memory-Based

Single-Case Centered

Process-Oriented

Fig. 1.

Physician transmuted information is the most reliable of medical record data, and where that physician is a specialist in an academic setting that data is the most objective. Vital patient management data consists of biomedical terms that are buttressed by laboratory specifics.

These premises are shared by a majority of clinicians and are in turn derived from a biologistic paradigm (Engel 1977) embedded in the allocated physician role in the United States. Engel claims the medical model is predicated on two separately conceived dichotomies: (1) the Body versus the Mind, and (2) Biology versus Social Behavior. Thus, medicine can logically equate, as it does, body and biology and not be concerned with mind and social behavior. Resulting from this split are different discourse styles — medical and psychiatric languages (Fabrega 1972).

The biomedical model assumes that disease reality is to be accounted for by aberrations from measurable biologic parameters. Therefore disease can and should be dealt with apart from sociobehavioral dimensions. The search for causes must therefore be neurophysiologically or biochemically anchored; otherwise, it is a less than legitimate endeavor.

The model sketched above purports to explain the views of a majority of practicing clinicians and applies best to academic subspecialists. Many physicians have had some exposure to psychosomatic medicine although usually apart from the core arena with the most highly valued role models where they acquire their clinical mentality. Psychosomatic medicine is even perceived by advocates as confused, as uncertain whether it is an approach or a discipline, and unclear as to a basic definition (Lipowski 1977). Some psychosomaticists are optimistic about the future growth of consultation-liason psychiatry, although I have seen no reports illustrating the extent and the impact of this psychiatric subspeciality on general medicine.

CULTURE AS GROWTH

Barbour cites a hypothetical case study contrasting the disease model with the "growth" model (a model searching for the patient's explanatory world and the meaning of illness to him) that fits nicely with a clinical anthropological approach.

A fifty year old, white male presents with a history of dizzy spells. His physical exam is negative except for a blood pressure of 150/100. The diagnosis of essential hypertension is made. Laboratory orders include a routine CBC, SMA 6/60 and 12/60, urine, EKG, chest X-ray. Special workup includes a hypertensive IVP, 24 hour urine for VMA, sodium and plasma renin assays. In the following year, while on Chlorothiazide B.I.D., he has six office visits, and five electrolyte panels to monitor potassium. Rx additions include KCL, D.C. Chlorothiazide, and Aldactazide. The patient is assessed as having chronic hypertensive disease, and his blood pressure is satisfactory at 130/85. (Both the patient and his physician regard the treatment as successful — the blood pressure is normal.) (Barbour, 1975:45ff.)

The same patient was taken to a culturally sensitive physician, one motivated by the theme, "If you listen to the patient you will begin to understand the meaning of his illness."

The physician asked, "Why does he have dizzy spells, are there other factors in his life that cause this symptom?" (The doctor presumed that the blood pressure was not sufficient to cause them).

The doctor elicited a recent business failure, some marital problems, compulsive eating, drinking and smoking, and poor sleep cycles. These stress factors could produce reactive hypertension and dizziness.

The interpretation was offered to the patient in order to actively involve him in treatment. A routine laboratory survey is ordered but the special tests for exotic hypertension factors are deferred. Subsequent to this interaction the patient implemented changes in his lifestyle. His dizzy spells disappear and his blood pressure returns to normal. Two follow-up visits corroborate the normalizing of his blood pressure. No further laboratory tests are necessary, nor are drugs ordered (with their potential side-effects and the need for physician monitoring). Both the patient and the doctor regard the problem as closed; *the patient perceives himself as well.*

As Barbour describes,

Both approaches result in normalization of the blood pressure. However, when the disease model is applied strictly, as in the first approach, the patient becomes a normotensive person who sees himself as sick with chronic illness, a reduced life expectancy, a limited potential, a dependency on doctors and continuing drug therapy (1975:48).

If one charts the two approaches a dramatic difference in cost is evident:

Patient:	Male, age 50
History:	Dizzy spells
Physical Exam:	Negative except BP 150/100

DX:	DX:
* Essential Hypertension	* Nervous tension
First Exam: . . . . $ 50	First Exam: . . . . $ 50
Lab: 206	Lab: 88
Drugs:. 100	Drugs:. 0
Follow-up Visits:. 90	Follow-up Visits:. 30
Additional Lab: 52	Additional Lab: 0
$498	$168
Result:	*Result:*
Chronically ill person.	Well person.

From, Allen Barbour, M.D., 1975:49

Barbour's growth model sounds easy to apply, and if it were that easy doctors should readily adopt it. That does not appear to be the case. Doctors find it difficult to embrace the growth model because they have not encountered much modeling of that kind of practice, seen statistics to validate its success, or been willing to work hard at activating patient responsibility. Patients find it difficult to embrace the model because they have few patient or physician role models, perceive a personal loss if their physician rejects their participatory efforts, and also are hesitant to assume responsibility, which in any case runs counter to the authoritarian model of health care most of them have experienced.

MEDICINE AS A SOCIAL MIRROR

If physicians apply a narrow disease model — a belief system is a model — implying that all disease should be conceptualized in terms of an aberration of underlying physical mechanisms then they can only search for the fit between their observations and physiochemical principles (Engel 1977). Their belief system acts as a dogma and is culturally imperative (ibid.). Other explanations of phenomena not easily reconciled are excluded and questions concerning the meaning of illness are considered unorthodox. The folk belief of biologistic reductionism is the clinician's model and with it clinicians effectively limit their sensory input. They filter out as noise information on the meaning, experience and context of illness.[2] They impoverish their ability to create unique person-specific treatment options. Communication between doctor and patient suffers and the healing relationship retreats from easy realization.

Healers who adopt the disease model as their folk belief, their dogma, become transformed into technocrats and technicians. The physician who wishes to enrich his life through healing relationships loses and the patient gains ammunition for anger at the medical system. As Lander has written, "... for social purposes a malpractice claim represents the intersection of patient injury and patient anger" (1978:6–7).

Substantial evidence exists that the obverse relationship, a healer relationship rather than a technocratic relationship, immunizes against anger and malpractice (Lander 1978; Gazda et al. 1975).

Medical technology, the result of scientistic, reductionistic behavior increases risk for unfulfillment by patient and provider. Technology increases iatrogenic risk and the social distance between doctor and patient. The patient retreats into environmentally induced passivity and reduces the opportunity to be actively involved in his/her own health treatment. By being passive the patient also reduces the opportunity for acting as an honest audit system for the physician. In my experience, physicians receive sub-optimal feedback either from patients, peers, faculty or nurses. Evaluation tends to be judgemental, more negative than positive, and removed from the immediate clinical experience. Housestaff are constantly waiting for the rules of the game to be explained but the time never seems to arrive. The absence of clearly defined rules for patient care, opportunities for feedback, and for expectations in the physician role leaves the housestaff feeling stressed and compounds their insecurity. Technological, superspecialized medicine and payment mechanisms that reward the untested and the quantifiable create a medicine that is best described as commodity oriented. When medical students see commodity models, feel commodity teaching, and are financially reimbursed for commodity practice why should they become capable of initiating a healing, caring relationship?

As anthropologists view the world through sociocultural lenses they see commodity medicine as very much a creature of a curative technology, itself a part of a distinctive American political economy. (cf. Ingelfinger 1978 for a curiously parallel view.) If medicine is technological, objectified, and curatively oriented it cannot systematically address the social etiology of so many presenting illnesses. Thus physicians cannot become advocates of sociopolitical activities that will prevent future social ills that present in the clinical setting. I often ask the residents I work with, "Why has that patient presented now, with that constellation of symptoms?" All too often the response is, "I never thought of that." A patient is in the medical setting only rarely just for a medically appropriate reason: it is usually a socially appropriate resort path.

As Ingelfinger has astutely noted,

If doctors are technologically oriented, hurried, and impersonally distant in their behavior, it is only because they, as a group, mirror the society of which they are an integral part (1978:942).

As an anthropologist analyzing doctors I find Ingelfinger, the editor emeritus of the *New England Journal of Medicine*, a remarkable apologist. Doctors are not "ordinary if specially educated folk" (ibid.), they are a cultural minority with extraordinary invading, labeling, and biology transforming capabilities. They are deprived, by their leaders (medical educators), of social and psychological growth through the primacy of the biomedical, technologic template. They deal with intense experiences and are given minimal opportunity to reflect and mature through these experiences. Their outward, commodity manifestations may parallel American technological addiction but they are systematically denied maturity during a lengthy adolescence (medical training).

Mastery of multifield content, technology and medical language leaves little time for the synthesis and self-reflection necessary to the humanist physician. They are deprived of the coordination resources, available to corporate industry via computers and information systems, because of an outmoded dependency on memory — the most common activity of medical students.

They are denied an opportunity to perceive the logic behind faculty decision-making, and the resultant growth and scientific advances, because the logic is rarely made explicit.

As a sensitive pediatrician has written to me, "physicians focus their attention on data about patients rather than on patients directly." Medical students must constantly unlearn moral, legal, and street language perspectives. They must learn the language of disease: a crucial ritual separating the healer from the patient.

Physicians are educated to be a separate co-culture within American society and thus systematically trained to be divergent from their patients. In the following section I would like to share a series of insights borrowed from Lipowski (1970) that deal with the meaning of illness. It is my feeling that biomedical training fosters among providers a single meaning of illness: illness as challenge.

Physicians' understanding of their divergent socialization will enhance their awareness of co-cultural status, and should prepare them for dealing with the varieties of meanings of illness that present in the clinical encounter.

COMMON MEANINGS OF ILLNESS: AMERICAN PATIENTS

Several authors have hypothesized that the meaning of illness directly affects a person's coping behavior to that episode. The meanings of illness to an individual vary from episode to episode (and the length of the episode is differently conceived by patients in different cultures), but most people have certain characteristic attitudes towards their illness. These attitudes reflect their past personal experience, knowledge and cultural background. These meanings may be conscious or out-of-awareness to the individual, (Janis 1958; Lazarus 1966; and Lipowski 1970).

Lipowski has attempted to list frequently identified meanings of illness found in his clinical experience (see Figure 2) (1970:98ff.). It is his thesis that specific coping strategies are directly related to the patient's meaning of and attitude toward his experience of disease (illness), injury or disability.

COMMON STYLES OF ATTRIBUTING MEANING
TO ILLNESS

ILLNESS AS CHALLENGE

ILLNESS AS ENEMY

ILLNESS AS PUNISHMENT

ILLNESS AS WEAKNESS

ILLNESS AS RELIEF

ILLNESS AS STRATEGY

ILLNESS AS IRREPARABLE LOSS OR DAMAGE

ILLNESS AS VALUE

Fig. 2.

I offer this list as a useful, sensitizing item that will help the clinician to be prepared for particular coping behaviors that seem inappropriate from the provider view. When I have asked clinicians to reflect upon this list in reference to *their* personal meaning of illness and their "difficult" patients, they usually gain insight into unexplained patient discomfort. For example, clinicians, in my experience, perceive *illness as challenge*. This view inspires them to actively adapt to the illness episode. They need to master the episode and get on with the business. This view of illness generates rational, task-oriented behavior that is situationally determined. The patient using this meaning-set seeks advice in a timely fashion, is cooperative and actively seeks further illness-specific facts.

The physician who views illness as challenge is often baffled when s/he confronts a patient with another view: *illness as punishment*. This person sees the punishment, via the illness, as either just or unjust, and either allowing an opportunity for atonement and redemption or not. Commonly, according to Lipowski, these patients are anxious, depressed and/or angry. This anxiety is associated with the illness episode. If they regard the illness as just and final then they are model, passive patients. They offer little resistance. On the other hand they may perceive illness as a chance for atonement and be elated by the opportunity. Subsequent to the episode, if they recover, there may be a perceived major personality change. They may have made vows during the crisis and now they must carry out those promises. If they view the illness as unjust punishment their depressive affect may be perceived by the clinician as totally out of proportion to the severity of the episode. But severity is judged differently by a person with this model than someone with illness as a challenge model.

Other American patients view *illness as enemy*. Their episode of illness confirms an invasion by exogenous or endogenous forces. They commonly speak of "conquering or combating their enemy." They may be anxious, fearful or hostile. They may be ready to fight, to flee or to surrender. They may cope by defending themselves vigorously from danger and attack. They may be ready to blame others for their illness, or their vulnerability. Their aggressiveness or hostility may be used by the astute clinician who mobilizes their energy for "conquering the enemy" (many oncologists have profound anecdotes about hyperaggressive patients).

Patients who perceive illness as enemy may cope by a denial of their capacity to resist, or may resist with tremendous hostility. When clinicians view illness in this way, with a primary coping strategy of combat, and their patients appear helpless (the extreme flight response) the physician may view the patient with extreme hostility. Communication problems between physician and patient can easily be produced.

Some physicians and some patients view their *illness as weakness*: a sign of moral loss of control. They feel ashamed of their failure to control their person. This internalized meaning may cause them to deny or conceal their illness. Often these individuals overreact by working hard at projecting a model patient image, thus covering their "weakness." In interviewing residents about their illness experiences I recall one resident who said, "I was sick the first month of my residency; I had constant guilt wondering what the chairman would think of me." Another resident described his regression, when he was sick, with a resultant self-deprecation, "How could I be so weak, what kind of a doctor is that?"

For some patients, and also for some doctors, being ill means a time of removal from other responsibilities. Being ill means that one does not have to face up to difficult decisions and/or daily demands. This view generates the meaning of *illness as relief*. Illness offers a role that reduces other obligations and excuses unfullfilled transactions. (A classic description of this role has been presented by Talcott Parsons and reconsidered in his 1975 paper, "The Sick Role and the

Role of the Physician Reconsidered.") Our language has a whole host of labels for those patients who cling to their sick role when they "should" be well: malingerer, hypochrondriac, crock, somatizer, psychogenic, and so on. It is well known that patients who present with complaints for which no adequate organic pathology can be found are serious management problems (Lowy 1977). It is my suggestion that one of the reasons they do not receive adequate treatment, enjoy the benefits of a good doctor-patient relationship, and get labeled but not cared for is because their prevailing meaning of illness is that of relief. Their physicians are heavily motivated to dislike, be easily frustrated by, and to fear pollution from these patients. If physicians are socialized to fear the contagious patient with the model of illness as relief then these patients should be in double jeopardy. Firstly, from physicians who view as acceptable the *model of illness as challenge*, and secondly, from physicians who themselves find *illness as relief* ideologically comfortable, but who are reinforced in denying this model.

Lipowski (1970) sees another meaning of illness, commonly used by American patients, related to but different from illness as relief: *illness as strategy*. These individuals use their illness experience as a strategic ploy in dealing with their social environment. They can manipulate others to secure attention, compliance, and nurturance when they are in the sick role. Persistent somatizers secure physician attention by playing into the doctor's fear that s/he will miss an organic etiology. Patients who are viewed as "interesting" cases quickly learn medical center values and may embellish their illness to remain the center of medical attention. Parents often cling to their dependent role in order to control their children's ties to them. As Lipowski generalizes, "For some patients coping with illness amounts to maintaining it at any cost and displaying it prominently" (ibid:99).

For some individuals the loss of a body function, organ, or range of activity may be processed as an overwhelming loss. They may view their person as irreparably changed and damaged. The physicians involved in the episode may consider the loss as "minor" and disregard the emotional impact the loss appears to have on the patient. These patients may gain negatively valued labels from the medical care team, such as "overreactor," "hypochondriac," etc. Lipowski views this model as *illness as irreparable loss or damage*. He sees patients with this view as particularly prone to depression, hostility, and resistant to rehabilitation. They would also be preadaptive to suicide. Physicians who receive the sudden notice of a malpractice suit, a letter of audit from their peer review board, and who "overreact" may be demonstrating this meaning of illness. Early intervention by State Medical Societies' Peer Review Committees in the case of a pre-alcoholic or drug-dependent physician may be more successful than expected because physicians may perceive the eventual loss of a license as irreparable loss.

A final category listed by Lipowski is *illness as value*. To individuals with this model illness has an intrinsic, enriching value. These individuals perceive the experience of illness as an opportunity to deeply reflect and subsequently expand their personality. Medical historians view this mode of coping as a superior adaptation and anecdotes of famous cultural and medical personalities evidence this view (Sigerist (1952) has written an autobiography detailing his post-coronary aesthetic sensitivity.) Illness is thus seen as a creative catalyst, perhaps necessary and sufficient for some leaps of creativity.

These categories are suggested to reflect underlying models of meaning that individuals carry with them into the clinical encounter. Lipowski proposes that concrete strategies used by patients to cope with the experience of disease are predicated on the underlying meaning that illness has to them. His formulation needs to be tested and validated. I find his ideas useful and illuminating. I also find his categories relevant in viewing physicians' reactions to both their own illnesses, and to particular frustrations about their patient interactions.

When one views other prevailing meaning attributions, in other cultural groups, these ideas seem intuitively accurate. For example, among most Hispanic-American populations certain body fluids are considered nonrenewable; loss of such substances means the permanent removal of an integral spiritual component. It is easy to see why Hispanic-Americans are poor blood donors. Blood is also intimately related to one's spirit, a kind of genome. Unexplained personality changes, after transfusion, have resisted explanation because the medical writer failed to take into account the patient's underlying meaning of illness. Obstetricians complain bitterly about their patients' refusal to use anesthetic agents. Is it because many young pregnant Americans are adopting a new meaning of illness: as value?

Clinical Lessons from the Meaning of Illness

By conceptualizing frustrations in the clinical encounter with an eye toward the patient's, and the physician's, meaning of illness we are likely to make progress in reducing the prevalent dissatisfaction with American medical care (Kleinman 1978). American health culture is pluralistic, with multiple ideologies and priorities of health practices. Patients and providers have differential concepts about every step in the clinical sequence. These underlying models of clinical reality generate behavior in the provider-layperson transaction. Each party to the transaction has highly valued models (what Kleinman has called mediocentric views (op. cit.)). Divergent communication often ensues when there is discordance between the realities. This discordance can be on every level: semantic referential meaning, etiologic theory, "disease" classification, vocabulary, and valued emotional consequences including perception of prognostic statements. This essay has been an initial step in detailing differential views carried to the clinical encounter, outlining strategies that I have found useful in sensitizing physicians to clinical *realities*, assuming that efforts in these directions will enable both patients and providers to accommodate to each other's cultural premises.[3]

ACKNOWLEDGMENTS

I would like to thank Teresa Graedon, Ph.D., Joe Strayhorn, M.D. and John

Crellin, M.D., Ph.D. all at Duke University Medical Center for comments on an earlier draft of this paper. I am indebted to Arthur Kleinman, M.D. for editorial suggestions and needed encouragement. My optimism is derived in large part from interacting with the following physicians, all of whom model attributes of a culturally sensitive practitioner: Drs. William Jeffries (Neurology), William Wilson (Psychiatry), Ronald Wintrobe (Psychiatry), David Larson (Psychiatry), David Elpern (Dermatology), Virginia Soules (Family Practice), Laney Prichard (Family Practice), Irvin Cronin (Family Practice), Ramon Velez (Internal Medicine), and Andrew Greganti (Internal Medicine).

NOTES

1. Although culture is the unifying concept shared by anthropologists, a unanimously agreed upon definition of culture does not exist. I find that the notions of templates and models for behavior and thought, shared by individuals in a community and applied in daily situations contains the essence of the cultural concept. Culture is not innate but learned in a social setting; the various facets of culture are integrated (if you manipulate a cultural item multiple others are effected): it is shared by people in a group and defines their boundaries vis-à-vis other groups (cf. Hall 1976:7–21 for a fuller analysis). Culture is embedded individual knowledge. It consists of conceptions implicit and explicit, latent and manifest, of "what is, . . . what can be, . . . how one feels about it, . . . what to do about it, . . . and how to go about doing it" (Goodenough 1961:522, quoted in Keesing 1979:16).

2. The field of Family Medicine claims to be oriented toward holistic treatment emphasizing continuous and comprehensive family-centered care, but in four years of observing different family practice programs I found little systematic teaching, feedback, evaluation, and prestige value allocated to continuously monitoring the residents as they applied behavioral or psychosomatic skills in the clinical setting. Their faculty allowed behavioral science teaching in a lecture setting but maintained the sacrosanctity of the examination room; it was a rare occurrence when a behavioral scientist conferred with the resident during the clinical decision-making process. Some residents attempted to more actively use the anthropologist – but the faculty dissuaded each attempt.

3. Very useful efforts in identifying divergencies and suggesting strategies for negotiation have been undertaken by Harwood (1971, and personal communication), Korsch and Negrete (1972), Davis (1971), and Kleinman (1978).

REFERENCES

Bandler, Richard and John Grinder
   1975 The Structure of Magic, Vol. I, II. Cupertino, California: Meta Publications.
Barbour, Allen B.
   1975 Humanistic Patient Care: A Comparison of the Disease Model and the Growth Model. In Dimensions of Humanistic Medicine. S. Miller, N. Remen, A. Barbour, M. Nakles, S. Miller, D. Garell, eds. San Francisco: Institute for Humanistic Medicine.
Becker, Marshall H.
   1976 Sociobehavioral Determinants of Compliance. In Compliance with Therapeutic Regimens. David L. Sackett and R. Brian Haynes, eds. pp. 40–50. Baltimore: Johns Hopkins University Press.

Bryan, James E.
    1979 View from the Hill. American Family Physician 19:239–247.
Carlton, Wendy
    1979 In Our Professional Opinion . . . The Primacy of Clinical Judgement Over Moral
          Choice. Notre Dame, Indiana: University of Notre Dame Press.
Charney, Evan
    1972 Patient-Doctor Communication. Pediatric Clinics of North America 19(2):263–
          279.
Davis, M. S.
    1971 Variations in Patient's Compliance with Doctor's Orders: Medical Practices and
          Doctor-Patient Interaction. Psychiatry in Medicine 2:31–54.
Donnelly, Julie C.
    1979 The Internship Experience: Coping and Ego Development in Young Physicians.
          Unpublished Ph.D. dissertation. Harvard University.
Drossman, Douglas A.
    1978a The Problem Patient, Evaluation and Care of Medical Patients with Psychosocial
          Disturbances. Annals of Internal Medicine 88:366–372.
    1978b Can the Primary Care Physician be Better Trained in the Psychosocial Dimensions
          of Patient Care? International Journal of Psychiatry in Medicine 92:169–184.
Eddy, Elizabeth and William Partridge, eds.
    1978 Applied Anthropology in America. New York: Columbia University Press.
Engel, George L.
    1977 The Need for a New Medical Model: A Challenge for Biomedicine. Science 196
          (4286):129–136.
Fabrega, Horacio
    1975 The Position of Psychiatry in the Understanding of Human Disease. Archives of
          General Psychiatry 32:1500–1512.
Favazza, Armando
    1978 Overview: Foundations of Cultural Psychiatry. American Journal of Psychiatry
          135(3):293–303.
Fink, D. L.
    1976 Tailoring the Consensual Regimen. *In* Compliance with Therapeutic Regimens.
          David L. Sackett and R. Brian Haynes, eds. pp. 110–118. Baltimore: Johns
          Hopkins University Press.
Gazda, G. M., R. P. Walters, and W. D. Childers
    1975 Human Relations Development: A Manual for Health Sciences. Boston: Allyn
          and Bacon.
Goodenough, Ward H.
    1961 Comment on Cultural Evolution. Daedalus 90:521–528.
Green, Lawrence W., Stanley Werlin, Helen Schauffler, and Charles Avery
    1977 Research and Demonstration Issues in Self-Care: Measuring the Decline of Medico-
          centrism. Appendix D. *In* Consumer Self-Care in Health. National Center for
          Health Services Research, Research Proceedings Series. DHEW, HRA 77–3181.
          pp. 20–36.
Hall, Edward T.
    1976 Beyond Culture. New York: Anchor Press.
Harwood, Alan
    n.d.   Communicating about Disease: Clinical Implications of Divergent Concepts
          among Patients and Physicians. Personal communication, manuscript.
    1971 The Hot-Cold Theory of Disease: Implications for Treatment of Puerto Rican
          Patients. Journal of the American Medical Association 216:1153–1155.
Ingelfinger, Franz J.
    1978 Medicine: Meritorious or Meretricious. Science 200(6):942–946.

Janis, I. L.
   1958 Psychological Stress. New York: Wiley.
Keesing, Roger M.
   1979 Linguistic Knowledge and Cultural Knowledge: Some Doubts and Speculations.
         American Anthropologist 81(1):14–36.
King, Lewis M.
   1978 Social and Cultural Influences on Psychopathology. Annual Reviews in Psy-
         chology 29:405–433.
Kleinman, Arthur
   1978 Clinical Relevance of Anthropological and Cross-Cultural Research: Concepts and
         Strategies. American Journal of Psychiatry 135(4):427–431.
Kleinman, Arthur, Leon Eisenberg, and Byron Good
   1978 Culture, Illness, and Care. Annals of Internal Medicine 88:251–258.
Korsch, B. and Negrete, V. F.
   1972 Doctor-Patient Communication. Scientific American 227:66–74.
Lander, Louis
   1978 Defective Medicine: Risk, Anger and the Malpractice Crisis. New York: Farrar,
         Straus and Giroux.
Lazurus, R. S.
   1966 Psychological Stress and the Coping Process. New York: McGraw Hill.
Lipowski, Z. J.
   1970 Physical Illness, the Individual, and the Coping Process. Psychiatry in Medicine 1
         (April):91–102.
Lipowski, Z. J., Don Lipsett and Peter Whybrow, eds.
   1977 Psychosomatic Medicine. New York: Oxford University Press.
Lowy, Frederick H.
   1977 Management of the Persistent Somatizer. In Psychosomatic Medicine. Z. J.
         Lipowski, Don Lipsett and Peter Whybrow, eds. pp. 510–522. New York: Oxford
         University Press.
Mawardi, Betty H.
   1979 Satisfactions, Dissatisfactions, and Causes of Stress in Medical Practice. Journal
         of American Medical Association 241(14):1483–1486.
Pfifferling, John-Henry
   1975 Some Issues in the Considerations of Western and Non-Western Practices as
         Epidemiologic Data. Social Science and Medicine 9:655–658.
   n.d.   Present Medical Education is Obsolete. Mimeograph, Dept. of Anthropology,
         University of North Carolina, Chapel Hill.
   1977 Records and Revitalization: The Problem-Oriented Medical Record System in
         a Clinical Setting. Ph.D. dissertation. The Pennsylvania State University. No.
         7808408. Ann Arbor: University Microfilms International.
Pattison, E. Mansell
   1977 Psychosocial Interpretations of Exorcism. Journal of Operational Psychiatry VIII,
         No. 2:5–21.
Roter, Debra L.
   1977 Patient Participation in the Patient-Provider Interaction: The Effects of Patient
         Question Asking on the Quality of Interaction, Satisfaction and Compliance.
         Health Education Monographs 5(4):281–315.
Sackett, David L. and R. Brian Haynes, eds.
   1976 Compliance with Therapeutic Regimens. Baltimore: Johns Hopkins University
         Press.
Sigerist, Henry E.
   1952 Living Under the Shadow. In When Doctors Are Patients. Max Pinnel and Ben-
         jamin Miller, eds. New York: Norton.

Somers, A. R., et al.
  1976 Preventive Medicine USA: Health Promotion and Consumer Health Education.
         New York: Prodist.
Spiegel, John P.
  1959 Some Cultural Aspects of Transference and Countertransference. *In* Individual
         and Family Dynamics. Jules Masserman, ed. pp. 160–182. New York: Grune and
         Stratton.
  1976 Cultural Aspects of Transference and Countertransference Revisited. Journal of
         the American Academy of Psychoanalysis 4(4):447–467.
Wallston, Kenneth A., and Barbara S. Wallston
  1978 Health Locus of Control. Health Education Monographs 6(2):101–170.
Weed, Lawrence L.
  1978 Your Health Care and How To Manage It. Vermont: Essex Publishing.
Zborowski, Mark
  1969 People in Pain. San Francisco: Jossey-Bass.

JOHN D. STOECKLE AND ARTHUR J. BARSKY

10. ATTRIBUTIONS: USES OF SOCIAL SCIENCE
KNOWLEDGE IN THE 'DOCTORING' OF PRIMARY CARE

> "The process is not physical, it's mental, and if your mind
> says you're weak, you'll be tired physically. Your mind is
> where you control everything. What you think is what
> you are."
>
> Alex Grammas,
> Manager, Milwaukee Brewers

I. WHY CONNECT SOCIAL SCIENCE KNOWLEDGE TO PRIMARY CARE?

As primary care medicine assumes greater stature, so increase public and academic pressures for its improvement. The same scientific rationalization of the doctor's interventions for acute medical disease in the hospital is now expected of the doctor's acts in medical practice. These represent new pressures because, in the past, the doctor's job outside the hospital was regarded as mere vocational work, quite apart from, and of little concern to, the academic and scientific enterprise of the university medical school. The current modern renewal of primary care is now within the medical school. In this new setting, it is argued, the traditional clinical sciences alone cannot rationalize the doctor's tasks of care and application of the behavioral sciences becomes necessary. Thus, both behavioral scientists and clinical teachers are trying to make "doctoring" more scientific, struggling to relate social science knowledge to the doctor's job. By doing so, they hope to improve, as the public expects, the care of patients. Yet such knowledge and clinical work cannot be automatically linked when that social science knowledge has often been developed out of interests other than what the doctor does and when the doctor's own reflective analyses of the processes of care have been scant indeed — hence the struggle to make useful connections. This paper is one example of such an effort, an exercise in relating social science knowledge and clinical action. It identifies the doctor's tasks of primary care, illustrates the use of attributions in these tasks, and then reviews the literature about attributions from anthropology, medical sociology, social psychology, and clinical medicine.

II. THE USE OF ATTRIBUTIONS IN THE CLINICAL TASKS OF
PRIMARY CARE

Clinical teachers and behavioral scientists regularly admonish medical students to examine patients' perspectives on their illness: their views are essential for proper patient care. Yet one feature of that perspective, their illness attribution,

223

L. Eisenberg and A. Kleinman (eds.), The Relevance of Social Science for Medicine, 223–240.
Copyright © 1980 by D. Reidel Publishing Company.

what patients think has caused their illness, is often neglected when doctors question, listen and respond to patients. If practitioners neglect what the patient thinks has made him sick, however, the same cannot be said for anthropologists, medical sociologists and social psychologists, all of whom have carefully studied illness attributions. Regrettably, their perspectives are not always directly related to patient care. Concerned with the diffusion of innovation, anthropologists note how folk medical beliefs may impede the adoption of modern public health practices; medical sociologists, concerned with the use of services, report how popular medical ideas may account for doctor visits; while social psychologists have analyzed the dynamics of attributions, the process by which notions of causation develop to explain everyday human experiences, only some of which may be illness. Most practitioners and students find these contributions, however interesting, not particularly useful in their personal work with patients.

If attributions are often ignored despite pedagogical advice and social science knowledge about them, it is because their uses in everyday medical practice have not been made explicit: in what tasks of care, for what patients, and in what clinical disorders might attributions be important?

To connect the body of knowledge about attributions specifically with vocational use in medical practice, this paper first defines the several tasks of primary care and then demonstrates by case examples how the patient's attributions can be used in those tasks of "doctoring": (1) medical diagnosis and treatment, (2) personal support, (3) communication of information about illness, (4) maintenance and rehabilitation of the chronically ill, (5) psychological diagnosis and treatment, and (6) prevention of disability and disease through education, persuasion, and preventive treatment (Stoeckle 1979).

III. ATTRIBUTION, A PROCESS AND CONTENT

Before any illustrations, a word about definitions. Attribution theory from social psychology is based on the common observation that *human beings try to understand their experiences and perceptions by assigning causes to them* (Shaver 1975). One example is illness. Persons respond to a bodily discomfort by attributing it to a cause that may fall into one or more of four general categories: events prior to the onset, actions of the individual or of another person, the physical environment, or medical disease and its presumed biophysical basis. The first step in deriving an attribution is the patient's explanation of what he believes is "wrong" with him, what he thinks he "has," an attribution that others might call the "self-diagnosis" or "label." This is then followed by the patient's etiologic notions of what has caused the illness. Causes often involve the assignment of blame which may be directed internally to the self, externally to another person or to the physical environment (Bard 1956; Lipowski 1969; Young 1976). In this paper the *illness attribution* refers both to the cognitive processes by which an individual arrives at an explanatory belief and also to the explanation itself.

Given the interactional nature of the doctor-patient encounter it follows that attributions are important to each. For the patient distressed by bodily feelings, a causal explanation provides some control of them. First, knowing a cause can reduce the anxiety aroused by the discomfort. Even in situations in which the information cannot be used to alter the cause, the explanation of "what is it" and "what is it from" can, *by itself*, reduce anxiety (Vernon 1971; Fox 1959). When the causal "blame" of car accidents, machine breakdowns, or natural disasters is assigned to an agent over which the individual has some control, helplessness is reduced; one is no longer the unsuspecting victim of senseless catastrophe (Walster 1966). Second, causal explanations indicate activities, self-treatment, lay and medical consultation that may also be pursued to control the discomfort and decrease helplessness (Martin 1967). In effect, *causal explanations provide control because they give personal meaning to bodily discomfort as well as suggesting actions to take.*

For the doctor's work, illness attributions are important precisely because they reveal the meanings patients attach to those symptoms, disabilities, or diseases which they bring to the medical visit. And it is this meaning of illness that determines, in turn, the patient's illness behaviors, coping responses, and emotional reactions (Lipowski 1969; Lipowski 1974) which also may be brought to the doctor's attention (Engel 1973). Taking the patient's attributions into account by acknowledgement, interpretation, or redefinition, facilitates the several caring tasks of the doctor as the following reports of visits between doctors and patients illustrate. These visits are reported from two medical practices, the Ambulatory Screening Clinic, a walk-in service, and the Internal Medicine Associates, a teaching group practice of the Massachusetts General Hospital.

Personal Support

Patients are more likely to feel genuinely supported when they sense that the doctor's behavior expresses a concern based on a personal understanding of them than when it only shows authoritative medical competence. Because attribution is a sensitive indicator of the patient's perceptions, its recognition is one demonstration of that understanding.

On initial contact patients may be reluctant to divulge their ideas for fear these will be regarded as unsophisticated, foolish or so irrational that they themselves will be met with amusement, disrespect, or even reproach. Yet after a relationship has been established, a respectful, persistent inquiry and non-judgmental stance will typically elicit the patient's ideas. Patients can be directly asked what they think is causing their distress. The initial blank response of "I don't know," or "You're the doctor," as if the doctor is giving up his expected competence to the patient, may well vanish when the doctor answers, "Well, most people have some ideas of their own about what brought on their sickness." Indirect questions may also be revealing, as for example, "Well, what does your husband, wife, or family think is the cause?"

That attention to the patient's attributions can be an expression of personal support is illustrated by the following visit.

Encounter 1: Elicitation and Acknowledgement
A 50-year-old engineer with chronic obstructive lung disease complained of increased dyspnea and a sensation of "bubbles" felt in his lower chest. Asked what he thought prevented his improvement, he attributed his dyspnea to the physical condition of "bubbles" in his "mucous" which prevented expectoration. He mentioned this to his previous physician whom he perceived "making fun" of the idea. The patient resented the doctor's response but did not mention it. Instead, he requested a referral. After eliciting this attribution and the patient's report of the referring doctor's response, the consulting doctor acknowledged that this perception and condition might well exist, but that other factors could also explain the difficulty. The patient then remarked he felt "someone" was interested in him and in "why he wasn't getting better."

In this encounter the doctor elicited the patient's attributions and did not reject his physical-anatomical explanations; the patient, in turn, expressed confidence that he was accepted along with his ideas.

The Communication of Information about Illness

Looking at such other tasks as information transmittal, anthropologists, in particular Kleinman (1973; 1975), an anthropologist and psychiatrist, have noted that *explanation* is one of the major functions of any system of medical care (and its practitioners) whether it be scientific, folk, or primitive medicine. Moreover, general agreement exists that explanation of illness enhances the patient's autonomy, cooperation and capacity for self-care (Waitzkin 1972; 1976). Yet information about illness is the most common unmet request that patients make of doctors (Reader 1957). Effective explanation requires that the patient's conceptions of illness be explored and differences with the doctor be acknowledged, interpreted, and, if possible, resolved. The following visit is illustrative.

Encounter 2: Redefinition
An 18-year-old female student was found to have albuminuria. Studies of renal function were normal. She reported being told she had "kidney trouble." Without apparent explanation, she became depressed. Another opinion was obtained. For what was diagnosed as postural albuminuria, only periodic examination of urine for albumin was recommended. With this advice the patient's mood rapidly improved. She reported relief because she now knew she "wasn't going to die." Further questioning revealed she had read about "kidney trouble" and concluded all such patients were "doomed," or subject to dialysis or transplants. With adequate explanation of the variety of renal disorders and discussion of the goals of her management, she felt greatly relieved.

In this everyday practice situation failure to elaborate explanation of diagnosis and prognosis by eliciting the patient's conceptions of "kidney trouble" led to a frightened and depressed patient.

Maintenance of the Chronically Ill and Prevention

That prevention and maintenance treatment of chronic medical disorders depend on the patient's cooperation is now a widely-acknowledged popular theme, and in that cooperation attributions may prove essential. Since the patient's etiologic notions often radically differ from the doctor's a prescribed regimen may thereby seem illogical, to be ignored by the patient's "common sense." Examples are common enough in the literature on compliance and patients' beliefs. Thus, some peptic ulcer patients are reported to believe that acid (which they feel brings on ulcers) comes from ingested foods rather than gastric secretions (Roth 1962), so they do not take the usual between-meal snacks and antacids. Here ethnicity and religious beliefs complicate matters. The Puerto Ricans' humoral theory of disease dictates diets and activities often contradictory to those medically prescribed (Harwood 1971). For such patients with heart failure, orange juice advised as a potassium supplement with diuretics seems harmful since oranges are believed to exacerbate, rather than improve, the imbalance of "hot and cold humors" from which the patient suffers. Other wide discrepancies between advice and beliefs have been observed among Mexican-Americans who believe that suffering is intimately related, via religious design and interpersonal interaction, to the illness of others in their social network (Kiev 1968). This group of patients may not take medication because they are skeptical of "scientific" medical advice which only focuses on their medical history without acknowledging aspects of their religious or social life that they believe may also be causative.

Despite these conflicting ideas about causation between doctors and patients, successful treatment may still be accomplished. By eliciting the patient's etiological and pathophysiological ideas, the doctor and patient can then discuss, negotiate and bargain for cooperation.

In the following visit a misattribution that interfered with preventive treatment was elicited.

Encounter 3: Reinterpretation

A 58-year-old white male returned for a routine blood pressure check having been well controlled on diuretics when seen six months before. His blood pressure was once again elevated. He disclosed that he had discontinued his "water pills" because he felt he no longer had any serious problems with his "urine." The medication no longer produced a diuresis as it had at the beginning of treatment. The patient believed that diuretics prescribed for his hypertension were only needed when producing more "water." Actually, he was having nocturia, and on further questioning, hesitancy and dribbling as symptoms of bladder obstruction from benign prostatic hypertrophy. He accepted the explanation that his nocturia was due to prostatic enlargement and the reinterpretation of the use of diuretics for his "blood pressure." He then took medication regularly and regained his improved condition.

In giving a common chronic medication this patient's attributions had not been explored. Once his ideas were elicited and corrected, he again took the required medication.

Psychological Diagnosis and Treatment

Attributions are helpful too in the doctor's psychological diagnosis and treatment tasks. They assist him in managing symptomatic states, emotional reactions to disease, and in understanding the patient's psychology.

Managing Symptomatic States

Much of ambulatory care involves patients who have bodily complaints for which no organic etiology is found. In caring for such patients, often perjoratively labeled the "worried well," both the complaint and the attribution require attention. The attribution is a useful focus of treatment since it alone may produce an anxiety state more discomforting than the bodily distress itself. In many instances, the patient only seeks help because of his worry over his "own diagnosis," not his distress: "Doctor, I want to know if it's my nerves or my heart." Many other patients are too embarrassed to mention such concerns spontaneously. These issues are illustrated by the following visit:

Encounter 4: Redefinition
A 30-year-old unemployed printer complained of aching distress in his left axila for four weeks. He had a past history of pneumothorax. Physical exam was normal. He had attended the Emergency Ward because he thought he might have a recurrence of pneumothorax. After a complete examination and chest X-ray, his distress was explained as "muscular strain," but his symptoms did not go away with the local treatment and restricted activity were advised. He again sought medical aid. Questioned on his "other ideas" about what might cause his symptoms to persist, he volunteered he might have enlarged glands or lymphoma. In explaining how he arrived at this attribution he revealed that in the last year he experienced several events that seemed to him signals of "serious disease." First, pneumothorax developed spontaneously, followed by the "flu," then he lost his job, and, during his recent physical exam, he was told he had "muscular strain" that did not "go away." These events led him to think he must have a "serious disease" like lymphoma that his father had died from several years previously. The patient was quite relieved after recounting these past experiences and receiving specific reassurance about not having lymphoma. When he called several weeks later, he was completely "cured" and was optimistic about himself.

Looking for this patient's attributions led to specific redefinition, reassurance and clarification of the underlying emotional distress. By contrast, use of only general reassurance, e.g., "you're all right," is often ineffective, because, as Sapira notes, it does not acknowledge the patient's specific understanding of his condition (Sapira 1972). Mechanic's interpretations of the bodily complaints observed in medical students also confirm Sapira, especially his observation that complaints may result from the reattribution of significant pathology to common bodily feelings previously considered minor, transient, and insignificant (Mechanic 1972; Sapira 1972). This occurs for two reasons. Initially the stress of medical school heightens the awareness of bodily feelings and evokes the somatic symptoms of anxiety. In the process of acquiring new and detailed, but as yet incomplete knowledge about disease, the student then identifies and gives meaning to these previously neglected bodily feelings. Successful management consists of eliciting attributions and then of correcting the misattribution that benign transitory bodily sensations are due to serious disease.

The attributional perspective is also useful in taking a fresh look at the literature on symptom perception and tolerance, pain in particular, since it is known that experimentally induced pain differs significantly from that caused by disease. Individuals show less tolerance for, more vasomotor signs with, and less analgesic relief from pain produced by a disease, than from pain produced by an experiment (Beecher 1959; Weisenberg 1975). Pain responses are more intense with the threatening question of attribution – of underlying disease with possible serious prognosis. Experiments demonstrate that subjects could better stand painful electric shocks when they believed the induced vasomotor symptoms were due to a placebo taken before the experiment than when they attributed them to the emotional tension of the pain experience itself (Jones 1972).

In Zborowski's much-quoted study of cultural factors in pain both Jews and Italians responded to pain in an expressive, emotional fashion (Zborowski 1952), yet their treatment differed because of their attributions. Italians ceased complaining once analgesia was obtained since their concern was the pain experience itself. Jews were reluctant to take medication, since they were concerned with the meaning of pain – with its implications of serious pathology. It follows that the control of pain in chronic disorders can be improved when the attributions attached to it are understood. Asking what is causing the pain *and* what the cause means about the patient and his future health often uncovers deeply held concerns. As a result of the shared information both patient and doctor have greater engagement in the therapeutic relation in which the doctor can then try to deal realistically with the patient's concerns, providing information and reassurance that may alter the meaning and, in turn, the experience of pain.

Managing Emotional Reactions to Disease

The emotional reactions that occur with chronic medical disorders are also amenable to a therapeutic approach that explores attributions. General or "constitutional" symptoms such as fatigue, weakness, and malaise that occur in patients with chronic disease may be misattributed by the patient (and frequently by the doctor as well) to the continued activity of the disease rather than to a depressive or anxiety reaction. Because of the misattribution the patient may restrict activities and prolong convalescence.

For example, clinicians have noted that patients with myocardial infarction perceive their disorder not only as a potential threat to life but also as an indication of persistent bodily fragility. They may become fearful of physical activities and emotions which they see as capable of precipitating sudden death. In such patients, Klein et al. (1965) have described prolonged invalidism when palpitations, dyspnea and fatigue are misattributed to continued cardiac disease, when in fact there was no evidence for it. In the rehabilitation of cardiac patients, others have noted the importance of specifying which symptoms are actually somatic symptoms of anxiety rather than of persistent cardiac disease (Bellak 1956). With infectious diseases the recovery may similarly be delayed. In cases of brucellosis and influenza, Imboden and colleagues observed that some patients recovered without any objective evidence of active infection yet continued to have symptoms (Imboden et al. 1959; Imboden, Canter, and Leighton 1961), experiencing malaise, fatigue, lack of interest and other symptoms of depression. The authors observed that recovery was delayed because patients and their physicians tended to misattribute these symptoms to continued active infection.

Recuperating patients cope not only with their symptoms and disability but with their etiologic beliefs as well. It then becomes crucial to elicit attributions and to arrive at the correct explanation for the troublesome symptoms. These steps themselves may provide emotional relief or uncover disabling depression and anxiety states that may be treated in medical, social work or psychiatric practice. The following patient was treated in medical practice.

Encounter 5: Reinterpretation
A 60-year-old woman with known arteriosclerotic heart disease and mild hypertension returned with new complaints of weakness, anorexia, weight loss and insomnia. She knew what medical disorders she had and attributed her new symptoms to worsening of her condition. A careful physical examination, laboratory and X-ray studies were carried out over three visits. These studies, which reassessed her heart disease, revealed that her objective physical status was unchanged. Although informed about the medical findings this information and communication was only partially successful in relieving her symptoms. Questioned about her "other ideas," she noted that "nerves" might be an explanation of her condition because of a recent death in the family. She agreed to discuss her personal concerns about it. When her continued grief from the loss of a relative was explored, she had further improvement to her usual status.

In this encounter elicitation of attributions suggested another explanation of the patient's symptoms and their treatment. Once this clarification was made, improvement followed.

Understanding the Patient's Psychology

Since attributions are beliefs which are elaborated as a means of coping with the stress of being ill, their specific content, then, is shaped by the patient's personality, prior knowledge and experience, cultural beliefs and characteristic defense mechanisms.

A clue to a patient's predominant defenses may be suggested by his attributions. For example, persons who tend to blame themselves when things go wrong also view illness as their own fault as something they have brought upon themselves; those who typically see themselves as helpless and at the mercy of their environment tend to see illness as something externally inflicted upon them.

Encounter 6: Uncovering Defenses
A 50-year-old delivery man developed a myocardial infarct. He attributed this to his work and to the manipulation of a joint that was done four weeks prior to his illness. Despite education about the risk factors in coronary heart disease, he persisted with his own attributions. Even though he did not have functional or symptomatic impairment he insisted on retiring from work because of his belief about its ill effects on his heart; he also pursued legal action concerning the manipulation prior to his illness. The patient's explanations were

in keeping with other tendencies he displayed, such as suspiciousness, readily imagined insult and quick hostility. Not surprisingly, intravenous fluids and the placement of a temporary pacemaker were refused and viewed as harmful.

The attributions here were external. Knowledge about them was not specifically used in treatment; however, they were signals to the doctor to adapt a very formal relationship with the patient to avoid becoming an object of the patient's suspicions.

Though it is speculative, we are impressed with the possibility that the individual who forms external illness attributions is more likely to resort to anger and projective behavior under stress whereas the individual who tends to blame himself for his disorder is more prone to depression. These observations are consistent with intrapsychic theory. The tendency to see malevolent external forces as responsible for one's unhappiness is basically a paranoid mechanism, while a postulated mechanism of depression is the notion of diminished self-esteem from seeing oneself as unworthy.

If reviewing the clinical vignettes reported here, strict attribution theorists in the social sciences — whether social psychologists, anthropologists or medical sociologists — might complain that the causal notions we observed have been confused with what strict labeling theorists in those same disciplines would call labels or self-diagnosis. Or, put another way, what the patient thinks has *caused* his illness is confused with what he thinks his illness *is*. In medical practice these usual analytic distinctions disappear since what the patient thinks he has carries its own etiologic ideas. Thus, the patient's initial "self-diagnosis" response that "I think my pain is heart trouble" is an illness attribution (not only self-diagnosis) that itself contains more causal notions, e.g., "smoking did it." In effect, "self-diagnosis," if that term is used, is the first step in the attribution process of explaining illness.

These several medical visits illustrate that the patient's illness attribution and its logic can be learned in the clinical encounter to useful effect in the tasks of care. Clinical teachers can thus demonstrate practical use of this information that is social, cultural, and personal, constructed out of the patient's medical knowledge, beliefs, and personal meanings. Even though teachers demonstrate practical clinical uses of attributions, this alone is insufficient instruction. Pedagogy also requires that patients' ideas have a scientific explanation of their origin and development. For understanding these important cognitive notions of patients in "the clinical science of care," teachers and beginning practitioners need to know the correlative behavioral science knowledge that has been learned about attributions from anthropology, sociology, and clinical practice. So that teachers may illustrate the behavioral science of attributions, this paper selectively reviews the literature.

IV. WHERE DO ATTRIBUTIONS COME FROM?

Unlike the current scientific explanations of disease which are organized in up-to-date medical texts, the patient's cognitive notions about the cause of illness are often reported under headings other than attribution and are scattered in both the social science and clinical literature. When, for example, sociologists write about *lay knowledge of illness*, when anthropologists record the health and *illness beliefs of other cultures*, and when clinicians retell their colleagues the *personal meaning of illness* in the course of what they have learned from patients, the content of each of these topics is illness attributions. These three topics are selectively reviewed because they contain facts about the social, cultural, and personal origins of patients' attributions.

Knowledge about Illness

Many populations have been surveyed to determine their etiologic and pathophysiological knowledge of common symptoms and diseases. Some studies, for example, Mabry's (Mabry 1964), used samples of the general population, questioning rural and urban residents as to their causal notions. Answers varied with residence, age, sex, marital status, but typical attributions in both groups included exposure to the "elements," "germs," "allowing myself to become rundown," "nerves," and "diet." Other field studies have reported the public's knowledge about heart disease and cancer. In a work typical of this approach, Samora and others sampled causal knowledge about ten common chronic diseases in both patient and general population samples (Samora 1962). Here level of knowledge depended on the particular disease in question and varied positively with the respondent's socio-economic and educational level. More recently, Monteiro has reviewed the literature pertaining to heart disease (Monteiro 1979).

In general, such studies only report the "correctness" of the respondent's answers, that is, the degree of congruence between lay explanations and those generally held to be correct, or between the patient's explanations and those of the doctor. In the first instance, the incongruence has been used to explain why the public's health practices may diverge from professional recommendations and therefore implies a need for improving the public's education about disease in order to reduce the divergence between lay and professional knowledge and common action for prevention. In the second, the patient's knowledge may be found "inadequate for optimal patient-physician cooperation in the management of illness" (Seligman 1957), hence an argument for the doctor (or others) to provide more health education in their encounters with patients.

Besides these field surveys of lay and patient knowledge, researchers have examined the beliefs of patients with specific diseases. Elder (1973) found rheumatoid arthritics offering such etiological explanations as aging, climate, working conditions, and "exposure to the elements." In another study of arthritic patients, Markson (1971) discovered that they gave similar explanations of their joint disease. He also observed a pervasive notion of victimization by external agents as an attribution. Patients felt that because of their own frailty, these events were not successfully withstood and they became ill. Among cancer patients, Bard and Dyk (1956) noted somewhat different attributions, often of blame directed at themselves or at an external force. The explanation often took one of two forms, either acts, habits, or thoughts for which that patient felt guilty or responsible (and for which he blamed himself), or external occurrences, such as interpersonal friction, the hostility of others, or supernatural or environmental events. Abrams and Finesinger (1953) also reported the attribution of blame by cancer patients to either themselves or others. Among the reasons for self-blame were previous venereal disease, "sin or misdeed," "own negligence," "not smart enough to recognize cancer," an old injury; among the reasons for blaming others were inheritance or contagion, strenuous care of another, blow by relative or spouse, failure of doctor. Besides these external notions other researchers have observed that being "hexed" by someone may cause illness, disease, or even death (Tingling 1967; Hackett 1961).

Another helpful approach to patient knowledge of illness has been to ask in open-ended, non-structured fashion about their mechanical and biophysical conceptions of the bodily changes of disease. Thus Bellak, for example, notes that peptic ulcers are often viewed as putrid and festering, that a purulent cough is indicative of something dirty or hidden inside, and that infections are often seen as an irresistable attack by "bugs" which are often anthropomorophized. A malignant tumor may be viewed as an invading enemy of cells that renders the patient passive and helpless (Bellak 1952). Cassell (1976) has noted that most diseases and symptoms are viewed as intrusive objects, rather than as a part of the sufferer. This view is revealed in the language patients used when speaking about their illnesses. Aside from attention to their diction and use of metaphor by patient, their using "the" and "it," rather than "I" and "my" indicated how patients had separated themselves (and their bodies) from their illnesses.

Health and Illness Beliefs

Despite the widespread publicity given to the "scientific" conception of disease in our society, a patient's particular illness attribution is often embedded in older culturally determined systems of belief about health and illness. King, Fabrega, Kleinman, to name three, have described the content of key general belief systems – the scientific, primitive, and folk (King 1962; Fabrega 1973; Kleinman 1973).

Among these systems, scientific medicine assumes "natural" causes which can be elucidated through the scientific method of observation, description, and classification; hence it takes on machine or mechanical images or more recently, chemical ones. Primitive medicine is founded on the belief that both animate and inanimate objects have the power to produce good or evil so that disease is then magically caused by the malintent of an individual or supernatural power. The etiological and therapeutic beliefs of folk medicine rest upon their promulgation by authoritative and respected members of the social group.

Folk and primitive beliefs persist today, even in the attributions offered by the modern "well-educated" patient, not only in those of the less educated, ethnic minorities. In a small sample of middle-class French professionals, Herzlich

(1973) found that illness attributions were either exogenous social forces such as "way of life," "crowded cities," "bad" air and food, or endogenous individual factors such as "temperament," "constitution," "disposition," and "resistence."

It may come as a shock to learn that patients may hold other beliefs simultaneously with scientific explanations. The former are seen most clearly when the seriousness, threat, and ambiguity of the illness (e.g., colds, backache, headache) are relatively low; they are seen more often among patients from unassimilated ethnic groups (Snow 1975). These simultaneous attributions may lead to self-treatment, such as the use of poultices, the "laying on the hands," and the consumption of household remedies and patent medicine that may be discrepant with professional advice.

In addition to documenting the persistence of primitive and folk medicine in modern cultures, anthropologists, in particular Kleinman, have noted the central function of all medical systems: that they give meaning to illness by naming and defining its cause (Kleinman 1973). Despite the technological character of modern "scientific" medicine, this explanatory function remains significant. In her study of the social functions of medical practice, Shuval reports that patients seek medical aid specifically for the doctor's "scientific" explanation (Shuval 1970). Finding out that the modern doctor thinks the cause is environmental or biochemical may be as comforting as a similar external explanation from folk or primitive medicine, since both, in effect, remove personal responsibility.

The Personal Meaning of Illness

Attributions not only reflect knowledge or a particular system of prevailing cultural beliefs about health and disease but they also contain highly personal meanings. As Herzlich (1973) notes, "the person as a subject of illness constitutes a mechanism for the illness to develop and so illness takes on a personal meaning." Meaning has clinical pertinence since it is a basis for the patient's affective, cognitive, and behavioral response to illness.

Among the most prevalent categories of personal meanings Lipowski considers five: illness as an enemy, as weakness, as punishment, as loss or damage, and as challenge (Lipowski 1979). It is important to remember that for the patient, each meaning has psychological and behavioral consequences. When illness is experienced as an enemy, for example, the patient acts through the use of denial, projection and paranoid thought as if he were in danger and subject to attack. This attribution may result in anxiety, fear and anger. Illness when viewed as weakness is taken as evidence of a personal failing with the result that the patient may attempt to conceal or deny his sickness. The predominant affective response here is shame. If illness is seen as punishment for the patient's actions (a meaning particularly common in children) (Langford 1961), it may be seen as just or unjust, and as allowing or not allowing atonement. Emotional reactions in this instance may reflect passive resignation, angry depression, or an elated sense of redemption. When illness means loss or damage the sense of loss may be so overwhelming and irreparable that the patient becomes hostile and deeply depressed. Should illness be seen as a challenge there is an appropriate and hopeful attempt to cope and adjust, along with moderate depression and anxiety.

Some of the psychological factors that shape the particular meaning each person makes of his illness, e.g. the symbolic significance of body sites, organs and functions, the character of the patient, and identification with significant persons who had similar illnesses (Silverman 1968), are familiar themes in the psychosomatic literature. The role of symbolic significance is illustrated by disorders which impair eating. Such impairment signifies an inability to obtain emotional support for which the patient may feel a desperate need and, in response, become especially demanding and dependent. The importance of character to meaning is illustrated by the narcissistic personality disorder in a person whose self-esteem so depends on physical appearance that even minor disfigurements hold deep meanings of diminished self-worth. Finally, meaning is often influenced by feelings a patient harbors toward someone significant in his past, especially if that person had similar symptoms or disability. If that prior relationship was ambivalent, the patient may perceive his own illness as a deserved punishment for his unacceptable, negative feelings toward that person.

For the doctor, teacher, and student, viewing the roots of illness attribution in lay knowledge, cultural beliefs, and personal meaning is a rational scheme by which they may be studied, understood, and possibly changed.

V. DOES CORRECTING MISATTRIBUTION MAKE A DIFFERENCE?

Though it seems that the transmittal of detailed information about etiology, pathophysiology, and treatment rationale improves patient compliance (Reader 1957; Francis 1969; Ley 1967; Davis 1968; Abramson 1961), satisfaction (Duff 1968; Korsch 1968), and doctor-patient communication (Waitzkin 1972; Brewerton 1971; Wishnie 1971), does correcting misattributions result in improved medical outcomes? Three studies may be cited to support the assertion that corrections do matter.

Egbert et al. (1964) compared the pain responses of two groups of surgical patients. Before their operations one group received explicit information about the cause, nature, and predictability of post-operative pain and, additionally, was instructed in relaxation techniques. A second group received the usual brief preoperative visit. After operation the first group exhibited lower narcotic requirements, less emotional and physical discomfort and received earlier discharges.

Skipper and Leonard (1968) randomly assigned child tonsillectomy admissions to a control or experimental group. Experimental mothers were given a supportive and informational program about what to expect from the hospitalization experience and what might produce differing reactions to the experience. These mothers experienced less stress and evidently communicated this to their children who, in turn, post-operatively, showed significantly fewer complications, lower blood pressure, pulse and temperature elevations, improved sleep and less frequent emesis.

Insomnia was improved when Storms and Nisbett (1970) treated two groups of chronic insomniacs with placebo in a more manipulative reattribution of symptoms. One group was told that the placebo itself produced increased alertness, arousal and heart rate (symptoms which the insomniacs had described), while the other group was told the placebo would abolish these symptoms and improve sleep. The first group showed improved sleep while the insomnia of the second in fact worsened. The explanation for this paradoxical result lies in the attribution of disturbing symptoms to an external agent rather than to some internal pathological process which then decreases anxiety sufficiently to permit sleep.

VI. IS MORE KNOWLEDGE OF ATTRIBUTIONS IMPORTANT?

Reflecting on several examples of the clinical use of attributions and on the social science literature about them, clinical teachers might now promote more systematic elicitations of and response to attributions in medical practice. But this would not be enough.

Besides this important clinical and pedagogical work, much more research remains. The lines along which it should continue are varied. It would be fruitful to identify those patients in whom attributions could be expected to be an important factor in their response to illness and in their response to their physicians. Strategies and dynamics must be worked out, beyond those of simple education, to modify attributions when they are obstacles to optimal care and to coping with illness. Attributions are also an important vantage point from which to study doctor-patient communication and interaction, patient adherence to medical regimens, and the implicit, covert cognitive processes occurring in physicians when they explain illness to patients. Hardly any work has examined the doctor's views. And in a more theoretical vein, research could elucidate the relationship between attributions and personality types or defense mechanisms and, in turn, the relationship between attributions and the patient's coping strategies in adaption to disability.

Perhaps some findings from research in these several themes may then find their way into teaching and practice, making the doctor question and then respond to patients with greater understanding of their perspective, obtaining information that would enhance their care. That future promises a rationale for the doctor's communicative acts of care — and not incidentally, the improvement of treatment.

ACKNOWLEDGEMENTS

We wish to thank Arthur Peltin, University of Arizona, and Shelley Taylor, Harvard University, for introducing us to the psychological literature on attribution; Arthur Kleinman, University of Washington Medical School, for his discussions when teaching students in our practice about the issues of attribution in clinical care; and Howard Waitzkin, University of California, Berkeley, for his formative influences on our thinking about communication with patients.

REFERENCES

Abrams, R. D. and J. E. Finesinger
  1953 Guilt Reactions in Patients with Cancer. Cancer 6:474–482.
Abramson, J.
  1961 What Is Wrong with Me? A Study of the Views of African and Indian Patients in a Durban Hospital. South African Medical Journal 35:690–694.
Bard, M. and R. B. Dyk
  1956 The Psychodynamic Significance of Beliefs Regarding the Cause of Serious Illness. Psychoanalytic Review 43:146–162.
Beecher, H. K.
  1959 Measurement of Subjective Responses: Quantitative Effects of Drugs. New York: Oxford University Press.
Bellak, L. and F. Haselkorn
  1956 Psychological Aspects of Cardiac Illness and Rehabilitation. Social Casework 37: 483–489.
Bellak, L., ed.
  1952 Psychology of Physical Illness. New York: Grune and Stratton.
Brewerton, D. A. and J. W. Daniel
  1971 Factors Influencing Return to Work. British Medical Journal 4:277–281.
Cassell, E. J.
  1976 Disease as an "It": Concepts of Disease Revealed by Patients' Presentation of Symptoms. Social Science and Medicine 10:143–146.
Davis, M. S. and R. P. von der Lippe
  1968 Discharge from Hospital Against Medical Advice: A Study of Reciprocity in the Doctor-Patient Relationship. Social Science and Medicine 1:336–342.
Duff, R. S. and A. S. Hollingshead
  1968 Sickness and Society. New York: Harper and Row.
Egbert, L. D., et al.
  1964 Reduction of Post-Operative Pain by Encouragement and Instruction of Patients. New England Journal of Medicine 270:825–827.
Elder, R. G.
  1973 Social Class and Lay Explanations of the Etiology of Arthritis. Journal of Health and Social Behavior 14:28–38.
Engel, G. L.
  1973 Personal Theories of Disease as Determinants of Patient-Physician Relationships. Psychosomatic Medicine 35:184–185.
Fabrega, H.
  1973 Disease and Social Behavior. Cambridge, Mass: MIT Press.
Fox, R. C.
  1959 Experiment Perilous: Physicians and Patients Facing the Unknown. Glencoe, IL: The Free Press.
Francis, V., B. M. Korsch, and M. J. Morris
  1969 Gaps in Doctor-Patient Communication: Patients' Response to Medical Advice. New England Journal of Medicine 280:535–540.

Hackett, T. P. and A. D. Weisman
    1961 "Hexing" in Modern Medicine. Proc. Third World Congress of Psychiatry 1249–
        1252.
Harwood, A.
    1971 The Hot-Cold Theory of Disease: Implications for Treatment of Puerto Rican
        Patients. Journal of the American Medical Association 216:1153–1168.
Herzlich, C.
    1973 Health and Illness: A Social Psychological Analysis. New York: Academic Press.
Imboden, J. B., A. Canter, and E. C. Leighton
    1961 Convalescence from Influenza: A Study of Psychological and Clinical Deter-
        minants. Archives of Internal Medicine 108:393–399.
Imboden, J. B., A. Canter, L. E. Cluff, and R. W. Trever
    1959 Brucellosis III: Psychological Aspects of Delayed Convalescence. Archives of
        Internal Medicine 103:406–414.
Jones, E. E., et al.
    1972 Attribution: Perceiving the Causes of Behavior. Morrison, NJ: General Learning
        Press.
Kiev, A.
    1968 Curanderismo. Glencoe, IL: The Free Press.
King, S. H.
    1962 Perceptions of Illness and Medical Practices. New York: Russell Sage Foundation.
Kleinman, A. M.
    1973 Toward a Comparative Study of Medical Systems: An Integrated Approach to the
        Study of the Relationship of Medicine and Culture. Science, Medicine and Man
        1:55–65.
    1975 Explanatory Models in Health Care Relationships: A Conceptual Framework for
        Research on Family-Based Health Care Activities in Relation to Folk and Profes-
        sional Forms of Clinical Care. In Health and Family, Washington DC: National
        Council for International Health.
Klein, R. F., A. Dean, L. M. Willson, and M. D. Bogdonoff
    1965 The Physician and Postmyocardial Infarction Invalidism. Journal of the American
        Medical Association 194:143–148.
Korsch, B.M., E. K. Gozzi, and V. Francis
    1968 Gaps in Doctor-Patient Communication. 1. Doctor-Patient Interaction and Patient
        Satisfaction. Pediatrics 42:855–871.
Landford, W.
    1961 The Child in the Pediatric Hospital: Adaptation to Illness and Hospitalization.
        American Journal of Orthopsychiatry 31:667–684.
Ley, P., and M. S. Spelman
    1967 Communicating with the Patient. London: Staples Press.
Lipowski, Z. J.
    1969 Psychosocial Aspects of Disease. Annals of Internal Medicine 71:1197–1206.
    1974 Physical Illness, the Patient and His Environment: Psychosocial Foundations of
        Medicine. In American Handbook of Psychiatry, Vol. IV., 2nd Ed., Eds. S. Arieti,
        M. Reiser, New York: Basic Books.
    1979 Physical Illness, the Individual and the Coping Process. Psychiatry in Medicine
        1:91–102.
Mabry, J. H.
    1964 Lay Concepts of Etiology. Journal of Chronic Disease 17:371–386.
Markson, E. W.
    1971 Patient Semeiology of a Chronic Disease. Rheumatoid Arthritis. Social Science
        and Medicine 5:159–167.

Martin, H. L.
  1967 The Significance of Discussion with Patients about their Diagnosis and its Compli-
        cations. British Journal of Medical Psychology 40:233–242.
Mechanic, D. L.
  1972 Social Psychologic Factors Affecting the Presentation of Bodily Complaints. New
        England Journal of Medicine 286:1132–1139.
Monteiro, L.
  1979 Societal Views of the Cardiac Patient. In Cardiac Patient Rehabilitation. New
        York: Springer-Verlag.
Reader, G. G., L. Pratt, and M. C. Mudd
  1957 What Patients Expect from Their Doctors. Modern Hospital 80:83–95.
Roth, H. P., et al.
  1962 Patients' Beliefs About Peptic Ulcer and Its Treatment. Annals of Internal Medi-
        cine 56:72–80.
Samora, J., L. Saunders, and R. F. Larson
  1962 Knowledge About Specific Diseases in Four Selected Samples. Journal of Health
        and Human Behavior 3:176–185.
Sapira, J. D.
  1972 Reassurance Therapy: What to Say to Symptomatic Patients with Benign Diseases.
        Annals of Internal Medicine 77:603–604.
Seligman, A. W., N. E. McGrath, and L. L. Pratt
  1957 Level of Medical Information Among Clinic Patients. Journal of Chronic Diseases
        6:497–509.
Shaver, K. G.
  1975 An Introduction to Attribution Processes. Cambridge: Winthrop Publishers, Inc.
Shuval, J. T., A. Antonovsky, and A. M. Davies
  1970 Social Functions of Medical Practice: Doctor-Patient Relationships in Israel. San
        Francisco: Jossey-Bass.
Silverman, S.
  1968 Psychological Aspects of Physical Symptoms. New York: Appleton-Century-
        Crofts.
Skipper, J. K., and R. C. Leonard
  1968 Children, Stress and Hospitalization: A Field Experiment. Journal of Health and
        Social Behavior 9:275–287.
Snow, L. F.
  1975 The Humoral Pathology in Black and Southern White Folk Medicine. Paper
        presented at Southwestern Anthropological Association meeting, March 27–29,
        1975, Santa Fe, New Mexico.
Stoeckle, J. D.
  1979 The Tasks of Care: The Humanistic Dimensions of Medical Education. In Dimen-
        sions of Medical Education, Eds. W. R. Rogers, D. Barnard, Pittsburgh: University
        of Pittsburgh Press.
Storms, M. D., and R. E. Nisbett
  1970 Insomnia and the Attribution Process. Journal of Personality and Social Psychol-
        ogy 16:319–328.
Tinling, E. C.
  1967 Voodoo, Root Work and Medicine. Psychosomatic Medicine 29:483–490.
Vernon, D. T. A.
  1971 Information Seeking in a Natural Stress Situation. Journal of Applied Psychology
        55:359–363.
Walster, E.
  1966 Assignment of Responsibility for an Accident. Journal of Personality and Social
        Psychology 3:73–79.

Waitzkin, H. and J. D. Stoeckle
   1972 The Communication of Information About Illness. Advances in Psychosomatic
         Medicine 8:180–215.
   1976 Information Control and the Micropolitics of Health Care: Summary of an
         Ongoing Research Project. Social Science and Medicine 10:263–276, 1976.
Weisenberg, M.
   1975 Pain-Clinical and Experimental Perspectives. St. Louis, MO: C. V. Mosby & Co.
Wishnie, H. A., T. P. Hackett, and N. H. Cassem
   1971 Psychological Hazards of Convalescence Following Myocardial Infarction. Journal
         of the American Medical Association 215:1292–1296.
Young, A.
   1976 Some Implications of Medical Beliefs and Practices for Social Anthropology.
         American Anthropology 78:5–24.
Zborowski, M.
   1952 Cultural Components in Responses to Pain. Journal of Social Issues 8(4):16–30.

11. STRUCTURAL CONSTRAINTS IN THE DOCTOR-PATIENT RELATIONSHIP: THE CASE OF NON-COMPLIANCE

When I'm part of a medical group, and we get down to nitty-gritty issues, the most frequent question I'm asked is, "What can I do about the patient who won't take his medicine?" From a medical perspective this is what compliance is all about — how to get patients to follow a regimen which is "in their best interests." But in this seemingly straightforward task, all our best efforts seem to fail. Nearly 50% of patients stop taking their medications long before they are supposed to. Many take the wrong dose at the wrong time. And many more than we realize don't even fill their prescriptions. To paraphrase an advertising slogan, we must be doing something *wrong*.

And so *we* are. We, the health researchers and providers are doing at least two things which distort our understanding of compliance. We do not sufficiently appreciate what following a medical regimen means to an individual, nor do we fully acknowledge the role that health personnel have in contributing to the very non-compliance we seek to reverse. By examining both of these misconceptions I hope to shed some light on specific facets of the doctor-patient interaction which hinder patient compliance.

First, it is necessary to look at several disarming blind spots in regard to patient behavior.

We can start by looking at *when* people see doctors. While some people may go at the first sign of trouble, the far larger number delay and go quite reluctantly. Study after study shows that most people are fearful of seeing a doctor and that it takes a quite complex set of social events to make them go at all. (Anderson 1968; Freidson 1961; Suchman 1965; Zola 1973) Thus, patients cannot be assumed to be a group of willing supplicants, rushing with open arms to seek aid.

Secondly, the importance of the time dimension of most medical problems is too often neglected. Most problems are already chronic by the time a doctor is seen. This probably means that many people have already lived with, and perhaps adjusted to, many aspects of their conditions. It probably also means that they have done a number of things to cope with their problem, some of which have worked and some of which have not. Thus while the doctor may be expected to give some crucial aid, it will not be followed to the exclusion of all other methods. In short, it will rarely, if ever, be the only thing the patient will use.

Thirdly, disease in the modern sense is never a purely personal phenomenon, located in a single individual. It is always a social phenomenon, involving in varying degrees not only family and friends but many aspects of a person's life. Thus, to assume that an individual has the easy ability to make significant life

L. Eisenberg and A. Kleinman (eds.), The Relevance of Social Science for Medicine, 241–252.
Copyright © 1980 by D. Reidel Publishing Company.

changes without consulting others, is patent nonsense and often makes the
medical suggestion appear unrealistic. A specific example will clarify this point.
Many years ago my father, whose whole family had a history of heart disease,
was diagnosed as having 'angina.' The doctor who transmitted this information
to him was a specialist and recommended most strongly that he change jobs,
preferably to one with less physical exertion, perhaps at a desk. My father
thanked him dutifully as he left the office. The problem was that my father was
a bluecollar worker, a dress-cutter in the garment industry with a less than high
school education. He could no more get a desk job than he could climb Mt.
Everest. Unfortunately, because he regarded the doctor's basic suggestion as so
patently ridiculous, he treated the rest of his quite appropriate medical advice
with similar disdain. In other words, he non-complied.

Finally, it is no longer safe to assume that patients regard the treatment they
are asked to undertake as being entirely "for their own good" and "in their
best interests." Since the office hours, appointments, and location of visit, are
arranged for the doctor's convenience and not the patient's, the same may well
be seen for the very treatments the patients receive. I refer to all the publicity
about unnecessary surgery, the high salaries of medical personnel, the money
being made off of medicare and medicaid, the profit margins of pharmaceutical
companies, the adverse side effects of many drugs. Together they create an
unspoken suspicion in many patients' minds as to how much of what they are
receiving is really in *their* own interests.

What I am arguing in all these cases is that to "take one's medicine" is in no
sense the "natural thing" for patients to do. If anything, a safer working assumption is that most patients regard much of their medical treatment as unwanted,
intrusive, disruptive, and the manner in which it is given presumptuous.

In this sense the real work in patient care begins, not ends, when the physician
reaches for the prescription pad. The patient has to be made the ally in treatment
not the object of it. As such the instructions, the form and even dosage of
medicines must be integrated into his or her life style. If a four times a day
prescription is medically best but socially intolerable, then a one-a-day form
should not be second choice, but the best choice. What we need always to
understand is the place of the treatment in the everyday life of the patient.
Thus, we must seek analogs in people's lives compatible with taking medicine or
following a prescribed regimen.

Too much of this is done after the fact — *after* non-compliance becomes an
issue. Then it is often too late. The patient has already been disappointed and
is distrustful. The time to start is *before*. But it's hard to change, particularly
since health professionals have strong opinions about not letting the patient
know too much. In perhaps no other area of human contact has it been so
strongly and wrongly assumed that a little knowledge is a dangerous thing.

The strength and self-defeating nature of this attitude was brought home to
me at a conference I once attended on Essential Hypertension. This is one of
the most prevalent and untreated disorders in our country and one for which

there is a wide variety of available drugs. Yet this variety presents problems. It is often necessary that a sequence of medicines and perhaps even dosages must be tried until the most efficacious level is found and then it must be taken for the rest of one's life. Perhaps it is no great surprise that the non-compliance rate in regard to this disorder is extraordinarily high. When I asked my fellow medical panelists if they discussed with their patients the likelihood that the first course of treatment might not work, they answered emphatically, "NO!", arguing that such a statement would discourage their patients and stimulate non-compliance. To me it was hard to conceive that their patients' non-compliance could be any higher than it already was. My contention was that sharing with patients the possible treatment difficulties would not only be good preventitive medicine but an act of caring which would reinforce rather than erode trust. In short, if trust and confidence was not justified the first time the patient gives it, it can hardly be expected to improve the second time it is asked for.

Thus, to make the patient an ally in treatment, first we have to know where he or she is coming from, second we must regard her or him as an intelligent though anxious adult, and third we must look to their available resources.

In regard to available resources, I wish to make an important aside. For socioeconomic, and I would even say political reasons, there has been systematic neglect of an area of research — what people do to and for themselves to prevent, help, and cure a vast amount of physical and psychosocial conditions. The area is called self-treatment and the scanty data that does exist (Dunnell and Cartwright 1972, Zola 1972a) indicates that within any given 36-hour period from 67 to 80% of our adult population uses some sort of internal or external medication. The relevance of this data to the study of compliance should hopefully be obvious. For such a high prevalence of self-treatment indicates that the U.S. population as a whole is not averse to using drugs on a regular basis. What it must be averse to *is* the circumstances and purposes under which *some* drugs *must* be taken.

But as stated in my opening we need not only a better understanding of the recipient of help but also of the giver and their interaction. Too many investigations define non-compliance as almost entirely a patient issue. As such both research and programs emphasize what patient characteristics can be changed (cf. Becker and Maiman 1975 for general review). Study after study (such as Davis 1966) notes that physicians overwhelmingly attribute non-compliance to the patient's uncooperative personality or specifically blame the patient's inability to understand physicians' recommendations. In fact, the individual physician seems extraordinarily well-defended against closely examining the problems of non-compliance. Not only do doctors generally underestimate the rates of non-compliance in their practices but they are also inaccurate in identifying non-compliant individuals (Balint et al. 1970, Barsky and Gillum 1974, Davis 1966). Thus, while almost all clinicians agree that there *is* a problem, it seems to be someone else's.

The truth is, of course, closer to home. General studies of learning indicate the important role played by the transmitter of information. This role may not even be a conscious one. Several reports have noted that experimenter attitudes have even influenced the results of animal research (Freeman 1967). Surely, if the attitudes of an experimenter can effect the behavior of his rats, it is not too much to expect that the beliefs of prescribing physicians about their patients, their problems and their treatment must similarly influence the actions of those very patients.

My general contention is that there are certain structural barriers in the ordinary treatment situation which specifically impede communication. In short, the doctor-patient consult, as presently constituted, is an ill-suited one for learning to take place.

At the most general level, it is important to bear in mind that the doctor-patient encounter is perhaps the most anxiety-laden of all lay-expert consultations. Rarely does someone go for a reaffirmation of a good state. At best, they are told that they are indeed in good health and thus a previous worry should be dismissed (Zola 1972b). More likely they learn that a particular problem is not as serious as they feared. Moreover, given all the untreated medical complaints uncovered by epidemiological surveys, seeking a doctor's help is a relatively infrequent response to symptoms (Zola 1966, 1973). The visit to a doctor is likely approached with considerable caution. Delay is the statistical norm. Fear and anxiety the psychological ones. And while some anxiety has been found to be conducive to learning, the amount in the traditional doctor-patient encounter is surely excessive!

It is also not without significance that recall of the timing, if not the frequency, of doctor visitation is found to be notoriously inaccurate. In the large majority of instances the visit may well have been an experience to be finished as quickly as possible. And the most common way to deal with unpleasant events is to suppress them. In such a situation is it any surprise that a patient is likely to forget much that happened, including their physician's instructions?

But I can be more specific. At present I would contend that in the visiting of a physician, a negative context for answering and asking questions has been created — the result of both a witting and unwitting process of intimidation.

The negative context begins early. It starts with place. I am old enough to remember when the most frequent location of seeing a doctor was in my home. Whatever the 'good medical' reasons for the shift of almost all visits to hospitals, clinics, or the doctor's office (Gibson and Kramer 1965), it has resulted in a tremendous loss of the patient's power and security at a time when he or she is most vulnerable. The visit is no longer on one's home territory. Everything is now unfamiliar. There are now no social and physical supports, no easy way to relax, no private space to move around in or escape to. Moreover, while most examining rooms are physically closed to other patients and staff, they are often so audibly open that complaints and medical advice are easily overheard (Clute 1963, Stoeckle 1978). And little effort is made in medical settings to change this. If anything, the physical set-up emphasizes rather than reduces social distance between patient and the doctor, and heightens the strangeness of the encounter. Thrust amid suffering strangers one is assaulted by medical signs, equipment, uniforms and sterility. Let me be mundane. When I was a child, my mother, to make the situation more relaxed, would offer the doctor a cup of coffee or tea. Is there any remotely analogous experience to defuse or make more 'familiar' our current visits?

From place we can go to physical position. Whether it be horizontal, or in some awkward placement on one's back or stomach, with legs splayed or cramped, or even in front of a desk, the patient is placed in a series of passive, dependent, and often humiliating positions. These are positions where embarrassment and anger are at war with the desire to take in what the doctor is saying. In this battle learning is clearly the loser.

The standard gathering of essential information also brings in its wake a series of problems (cf. Waitzkin and Stoeckle 1972 for a general review). It often starts with the taking of the medical history. It's bad enough that I don't know all my family's medical diseases or of what my grandparents, whom I never knew, died, but I begin to feel positively stupid when at the mature age of forty-four I do not know whether as an infant I had the measles or chicken pox. I may do a little better with more recent conditions but the feeling sinks again when it comes to medications I've taken that have given me trouble. "Those little red pills" seems an insufficient answer and the recording physician's dubious look does not help much. It's with difficulty that I recall that prescription drugs have only been labelled within the last fifteen years. By this point in the interview when I am asked questions about the specific timing and location of my varying symptoms, I begin to answer with a specificity born more of desperation than accuracy. Any vagueness I report is responded to as related to my faulty memory than the very reality of the symptoms I am experiencing. The scenario may be different in detail from patient to patient. In short, confronted with a situation in which we already feel stupid not only sets a tone for the rest of the encounter but makes it very difficult, if not impossible, to ask the physician simple questions or admit that you do not understand certain things — no matter how much the physician may later encourage one to do so.

Another impediment to communication is the quantity of information to be transmitted in the doctor-patient encounter. Regardless of the potentially upsetting nature of the advice, there is quite simply the problem of *data-overload*. The patient is asked to remember too much, with too few tools, in too short a time. In most other teaching situations, the learner is encouraged to find ways of remembering (like taking notes). But the traditional position of the patient — without the 'set' or the implements — negates this possibility. Giving patients a printed sheet of instructions, as done occasionally in pediatric practice, is not the complete answer, but it is a start.

Next, there is the method of communication. For here is a situation where the physician attempts to distill, in several minutes, the knowledge and experience accumulated in decades. I have spent much of my professional life at

medical schools and teaching hospitals but have yet to see much explicit attention given to this problem. As is the case with college teaching, the degree is
regarded as sufficient guarantee of the ability to communicate what was learned.
But the task is not so simple. In fact, what few self-evident truths there are, are
soon forgotten. Experientially, we know that different subject matters, like
mathematics in contrast with literature, must be taught and learned in different
ways. By analogy, the same is true for a medical regimen, some things can be
told, some demonstrated, some only experienced, some written out, some stated
a single time, some repeated with variations. This in itself may lead to the further
realization that the teaching cannot be done all at once or by the same person.

On a rather mundane level, there is the matter of language which both in tone
and content often patronizes and thus further intimidates, and even confuses the
patient. First there is the manner of address. Whether it be to bridge the lack
of familiarity, physically or socially, or truly to establish authority and keep
distance, the use of first names and diminutives seems to have lost its endearing
charm. I will admit that it took the women's movement and a certain amount
of personal aging to make me realize how awkward it felt to be addressed by a
physician ten years my junior as 'Irv' while I could only call him by his attached
label, 'Dr. Smith'. But the ultimate ludicrousness was brought home by a colleague during a recent hospitalization. When visiting her I witnessed the following
interaction:

Looking down only at the chart and not at the patient in the bed, the physician said jocu-
larly, "Well Anne, how are you today?"

"Lousy, Robert how are you?"

Taken aback, he responded, "My name is Dr. Johnson, I only called you Anne to make you
feel comfortable."

"Well," my friend responded, "My name is Dr. Greene, I only called you Robert to make
you feel more comfortable."

While I'm not recommending the above dialogue as a general mode of response,
it did seem ludicrous to have my fellow colleague, herself a Ph.D. and several
years older than the M.D., addressed in such a manner. Few potential patients
would, however, be in such control as to handle the situation as did my colleague.
Given that the average time of doctor-patient interaction is so short (one estimate
is that the average visit is about five minutes with initial visits ranging to thirty,
Waitzkin and Stoeckle 1972) address itself sets a tone. Thus the use of the
diminutive and false familiarity further increases the already existing gap between
the helping provider and the anxious patient, making the latter feel even more
child-like, dependent, and intimidated.

A second aspect of tone that is worth reexamining is that most common and
important of the doctor's tools — reassurance. That even this cannot be given
without thought was illustrated in a recent study of pediatric practice (Pessen
1978). Confronted continually by what are often referred to as 'overanxious'

mothers, doctors often responded straightforwardly with, "There, there. You needn't have worried. Michael is fine." In general I've begun to realize that the admonition, 'not to worry' is perhaps the most overworked and useless advice in the English language (Janis 1958). But here in Pediatric consultation, it had a more dysfunctional effect. It was a truly double-edged sword. While, on the one hand, it did communicate to the mother that her child's condition was not medically serious, it also contained an implicit 'put down' of the mother's concern. It made her feel foolish for being bothered by something that turned out to be 'nothing'. As Pessen revealed, one of the lessons the mother learned was thus a negative one — to be more cautious in consulting a doctor, lest she look foolish. The mother, however, did not learn *what* to be cautious about, but rather in general to think twice about her next visit.

My guess is that in this situation, should the pediatrician try to correct the mother's perspective, she simply cannot take it in. Already feeling foolish for having bothered the doctor, the mother is not in a good position to learn any-thing — the information the pediatrician is trying to transmit just feels like a further scolding. What should have been communicated were *two* separate and distinct messages. First, the physician should state that the child's condition was not medically serious, i.e., nothing to worry about, then the pediatrician should probably tell her that s/he understood and appreciated her concern, i.e., given her newness as a mother and the inarticulateness of infants, a baby's signs and symptoms are naturally puzzling and disturbing. At this time, truly reassured as to both her being a good mother and the lack of medical seriousness of her child's illness, the mother can then 'hear' the pediatrician's instructions about medically appropriate 'worrisome' signs and symptoms.

My final comment on communications concerns the very words used. The technical jargon confronting a patient might be bad enough but the major confusion is the different meanings assigned to the same word by doctor and patient. I heard recently of a survey where, of all the patients who were told to take diuretics for fluid retention, over half believed that the drugs helped retain fluid and were, therefore, used to treat nocturia. They altered their use accordingly.

In many instances the process is equally insidious. For when heard by the patients, the dictionary meaning of the instructions is absolutely clear. The confusion sets in only after the consultation, when the patient is at home and must operationalize the instructions. Let me illustrate with several routine incidents.

1.   "Take this drug four times a day." Since this means taking it every six hours must I wake up in the middle of the night? What if I forget? Should I take two when I remember?

2.   "Keep your leg elevated most of the day." How high is elevated? Is it important that it be above my waist or below? How long is 'most'? What about when I sleep?

3.   "Take frequent baths." Are they supposed to be hot, cold or warm?
          Should I soak for a while? Is four times a day frequent? Does it
          matter when? Should I use some special soap?
4.   "Only use this pill if you can't stand the pain." What does "can't
          stand" mean? How long should I wait? Is it bad to take it? If I do,
          am I a weak person?
5.   "Come back if there are any complications." What is a complication?
          Must it be unbearable? What if my fingers feel a little numb? Which
          feelings are related to my problem and which to my treatment? Is
          it my fault if there are complications?

All of the issues in this paper I have delineated become even more complicated
when the health professional is treating a person wih chronic disease. When that
person is also poor and a woman they are triply cursed (Emerson 1970, Boston
Women's Health Book Collective, Cartwright 1964, Kosa and Zola, 1976). Everything becomes more complex — both in the telling and the hearing. Accordingly,
the instructions and teaching, like the disorder itself, is a long-term event. Thus,
the patient will, in the course of their disorder, inevitably have more questions,
more troubles, and more doubts. They must not be 'guilted' for things that are
just starting to bother them now. This should be regarded as the expected and
natural course of events and communicated thusly to the patient.

Finally, we come to what the reality of treating a person with a chronic
disease means for the provider of care. Particularly for physicians, this is a
frustrating task, one for which their training in acute care has left them largely
unprepared. Most of the diseases affecting us today cannot be cured, only
abated. Death cannot be defeated, only postponed. And these are realities that
both doctor and patient must deal with, not deny. Nor will the medical world's
previous defense against dealing with their own as well as their patients frustration
be any longer possible. The objectification of the patient as a disease state and
the distance this produced will no longer be tolerated. The appendicitis in Room
104 or the rheumatoid arthritis down the hall will not stand for it. There is at
long last in this country a consumer health movement. In its wake come many
demands: a demystification of expertise, a right to know everything about one's
bodies, and a sharing of power in any decision affecting one's life. Thus health
personnel are forced to look at their patients as people and in many cases
people who are quite different from themselves in gender, in class, race, ethnicity
and some of whom they may simply not like. There is no easy answer to these
new found feelings but they are there and must be dealt with.

While I have been detailed in my criticism of the present structure of the
doctor-patient relationship, I am by no means pessimistic that it will remain so.
As I just mentioned, there is a growing patient movement which will make them
continually more assertive of their rights. It is, however, necessary that the
medical world react not merely from a defensive posture. It can and should
realize that an altering of a position of dominance, while initially experienced as

loss, will in the long-run give us more freedom. (This is a lesson the women's movement is trying to teach men — that their 'liberation' will indeed help men in their own struggles to be free.)

Being mundane, a change in communication patterns with our patients can only improve our basic task. There is already research showing that the more information we share the greater is the likelihood of patient medical compliance (Davis 1968; Francis et al. 1969; Williams et al. 1967; Korsch et al. 1968). I believe that this sharing, including the sharing of uncertainty, will also decrease the psychological burden that physicians carry — a burden that I think is reflected in the alarmingly high rates of suicide, emotional breakdown, drug and alcohol addiction among health-care workers. A demystification of the doctor and his power, an opening up of communication, including angry communication between doctors and their patients, may also help stem the growing tide of malpractice suits. Part of the latter is, I believe, a response to dashed expectations. When there is no place to vent dissatisfaction within a system (i.e. the standard doctor-patient consult) the only recourse is to go outside (i.e. to seek redress in the legal system).

I am essentially arguing for more open communication between the doctor and the patient. As I have delineated in this paper, part of the barrier to such communication lies both in the unjustified assumptions about patient behavior held by the health provider as well as a series of socio-psycho-physical elements which currently structure the ordinary medical consult. Hopefully, my description of these misconceptions and these barriers has been sufficiently concrete to show how they can be dismantled.

There is, of course, much more that can be done within medical education (and health provider education in general) itself. It starts with an old truism, "Know thyself". I would expand it to say, "Know thyself and you will know your patient." Anything that will help providers be in touch with their own weaknesses as well as strengths, what upsets (as well as what satisfies) them about certain illnesses and certain patients, will contribute to this understanding. If I had to recommend a single psychological dimension with which every health provider should be in touch it would be a sense of vulnerability. A continual awareness of what it is like to be weak, dependent, scared, uncertain will do much to help us understand what it is like to be a patient and ill in Western society. There are psychological exercises which can sensitize one to this as well as role-playing. The use of video-taping is an excellent way in which we can monitor and understand how we 'come on' to patients. Continuing clinical seminars on "compliance" may also provide an important forum for understanding the frustrations of doctors and patients in dealing with this issue. And such seminars or case conferences might well include the recipients of care as well as the providers.

There are many elements of the clinical encounter itself which can and should be changed. While many changes are fairly explicit in my listing of barriers to communication let me deal with some that may not be. The patient's position within the consult must be strengthened. Some, as I have mentioned, must take place outside our purview but others we can at least encourage. We must look more explicitly at the encounter as a didactic one and thus analyze how learning can best take place. At least one suggestion is a more explicit separation in time if not space between the examination and the information that the patients must have to know about their diagnosis, their prognosis, and their care. Where, for whatever reason, there can be no substantial separation, then at least let us give the patient a chance to absorb what s/he has been through — some way of gathering themselves together before we proceed. In a workshop I am currently running, we are teaching patients 'relaxation exercises' so that they can 'center' themselves before (a) they receive more information and/or (b) they start asking questions.

A second element is a recreation in certain ways of the patient's territory. It may be impossible to shift the place of most medical encounters back to the home, though particularly in long-term care an occasional home-visit seems appropriate to keep health providers in touch with the reality of their suggestions. What we can do, however, is encourage a trend that is already beginning, what the self-help movement calls the presence of an advocate. To the degree that certain medical conditions as well as regimens involve patients' families and 'significant others' we should take this into consideration when we explain the implications of a particular diagnosis and its treatment. Without taking responsibility away from the patient we can encourage and allow the presence of others during all phases of the medical encounter. We have I think 'overprivatized' the medical interview to the detriment of all concerned.

This concludes my remarks on this contribution of health researchers and providers to the communication barriers in the doctor-patient relationship. In reference to non-compliance I am contending that part of what patients are responding to when they do not cooperate is not the medical treatment but how they are treated, not how they regard their required medical regimen but how they themselves are regarded. Unless we fully recognize this phenomenon, we will live out the warning of Walt Kelly's immortal Pogo, "We have met the enemy, and they are us!"

Hopefully, I have taken a step in this paper to reverse this process. It is time to reexamine many of the traditional assumptions of what it takes to heal and to help. I am naive enough to believe that knowledge and awareness are powerful tools. While acknowledging the dilemmas in the doctor-patient relationship will not be sufficient to make the problem of non-compliance disappear, it will at least change the context of discussion. The participants in deciding what is best must be patients as well as doctors. We must remember that giving up power is NOT the same as abdicating responsibility. There must be less talk of persuasion and more of negotiation. And when we do so, a change in philosophy will be reflected in a change in language. We will no longer speak of 'medication compliance' but rather of 'therapeutic alliance'.

REFERENCES

Anderson, R.
    1968 A Behavioral Model of Families' Use of Health Services Chicago: Center for
          Health Administration Studies Research, Series No. 25.
Balint, M., J. Hunt, D. Joyce, M. Marinker, and J. Woodcock
    1970 Treatment or Diagnosis — A Study of Repeat Prescriptions in General Practice.
          London: Tavistock Publications.
Barsky, A. and R. Gillum
    1974 The Diagnosis and Management of Patient Non-Compliance. Journal of the
          American Medical Association 228:1563—1567.
Becker, M. H. and L. A. Maiman
    1975 Sociobehavioral Determinants of Compliance with Health and Medical Care
          Recommendation. Medical Care 13:10—24.
Boston Women's Health Book Collective
    1976 Our Bodies Ourselves. New York: Simon and Schuster.
Cartwright, A.
    1964 Human Relations and Hospital Care. London: Routledge and Kegan Paul.
Clute, K. F.
    1963 The General Practitioner — A Study of Medical Education and Practice in Ontario
          and Nova Scotia. Toronto: University of Toronto Press.
Davis, M. S.
    1966 Variations in Patients' Compliance with Doctors' Orders. Journal of Medical
          Education 41:1037—1048.
    1968 Variations in Patients' Compliance with Doctors' Advice: An Empirical Analysis
          of Patterns of Communication. American Journal of Public Health 58:274—288.
Dunnell, K. and A. Cartwright
    1972 Medicine Takers, Prescribers, and Hoarders. London: Routledge and Kegan Paul.
Emerson, J. P.
    1970 Behavior in Private Places: Sustaining Definitions of Reality in Gynecological
          Examinations. In Recent Sociology, J. P. Dreitzel, ed. pp. 74—97. London:
          MacMillan Co.
Francis, V., B. M. Korsch, and M. J. Morris
    1969 Gaps in Doctor-Patient Communication: Patients' Response to Medical Advice.
          New England Journal of Medicine 280:535—540.
Freeman, N.
    1967 The Social Nature of Psychological Research. New York: Basic Books.
Freidson, E.
    1961 Patients' Views of Medical Practice New York: Russell Sage.
Gibson, C. D. and B. M. Kramer
    1965 Site of Care in Medical Practice. Medical Care, 3:14—17.
Janis, I.
    1958 Psychological Stress-Psychoanalytic and Behavioral Studies of Surgical Patients.
          New York: John Wiley & Sons.
Korsch, B. M., E. K. Gozzi, and V. Francis
    1969 Gaps in Doctor Patient Communication: Doctor-Patient Interaction and Patient
          Satisfaction. Pediatrics 42:855—871.
Kosa, John and Irving Kenneth Zola, eds.
    1975 Poverty and Health: A Sociological Analysis (rev. edition). Cambridge: Harvard
          University Press.
Pessen, B.
    1978 Learning to be a Mother: The Influence of the Medical Profession. Ph.D. disserta-
          tion, Department of Sociology, Brandeis University.

Stoeckle, J.
  1978 Encounters of Patients and Doctors — A Book of Readings with Commentary. Unpublished Manuscript.
Suchman, E. A.
  1965 Social Patterns of Illness and Medical Care. Journal of Health and Human Behavior, 6:2–16.
Waitzkin, H. and J. Stoeckle
  1972 Communication of Information about Illness. *In* Advances in Psychomatic Medicine, Vol. 8, Z. Lipowski, ed. pp. 180–215. Basel: Karger.
Williams, T. F., et al.
  1967 The Clinical Picture of Diabetes Control Studied in Four Settings. American Journal of Public Health 57:441–451.
Zola, I. K.
  1966 Culture and Symptoms — An Analysis of Patients' Presenting Complaints. American Sociological Review 31:615–630.
  1972a The Concept of Trouble and Sources of Medical Assistance. Social Science and Medicine 6:673–679.
  1972b Studying the Decision to See a Doctor: Review, Critique, Corrective. *In* Advances in Psychomatic Medicine, Vol. 8, Z. Lipowski, ed. pp. 216–236. Basel: Karger.
  1973 Pathways to the Doctor — From Person to Patient. Social Science and Medicine 7:677–684.

12. DOCTOR-PATIENT NEGOTIATION AND OTHER SOCIAL SCIENCE STRATEGIES IN PATIENT CARE

INTRODUCTION

The purpose of this chapter is to review certain clinical social science approaches that can be applied practically by physicians. They are designed to assess and treat psychosocial problems in sickness, problems which are neither adequately conceptualized nor managed within the narrow, biomedical model that currently dominates clinical practice. Eisenberg (1977, 1979), Engel (1977), Kleinman et al. (1978), among others, have explicated why the biomedical model is inadequate as a guide for patient care. The case for applying social science to clinical practice also has been well-made. We will describe several case examples which illustrate the importance of this perspective, and discuss specific concepts and strategies useful for clinical practice and teaching. In this way, we hope to contribute to the development of a "biopsychosocial" approach to patients (Engel 1979), one which integrates biomedical, psychiatric, and social science frameworks.

The following case vignette can be used to contrast biopsychosocial and biomedical approaches (See Figure 1).

CASE 1: Mrs. S. was a 42-year-old mother of four children who came to the Family Medical Center at the University of Washington with abdominal pain diagnosed as a duodenal ulcer. Over the last year the youngest of her four children developed juvenile arthritis. She and her husband had been having marital problems prior to the child's illness but the extra stress made things far worse. She had always felt that he offered little emotional support and she now felt completely overburdened by this new stress in addition to her usual duties of taking care of a household with four children. She became quite anxious and over the last two months developed abdominal pains. The pain then led her to feel threatened and depressed by her physical condition, and also increased her sense of being overwhelmed. Mrs. S. was diagnosed as having developed a duodenal ulcer by her family physician.

Using the traditional medical model, a physician might treat this case as one simply involving a woman with a genetic predisposition to gastric hyperacidity who now had developed a duodenal ulcer. The treatment would be an antacid regimen. If her ulcer failed to heal, the doctor might wonder about the patient's compliance.

In contrast, a clinician schooled in a biopsychosocial approach has an expanded view of the problem which requires a multilevel analysis of the biographical and ecological context of the problem. This yields a wider array of treatment options, beginning with the same biomedical interventions, i.e., antacids, cimetidine, hospitalization, but also including specific psychosocial interventions, i.e., marital counseling, family therapy and social work assistance (Figure 1).

253

L. Eisenberg and A. Kleinman (eds.), The Relevance of Social Science for Medicine, 253–279.
Copyright © 1980 by D. Reidel Publishing Company.

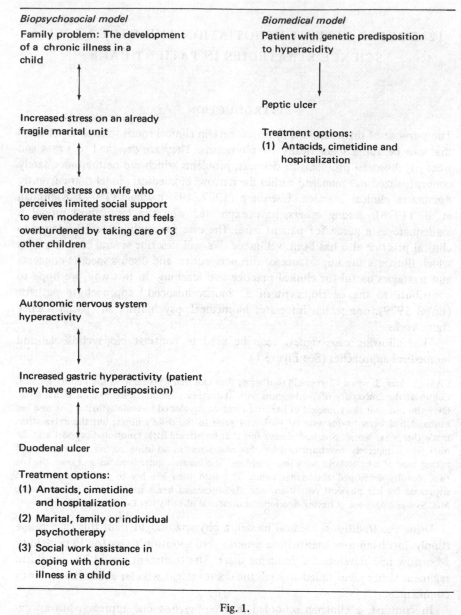

Biopsychosocial model

Family problem: The development
of a chronic illness in a
child

Increased stress on an already
fragile marital unit

Increased stress on wife who
perceives limited social support
to even moderate stress and feels
overburdened by taking care of 3
other children

Autonomic nervous system
hyperactivity

Increased gastric hyperactivity (patient
may have genetic predisposition)

Duodenal ulcer

Treatment options:
(1) Antacids, cimetidine
     and hospitalization
(2) Marital, family or individual
     psychotherapy
(3) Social work assistance in
     coping with chronic
     illness in a child

Biomedical model

Patient with genetic predisposition
to hyperacidity

Peptic ulcer

Treatment options:
(1) Antacids, cimetidine and
     hospitalization

Fig. 1.

Lacking a single explanatory system to unify our knowledge about the different levels of clinical reality relevant to patient symptomatology (i.e., physiological, behavioral, experiential, interpersonal, cultural), the physician who wishes to adopt a biopsychosocial approach is forced to apply alternative models (medical, behavioral, psychodynamic, social science, systems theory, etc.) to particular patient problems. For given problems, one model may be satisfactory in itself, but more often the clinician will need to employ several in an ad hoc integration that enables him to address a range of problems affecting different levels of clinical reality. Clinical judgment, then, involves the application of distinctive explanatory frameworks to generate relevant data, test hypotheses about contributing variables and types of problems, determine therapeutic resources, and decide on treatment courses which include both disease and illness interventions. Commitment to a pragmatic biopsychosocial approach should make the clinician equally intolerant of (a) simply reducing a complex human problem to a narrow biological issue requiring a single technological "fix", or (b) elaborating an abstract psychological or social science theory which is irrelevant to the clinical issue at hand, which calls for radical and far-reaching action infeasible in the clinical setting, or which cannot be integrated with other therapeutic models.

Anorexia nervosa is a clinical problem which illustrates the uses of a bio-psychosocial approach. In the last several years there have been reports that amitriptyline is an effective therapy (Needleman et al. 1976; Moore 1977), that behavior modification is the treatment of choice (Blinder et al. 1970), that psychodynamic psychotherapy is effective (Bruch 1978), and that family therapy is more effective than other approaches (Minuchin 1978).

The biopsychosocial approach, in contrast to this advocacy of single treatment interventions, encourages the clinician to evaluate a case of anorexia nervosa using each of these four therapeutic orientations concomitantly and thereby to select the one or more which seem most appropriate for the particular patient, problem, and situation. For example, from a biopsychosocial perspective a picture of anorexia nervosa can be synthesized out of the following interrelated points of view:

(1) Western culture has put tremendous pressure on women to maintain often unrealistically low body weights; thus, the incidence of anorexia is much higher in Western cultures than in Asian or African cultures (Bruch 1973).

(2) This pressure influences the family's attitudes toward food and eating; adolescents, who are most concerned with issues of acceptance in, and conformity to, peer group norms, are most subject to this pressure and consequently most likely to be affected by the disorder.

(3) The pressure of these cultural norms has its greatest impact on susceptible families which have specific modes of communication and behavior associated with a high prevalence of psychosomatic problems. Minuchin (1978) characterizes these families as rigid, lacking mechanisms to resolve conflict, overprotective, and organized to maintain the status quo and resist change despite high personal and interpersonal costs.

(4) Together cultural norms and specific family systems act to affect adversely certain children, perhaps those with genetic or early acquired traits of temperament like passivity and compliance. This may explain why only one child in such "psychosomatic families" is affected. That child frequently has been a "model

child," who always did what she or he was told (Bruch 1978:38–56). The psychodynamic pattern exhibited by these children again may be the result of genetic predisposition, specific family environment, early acquired behavioral repertoire, and cultural beliefs and behavioral norms. As Bruch notes, the anorectic child's only sense of control over his or her life is in the field of eating behavior, whereas there is often a lack of assertive behavior in other areas. The child learns that he or she can communicate distress and exercise control over self and others through the idiom of self-imposed starvation.

(5) Starvation itself has characteristic biological effects and leads to constant preoccupation with food, to depression and to cognitive-perceptual abnormalities, including distortions in body image which feed back to enforce the self-imposed weight loss. In turn, a reverse feedback system operates with the image of "a starving child in the midst of plenty" (Bruch 1978) reverberating back on the family system so that the child's eating behavior becomes the sanctioned metaphor for the family's system of communicating and manipulating power relationships.

Whether or not this expanded view of anorexia nervosa turns out in the long run to be scientifically "correct," at present it offers a more adequate and discriminating understanding of this complex problem based on the simultaneous interplay of biochemical, behavioral, psychodynamic, family and cultural systems rather than the limited picture based on only one of these determinants of clinical reality. This multilevel perspective generates specific hypotheses that can be tested in empirical research. More importantly, it suggests a number of practical therapeutic interventions to be applied together or in sequence to break the feedback loops maintaining anorectic behavior.

Most clinicians, however, faced with competing theoretical frameworks in the psychological sciences, elect to learn one therapeutic approach in depth. Like the proponents of each of the four therapies, they try to reduce a complex issue. They construct clinical reality in such fashion as to justify the use of their preferred intervention by defining what they consider to be clinical evidence and making it fit the Procrustean Bed of their theory. This professional ideological basis of clinical practice is well illustrated in psychiatry by the call to return to a narrow medical model to resolve psychiatry's "identity crisis" (Ludwig and Othmer 1977). Psychiatrists should first examine the problems other medical specialists are facing because of the limitations of this undimensional perspective, before they repeat the same mistakes (Engel 1977). Even in psychiatric disease – i.e., the schizophrenias, affective disorders, etc., in which there is strong evidence for core biological components – psychosocial variables play a crucial role. For example, among schizophrenic patients, Vaughn and Leff (1976) and Brown (1962) showed the likelihood of rehospitalization to be more determined by family strife than by medication compliance. Such patients also have been shown to do better when treated with psychotherapy and antipsychotic medication together than when given medication alone (Mosher and Keith 1979). Brown and Birley (1967) have demonstrated that 60% of relapses of schizophrenic patients have been associated with the death of a parent or a move to a new residence. Gunderson et al. (1974) have reported that 50% of institutionalized patients freed of their symptoms by the use of drugs discontinue medication after discharge because of a lack of continuing therapeutic contact that makes them feel uncared for. Recently Weissman et al. (1979) and Herceg-Baron et al. (1979) have published data from controlled studies disclosing that depressed patients do best with a combination of antidepressants and focused psychotherapy. Rush et al. (1977) have demonstrated that the efficacy of cognitive behavioral therapy in depression is as high as antidepressants. We could add many other citations to indicate that, while adherence to a traditional medical model may relieve the cognitive dissonance of the psychiatrist, it is an inadequate framework to conceptualize and treat his patients.

Moving from particular psychiatric disorders to disease generally, a very considerable literature indicts psychosocial stress as a pathogenic factor in disease onset; Holmes' work on life event changes as a general precipitant of disease (Holmes and Rahe 1967) has been extended to more discriminating understanding of the way the subjective significance of such changes and available social support systems for coping with them interplay to mediate their effects (Horowitz 1979; Henderson et al. 1978; Berkman and Syme 1979). Two recent studies which demonstrate the potential preventive significance of psychosocial support systems are worth noting.

Nuckolls and colleagues (1972) studied 170 pregnant army wives who were rated on the basis of life change scores and their level of social support. When they assessed the incidence of complications in these women, they found that the only group with excessive complications were women with high life changes and low support. Of special interest is their finding that those women at risk for high life change scores, but who also had high social support, had no higher rate of complications than the low support risk group. Medalie and Goldbourt (1976), in an elegant epidemiological study, performed a multivariant analysis of factors associated with the development of new cases of angina pectoris in a group of 10,000 men over a five-year period. Seven risk factors were discovered to be significantly associated with the development of angina pectoris; one was the presence of family problems. Of particular interest was their finding that, given a constant level of other risk factors, the subject's perception of his wife's love and support "protected" against the development of angina. The authors state "the wife's love and support is an important balancing factor, which apparently reduces the risk of angina pectoris even in the presence of high risk factors." Brown and Harris's (1975) finding that the presence of an intimate and a confiding relationship with a husband or boyfriend protects young women against depression is further evidence of the importance of psychosocial factors in illness and their clinical significance in patient care (see also the chapters by Berkman and McKinlay in this volume).

Sociocultural influences exert major effects through the categories patients and practitioners employ to construct sickness as a social reality and to choose and evaluate treatment interventions. For example, patients experience their problems as "illness" — the personal and social significance of, as well as the problems created by, perceived sickness — whereas doctors and other health care professionals, socialized in the biomedical model, are chiefly concerned with "disease" — maladaption or malfunctioning of biological processes (Kleinman, Eisenberg and Good 1978). Patients experience and react to illness as psychosocial problems — problems in daily living, work, family relationships, personal identity, sexual functioning, financial status, etc. — while doctors search for technical interventions to "fix" disease problems, i.e., fractures, infections, arrythmias, electrolyte imbalances.

These distinctive social perceptions of clinical reality readily yield discrepancies in doctor and patient evaluations of outcome. For instance, Cay and Phillips (1975) have shown that patients' assessments of successful surgical outcome peptic ulcer surgery were frequently different from those of their surgeons. Patients based their judgments of surgical outcome on psychosocial factors, but surgeons' clinical judgments of success or failure were concerned solely with technical issues (e.g., gastric acid reduction, absence of infection, ulcer recurrence, weight loss, etc.).

Hypertension offers another illustration of such systematic discrepancies or even conflicts in practitioner and patient perspectives. Hypertensive patients are often asymptomatic at the time of diagnosis. That is to say, they have disease without illness, and the disease may in future lead to serious impairment (i.e., stroke, heart attack, heart failure, kidney abnormalities) unless treated. Paradoxically, antihypertensive medication may make asymptomatic hypertensive patients symptomatic because of side effects. Treatment can lead to significant psychosocial problems such as poor concentration at work owing to sedative effects of medication, muscle weakness produced by drug-induced potassium deficits, impotence, dizziness, etc. As a result, patients may believe they have incurred iatrogenic illness at a time when they feel healthy. This paradoxical result of treatment may help explain the large percentage of hypertension patients who do not take their medication. Blumhagen (1980) found that many of these patients' popular interpretation of their disorder is that hypertension is "too much tension" rather than high blood pressure. Moreover, in sharp contrast to contemporary biomedical understanding of the chronic role of stress in their disease, such patients often rationalize noncompliance with the medical regimen because of the absence of acute stress and resulting tension in their lives.

In response to the miscommunications caused by the different professional and lay cultures, as well as to the crucial psychological and social influences on sickness and care, clinical social scientists have developed concepts and management strategies which can be integrated into a comprehensive biopsychosocial approach to patients. These ideas have been successfully taught to clinicians and integrated into the everyday practice of primary care physicians (Kleinman 1979; Kleinman and Smilkstein 1979; Katon and Kleinman 1980; Chrisman and Kleinman 1979). They are *complementary* to traditional psychological and psychiatric evaluation techniques. They can improve the quality of clinical relationships and the effectiveness of care, and offer feasible ways to provide culturally appropriate care and to increase patient satisfaction. For these reasons we would like to outline and illustrate practical social science methods directly applicable to clinical teaching and practice.

(1) *Explanatory Models*:

The initial step of our clinical method, which is an integral part of the general psychosocial assessment, is to elicit the patient's perception of his illness, or what we call *the patient's explanatory model* (Kleinman et al. 1978; Kleinman 1979). The explanatory model contains the patient's understanding of the cause of his illness, its pathophysiology, expected course and prognosis, and the treatment that he believes *will be* or *should be* administered. It must be elicited by openended questions in layman's terms, questions which do not contaminate the patient's perspective with the physician's assumptions. In order to elicit such information the physician must demonstrate warmth, empathy, and persistence; and he must be nonjudgemental. Most of all he must have genuine interest in the meaning the sickness has for the patient, and make explicit to the patient his intent to draw on this essential information in constructing an appropriate treatment plan.

Lazare et al. (1978) found that 99% of patients filling out a patient request form had at least one specific request for treatment. He also found that in a clinic interview 63% of patients expressed specific requests. The importance of persistence in the clinical interview was shown by the fact that there was a significant increase in stated patient requests after a second inquiry about what the patient sought from the clinic. Once the patient's explanatory model is elicited the physician then assesses the meaning of the illness for the patient. Here the physician can follow Lipowski (1969) who notes that though illness can have many particular meanings, there are only a few general significances of illness that have behavioral implications, i.e., (a) loss, (b) gain, (c) threat, (d) opportunity for growth or (e) no significance.

The following case illustrates the importance of eliciting the patient's explanatory model of illness:

CASE 2: Mrs. S. was a 27-year-old Native American female with a six-year history of systemic lupus erythematosis, and treatment with steroids, who was referred to the University Hospital in Seattle at 30-weeks' gestation with symptoms of preeclampsia. The patient had had four previous miscarriages in the last six years at early stages of gestation. She had one daughter, age 8, and strongly desired another child.

Due to severe preeclampsia, labor was induced during her second hospital day and a nonviable premature infant was delivered. Psychiatric consultation was obtained three days later due to "psychotic depression with hallucinations."

The following history was obtained from the patient. She was mourning the death of her baby and had "heard the baby cry" two days after the death. She stated that it was normal in Indian culture for loved ones to talk with close family members after death to try to bring relatives with them into the hereafter. Although she had no prior experience with this custom, many of her friends had spoken of their experiences with loved ones after death.

The staff reacted with anxiety and alarm on hearing that Mrs. S. had heard her baby cry after it was dead for two days and never bothered to elicit her cultural explanation. Thus, a psychiatric consultation was requested.

After talking with the patient and the staff, we recommended that the staff help the patient ventilate her feelings about the death of the baby and also enable her to perform any cultural ceremony that she and her husband would normally go through at home. During the next seven days of the hospitalization the patient "heard her baby cry" daily but with the help of the staff and her husband this became less alarming to the patient. She and her husband went through the cultural rites of destroying all traces of the baby's existence including blankets, baby clothes, and an echogram picture. The patient made an uneventful recovery both physically and emotionally. Reports of similar culturally constituted acute grief reactions abound in the ethnographic literature on Native Americans.

(2) *Illness Problems*:

The next stage of clinical social science evaluation involves the determination of the patient's illness problems: i.e., the experiential, family, economic, interpersonal, occupational, and daily life problems created by the disease and its treatment. For example, the onset of chronic back pain in a construction worker may require him to curtail his work activities or even change careers, lead to significant economic problems, decrease his sexual relations, interfere with life style and recreation, and perhaps result in marital discord, in disruption of his social network, in disability-related lawsuits, and in serious personal distress which may lead to seeking care from many physicians simultaneously.

If we are to effectively utilize a biopsychosocial approach in the practice of medicine, then these illness problems must receive systematic attention. They can be listed on the chart just as disease problems, i.e., the diagnosis of clinical status, complications, etc., are listed. In the example used above we might envision the following disease and illness problems:

Disease problems	Illness problems
1. chronic back pain	1. vocational disability
2. status post L_3L_4 laminectomy	2. marital discord
	3. disability related lawsuit
	4. maladaptive coping mechanism – i.e., doctor shopping

Just as for each disease problem, an analysis and plan can be worked out, by listing illness problems the physician can either treat or refer for appropriate intervention (vocational counseling, social work assistance, psychotherapy, relaxation therapy, etc.).

The accompanying table lists the major illness problems frequently encountered in practice (See Table 1). Although illness problems are as diverse as disease problems, we have attempted to list the major categories to assess how patient and family cope with the illness and respond to treatment.

TABLE 1

Illness problems

1. Family problems created or worsened by sickness.
2. Financial problems created or worsened by sickness.
3. Major changes in a patient's personal identity and social role in the context of a terminal sickness or a permanent disability.
4. Lack of compliance with therapeutic regimen due to the unusual nature of a procedure or its expected outcome.
5. Maladaptive coping responses that patients and families use to manage sickness, such as denial, passive-hostile behavior, "shopping" among different doctors, and manipulative suicidal attempts.
6. Conflict in personal beliefs between patients (and family) and practitioners concerning cause or nature of sickness and expected course and objectives for treatment.
7. Inappropriate resort to sick role and illness behavior owing to psychological or social gain.
8. Conflict in cultural values concerning treatment style and interpersonal etiquette between patients and practitioners due to substantial differences in social class, life style and ethnic norms.
9. Inappropriate use of alternative or indigenous health care agents and agencies.
10. Breakdown in communication between patient (and family) and practitioners.
11. Transference and countertransference problems in the doctor-patient or doctor-family relationship.
12. Life problems stemming from the particular stresses engendered by special treatment environments.

By examining illness problems the physician can also assess psychosocial factors in a patient's complaints.

CASE 3: Mrs. L. was a 70-year-old woman who presented to the Harborview Medical Center with an overdose of a sedative hypnotic. She was subsequently found to have a major depressive disorder with a history of two prior serious depressions. She had vegetative symptoms of insomnia, anorexia, twenty-pound loss, and a decrease in energy. Her disease problem, then, was a major depressive disorder and disease interventions included treatment with antidepressants and psychotherapy. Analysis of the patient's illness problems revealed: (1) progressive social isolation with the death of many of her close friends and a distant relationship with her family, and (2) declining economic status. Interventions in the psychosocial sphere included family counseling, helping Mrs. S. participate in a nearby geriatric center and enlisting her in a medical care outreach program.

Her psychosocial history also revealed that she always had been a very independent woman and despite declining physical health had refused to ask for more support from her family. They in turn had visualized her as a fiercely autonomous, strong-willed, and at times stubborn woman, and had not noted her progressive decline in health or economic status. With the help of family counseling both the patient and the family became more aware of her current life condition and the family was able to provide more support with mutual appreciation of the ensuing close relationship.

One of the essential implications of concepts like the patient's explanatory model and illness problems is that conflicts may arise in the doctor-patient relationship. These in turn cause patient dissatisfaction, noncompliance, and poor care. Patient compliance studies have indicated that there are two positive physician factors that enhance compliance (Svarstad 1976). The first is giving the patient consistant information and education, and the second is continual monitoring for patient noncompliance and dissatisfaction with care. The physician who is sensitive to signs of patient dissatisfaction and noncompliance and who responds appropriately to them and to the management issues that give rise to them obtains better results and provides more effective care. The physician skill required is the ability to negotiate between differing perceptions of illness, goals of treatment, and conflicts. The objective is neither to dominate patients nor convert them to the physician's value orientation, but to enlist the patient as a therapeutic ally and provide care for problems patients regard as important in ways that patients desire. That is to say, these clinical social science interventions aim at making care less doctor-centered and more patient-centered. Crucial to this shift in the structure of clinical relationships is recognition that clinical care should involve a genuine negotiation between physician and patient.

(3) *Negotiation*:

Nader and Todd (1978) have defined seven methods for dealing with conflicts or disputes cross culturally, including avoidance, "lumping it" and coercion which are all based on unilateral action by one party in the conflict, negotiation which is a bilateral arrangement in which the two principal parties attempt to work out a solution, and mediation, arbitration and adjudication which are all procedures involving third-party assistance in finding a solution to a problem. We will emphasize the negotiation model as crucial in the two party physician-patient relationship, but clinical social science consultants may also be called upon to assume the role of mediator or arbiter.

Negotiation is defined simply as "conferring, discussing, or bargaining to reach an agreement" (Guralnik 1968). In groups and industry negotiation is looked at as "a sequence of behavior occurring in which one party presents a proposal, the other evaluates it and presents a counter proposal, the first party replies with a modified proposal and so on until a settlement is reached"(Johnson and Johnson 1975). The goal is to reduce conflict in a way that promotes cooperation. Perhaps a definition closer to the doctor-patient relationship is "a process in which people who want to come to an agreement but disagree on the nature of the agreement try to work out a settlement; it is aimed at achieving an agreement that determines what each party gives and receives in a transaction between them" (Johnson and Johnson 1975).

There are several barriers to negotiation in medical care. To begin with, the roots of contemporary doctor-patient relationships are in the authoritarian power structure of traditional practitioner-patient interactions. Professional biomedical relationships have always been hierarchical. Although all patients in such transactions are accorded less power than practitioners, there can be no doubt that the social class and status of the patient also influence how much influence he is accorded in the clinical encounter. Perhaps all professional relationships differentially distribute power with the client at somewhat of a disadvantage, but the power differentiation of the doctor-patient relationship is most impressively unequal. This inequality can even be found in governmental laws regulating medical practice, although in recent years the rights of patients have received increasing protection. It is, however, the physician whose view of clinical reality is legitimated in professional clinical care settings.

In cross-cultural and historical perspective, one sees that clinical relations are so rarely conducted as a negotiation among equals (in socialist societies as well) that the negotiation model can only be understood as an aspect of the current social crisis in the West, where authority is everywhere under attack, professionalism is suspect, and individual rights and autonomy are at the core of cultural values. Moreover, today the status of the physician is decreasing, and there is general consumer dissatisfaction with the provision of health care; this is reflected in the increase in medical-legal suits as well as in frequent attacks in the media on the abuse of medical institutions, the excessive financial gains of many practitioners, and the political implications of the medicalization of social problems. This climate of criticism requires reform in the structure of clinical transactions. Doctors in the West can no longer take as their model an authoritarian doctor-patient relationship in which they dictate the terms of care to their patients and fail to take their patients views into account.

But we wish to argue for a more fundamental reorientation of care than this. In contemporary American culture, it is appropriate for doctor and patient to meet as equals, with the former rendering expert advice and the latter bearing ultimate responsibility for deciding whether or not to follow that advice. Moreover, we believe enlightened consumer opinion and the other factors we have mentioned now make it feasible to routinely structure clinical relationships in this way.

One criticism of negotiation is that "it takes too much power away from the clinician and inappropriately gives it to the patient" (Lazare et al. 1978). Lazare and his colleagues answer critics who believe that patients do not have requests, that the requests are irrelevant, that eliciting requests places the patient in the role of a shopper in a medical supermarket and thereby dilutes the physician's ability to influence the patient through his sanctioned authority — the feared outcome of which is clinical helplessness in the face of ceaseless consumer demands. Lazare et al. convincingly demonstrate that patients do have requests, the expression of which does not bind the clinician to fulfill them. In fact, eliciting them makes the physician more knowledgeable and empathic, and this in turn enables him to exert a more sensitive and sensible therapeutic influence. Specifically, Lazare and his co-workers (1978) found that 63% of patients expressed specific requests for treatment with 37% expressing them spontaneously and the remaining 26% verbalizing a request after the clinician's elicitation. Even when presented with a standardized written patient request form, 99% of patients stated at least one specific request. Negotiating with patient requests also appears to increase patient satisfaction and otherwise positively affects care. These investigators do not find that negotiation lowers professional standards nor leads to therapeutic surrender. Indeed, they discovered that patient requests are "usually a more modest statement of perceived needs than the clinician had anticipated."

Another criticism of negotiation proceeds from just the opposite viewpoint that it will give the physician even greater control than he already possesses over his patient and that this will eventuate in further abuses of the physician's power. But, as Lazare and his colleagues point out, the elements of negotiation are core clinical tasks — developing trust, establishing expertise, explaining to patients why one therapeutic approach is preferable to another, arguing against actions that from the clinical perspective appear dangerous, and the like. They conclude, "What is really at issue, we believe, is not the physician's skill at negotiating but the possibility that he may influence patients to accept treatments which are not responsive to their needs or which may even be deleterious to their well being. The solution to these abuses is not to discourage the negotiation process, which we regard as a part of the treatment, but to encourage patients to be more educated consumers and to encourage varied auditing of medical practice" (Lazare et al. 1978). They also recognize that safeguards to protect patient rights in clinical negotiations may have to come from outside the medical profession. But they argue that negotiation between patient and physician strengthens and otherwise improves the participation of both parties in the clinical transaction. We would add that there is no reason why specific rules for negotiation could not be formally established that specify the extent and limits of physician responsibility, that define the patient as the final arbiter of clinical decisions, and that protect patient rights. Indeed, there are already ethical and legal constraints which circumscribe the nature of clinical relationships, and these could be built on to establish a system of formal guidelines governing clinical negotiations which are publically articulated and monitored. Doubtless, like all therapeutic interventions, negotiation may yield potential toxicities that should be monitored, but we believe these are likely to be limited and of small consequence when compared with the substantial toxicities this procedure is meant to correct.

Certain of the structural power differentials basic to the doctor-patient relationship are unlikely to be significantly altered in the foreseeable future. Hence, though we support increased patient access to knowledge and technical resources, the absence of real structural equality need not prevent negotiation from occurring, if both parties to the clinical transaction desire it. The act of negotiating itself helps diminish the discrepancy in power actually constituted in particular doctor-patient relationships. But in all cultures patients expect that doctors, based on their special training and skills, possess "special powers" that will "cure" their problems; and this universal expectation is likely to be as crucial to the placebo response as it is to the assuaging of anxiety and fear that is central to the entire healing process. Thus, some degree of structural inequality, regulated and monitored to be sure, is not only inevitable but potentially desirable, as long as it is neither extreme nor abused to exploit patients, but rather allows the physician to maximize the clinical efficacy of his therapeutic mandate to act. Of course, pseudo-negotiations that camouflage coercion under the guise of dialogue are a potential toxicity that needs to be prevented and controlled. But all human relationships are threatened by such mystification in the service of exploitation. It is our view that the negotiation process is the single most expedient way to bring to bear the patient's and family's viewpoint as forcefully as possible, heighten the affective side of care, and assure that ultimately clinical decisions are controlled by lay participants.

Of course, in certain cultures and among particular ethnic groups in the West where doctor-patient relationships are expected to follow an authoritarian format and a negotiation model represents a culturally inappropriate imposition of contemporary Western values, it would not make therapeutic sense to alter the relationship along this line. The clinician needs to determine in a particular case whether negotiation is culturally and personally acceptable to his patient. He also needs to discover if the family and especially key family members, not the patient, is regarded as the appropriate party to the negotiation. Ethnic stereotypes often do not apply in individual instances and may cause mischief even when applied with good intentions. The clinician who is sensitive to ethnic differences can employ the explanatory model approach to determine patient beliefs and norms regarding doctor-patient relationships to see if negotiation is feasible or not. Our impression is that simply showing an interest in the patient's perspective of the expected and desired form of clinical interaction has positive therapeutic consequences. Like the ethnographer working in an alien culture, the clinician needs to show the patient he is aware that there are likely to be differences as well as similarities in their ways of construing social relationships and that he is interested in determining what these are in order to minimize misunderstanding and maximize productive collaboration.

(4) *A Model of Clinical Negotiation*:

We will next outline the stages of the negotiation model which we are advocating and discuss the conflicts which commonly arise in the doctor-patient relationship and provide the day-to-day subject matter for clinical negotiation.

The first step in the clinical negotiation model, as in any therapeutic relationship, is the development of the therapeutic or working alliance. Greenson (1967) has defined the therapeutic alliance as "the relatively non-neurotic rational rapport that the patient has with his analyst." The main feature of this more traditional doctor-centered approach is "the patient's motivation to overcome his illness, his sense of helplessness, his conscious and rational willingness to cooperate and his ability to follow directions." Meissner and Nicholi (1978), in a more egalitarian vein, stress that the working alliance is based on both the patient and physician's explicit and implicit agreement to work together toward a mutually desired objective, the improvement of the patient. These psycho-analytic explanations can be translated into a more general approach to medical care in which the therapeutic alliance is based on the ability of the patient and physician to establish trust and to utilize the rational aspects of themselves and positive feelings toward one another to work together to alleviate distress and/or disability in the patient.

Thus, in order to carry out a negotiation the fundamental characteristics of an effective doctor-patient relationship are essential. These include setting up and establishing a milieu that is warm and accepting and in which the patient can express troublesome feelings. Perhaps the central feature of this milieu is physician empathy. Indeed, we regard empathy as so crucial to the negotiation model that it is unlikely that the elicitation of the patient's model and subsequent negotiation is possible without such an affective bond between doctor and patient. We also believe that the negotiation model itself (by validating the importance of the patient's feelings and beliefs) will function to increase affective bonds between doctor and patient.

At times the formation of the working alliance is hindered by negative feelings arising either in the patient or physician. These feelings can be based on such things as the patient or physician's appearance, personality and behavior or on conflicts in perspectives and expectations that emerge and are not resolved. Many of these variables are strongly influenced by cultural differences. Secondly, negative feelings can be based on unconscious processes whereby the patient or physician transfer experiences and emotions they have had toward people in the past to the present situation. Thus, a patient or physician may react negatively to one another because they are reminded of unpleasant past experiences or individuals.

Fortunately the reverse is also true and helpful in that most patients have had positive experiences with authority figures like parents and physicians and thus have positive emotional feelings and associations toward doctors.

Balint (1957) believed that many of the unconscious negative feelings arising in the doctor-patient relationship could undermine primary care relationships. He found that resolution of these unconscious feelings in the seminar he developed for primary care physicians could facilitate care, especially with those patients clinicians find most difficult to treat.

The first level of conflict that we will discuss occurs in situations where a therapeutic alliance cannot be developed due to the patient's distrust of the physician or loss of cognitive function necessary for interpersonal interaction (e.g., in dementia or delirium). The former reaction may be the result of serious psychopathology. An example here would be a paranoid patient who feels that the physician may poison him or be plotting against him. The following case is illustrative:

CASE: Mr. T. was a 30-year old white man who presented to the Emergency Room with anxiety, insomnia, and paranoid delusions that people were out to kill him by poisoning his food. He had auditory hallucinations in which he heard people talking about him derogatorily. Although he came to the Emergency Room for medical help, when the psychiatrist suggested treatment with medication and hospitalization, he refused and became threatening.

He stated that he felt unsafe and afraid in the hospital and was worried that the psychiatrist was also going to poison him with medication.

In certain situations, such mistrust may be a function of particular social systems. Hence the relationships between psychiatrists and political dissidents in the Soviet Union, or between industry and insurance company doctors and patients with potential work-related disabilities in the United States, or between patients with chronic factitious illness and physicians aware of this problem in any society are unlikely to engender trust.

Patients with organic brain syndrome, dementia or delirium often refuse treatment or are not able to understand the benefits or risks of treatment. In these cases as well as with patients psychiatrically impaired the physician must weigh patients' right to refuse treatment with the risk of harm to themselves or other people. If the physician feels the person is at risk to harm himself or another person, then he is usually legally obligated to try to treat that patient often with legal assistance.

Mrs. J. was a 65-year-old white female brought in by the Seattle Police Department after her neighbors called due to her deteriorating physical condition and refusal to seek medical help. The neighbors had tried to get her to see a doctor after watching Mrs. J. lose weight progressively and most recently become acutely short of breath. She had been acting increasingly bizarre, refusing to open her door to former friends, and only rarely going outside. Mrs. J. was found to have severe congestive heart failure on examination in the Emergency Room and initially agreed to be hospitalized. On the ward she began refusing medications stating that she felt she was going to be poisoned and wanted to leave immediately. She had always been an introverted woman with few friends but after her husband left her two years previously she became reclusive and suspicious. She told this psychiatric consultant that she was convinced that there were people plotting to drive her insane in her neighborhood and that they often would sneak into her house when she went out. Mrs. J. denied that there was anything wrong with her physically despite spending the last 24-hours standing up due to extreme shortness of breath and she asked to leave the hospital against medical advice. Her cognitive testing on mental status examination revealed a moderate dementia. With her paranoid ideation and dementia the patient was unable to recognize the severity of her condition or care for herself. Therefore it was recommended that a psychiatrist be called to evaluate the patient for involuntary commitment. The patient was legally committed due to grave disability (she had a life-threatening medical illness and due to psychiatric impairment could not care for herself) and her congestive heart failure rapidly improved over one week. Her paranoid delusions also cleared up with neuroleptic medication, though she was left with a mild to moderate dementia.

The previous cases are examples of the difficulty establishing a therapeutic alliance in the occasional cases in which the patient's cognitive functioning is impaired or there is a thought disorder such as paranoid delusions. These cases are not rare but most of the instances where the therapeutic alliance has broken down are due to problems at the conceptual level. Here there is difficulty with doctor-patient communication "because of differences that exist between physicians and patients concerning the categories of objects and events in the world and the beliefs and feelings associated with these categorizations"

(Harwood in press). Differences at the conceptual level are often secondary to differing cultural values, cognitive sets and beliefs about illness and lead, at times, besides breakdowns in clinical communication, to negative feelings between patient and physician that can cause a dissolution of the therapeutic alliance.

Harwood (in press) divides the conceptual differences between patient and doctor into five groups.

(1) The patient and doctor use the same term but actually mean different things. This commonly occurs when the doctor and patient use the same biomedical term with the physician thus assuming that the patient understands it the same way he does. A common example here is in the doctor's history taking when he asks the patient about allergies to medications. Many patients claim they are allergic to a certain type of drug but if the physician asks them about the reaction in detail, it is often only a minor side effect, not an allergy as the doctor understands that term.

(2) The patient and doctor use the same term, apply it to the same phenomena but have different etiologic concepts. The implication here is that the patient who views the cause of his or her illness differently than the physician may have differing expectations of treatment. An example is the folk model of hypertension mentioned above. Hypertensive patients often view their illness as caused by acute stresses in their lives. The physician may view chronic stress as a component in the complex etiology of hypertension but usually views genetic predisposition and physiologic abnormalities as being primary. He prescribes diuretics and perhaps occasionally counsels patients about decreasing the stress in their lives; many patients believe, however, that stress is primary and may try to work on this aspect of their lives but do not take their medications.

(3) A similar problem is one in which the physician and patient share the same terms and referents but these terms are embedded in different nosologies. Harwood (in press) gives an example from his study from the Puerto Rican culture in which 23 of 28 adults interviewed stated that ulcers led to cancer. Obviously, the physician's diagnosis of peptic ulcer disease to many Puerto Rican patients may have far more serious connotations to the patient than to the physician. Moreover, these culture meanings are hidden to the physician.

(4) Patients may stigmatize certain diseases so that physicians and patients share the same term and the same referent for the term but may have very different emotive meanings attached to it. An example here is the stigmatization of mental disease. This often adversely affects the psychiatrist's history-taking. Patients frequently will not give an adequate family history during an interview due to the stigma of having mental disease in their family. The following is a case example:

Tom was a 15-year-old white male brought to the University of Washington's University Hospital after three months of progressive withdrawal, ideas of reference that people were talking about him, delusions that people were trying to hurt him, depression, and psychomotor retardation. The family initially denied any family history of mental illness except that one of the father's brothers had a "mild nervous breakdown" under the stress of combat in World War II. The attending psychiatrist during his interview pointed out the significance of family history to the diagnosis and prognosis of Tom's case and then again persistently inquired about the possibility of family members with mental disease. The father then admitted that two of his brothers had recurrent nervous breakdowns in their teens and 20's and had received ECT with complete recovery! One sister also had mood swings between depression and euphoria but had never been treated. This data led to the suspicion that the teen-ager's symptoms might be more in line with affective illness than schizophrenia and was quite helpful in the management of the patient's disorder.

(5) The last communication difficulty (Harwood labels it a "lexicon" level problem) is where the doctor and patient simply do not use the same terms. Here the patient may speak a foreign language or dialect of the standard language or the physician may use medical jargon. Sometimes this problem is resolved by asking for clarification of one another's unknown terms. At times, however, the same word may have totally different meanings in the two cultures or there may be no equivalent of a term in the other language. Although such problems may be resolved by use of interpreters, interpreters may unwittingly amplify these problems. Few interpreters are trained in biomedical terminology, few may have systematic knowledge of their own culture's folk medical concepts and terms, and some may be so acculturated or otherwise alienated from indigenous concepts and norms that they fail to adequately interpret the native perspective. Indeed it is our experience that clinicians can anticipate frequent misunderstandings when using clinically inexperienced or untrained interpreters and need to monitor work-ups carefully to make sure such misunderstandings do not distort diagnostic assessment and undermine therapeutic plans.

The explanatory model technique reviewed above should help detect and resolve potential or actual conflicts in doctor-patient communication. Mutual understanding of patient and physician explanatory models is absolutely crucial to the negotiation process. This is particularly important when patients and physicians come from distinctive ethnic and social backgrounds and therefore are unlikely to share illness and treatment expectations. But we would suggest that even clinical encounters among members of the same culture are best conceived as requiring translation between differing "cultural" interpretative systems for deciding what is clinical evidence, rationalizing treatment choice, and assessing outcome.

It is also essential that physicians evaluate illness problems in order to be able to negotiate treatment with the patient. We have listed twelve common illness behavior problems in Table 1, and certainly understanding these psychosocial factors in a patient's life enhances the negotiation process. Often it is the affective reaction to illness and the cognitive behavioral response to it that lead to doctor-patient conflicts (e.g., transference-countertransference problems, maladaptive coping reactions, such as major denial, depression, passive-hostile behavior, etc.). These affective reactions and cognitive coping responses are important to monitor and we will review them in more depth in the next section.

Where doctor-patient (or doctor-family) conflicts do arise we have found the following model of negotiation invaluable. Besides listing the stages of the negotiation model, we present several case vignettes to portray actual negotiations.

(1) The physician elicits the patient's explanatory model and illness problems.

(2) The physician, based on his knowledge of the patient's illness problems, and his biomedical knowledge of the disease problems, then clearly and fully presents in layman's terms to the patient his explanatory model of the disorder including his treatment recommendations. (He also invites questions from the patient to which he responds with as complete an explanation as is possible.) This step may involve patient education in biomedical knowledge, but where technically and ethically feasible the physician should translate his ideas into the patient's conceptual system and work within the idiom (psychosomatic, somatizing, social, cosmological, etc.) the patient employs to articulate his illness problems and treatment goals.

(3) Often the patient will respond to the doctor's explanations by shifting his or her explanatory model of illness towards the physician's model, thus making a working alliance possible. The reverse is also true, that the physician armed with a greater understanding of the patient's explanatory model and illness problems may change his recommendations shifting more toward the patient's expectations of treatment.

(4) At times, however, the discrepancies in the patient's or doctor's expectations of treatment will remain. Here the doctor should openly acknowledge and clarify the conflict between the two. He can provide references and data to argue on behalf of his perspective and the treatment interventions it entails. He should also provide the patient and family with ample opportunity to present their alternatives and assess their arguments in support of them.

(5) Perhaps as a result of understanding one another's conflicting explanations the doctor, the patient, or both will change their position so that a mutually desired treatment can be agreed upon. We feel that this is the end result in most cases.

(6) Where a conflict cannot be resolved through such an understanding, the physician should decide on an acceptable compromise of treatment based on his biomedical knowledge, knowledge of the patient's explanatory model and illness problems, and his own ethical standards. Here the physician can call upon input from the family, other agencies or health professionals (social workers, ethnic and pastoral counselors, psychiatrists) to help implement the compromise. (Similarly, patients must have the right to involve members of their

social network and key others familiar with their case in the negotiation process, if they deem this essential.)

(7)   Throughout this process it is essential to recognize that the physician's role is to provide expert advice and rationale for treatment recommendations but the patient is the final arbiter of whatever choice is made. There is nothing wrong with the physician arguing strongly on behalf of a particular course of action, as long as he clarifies to the patient and family that the ultimate choice is theirs. As in any negotiation the patient may counter the physician's offer with a counterproposal and the physician must again decide with respect to his technical knowledge and ethical standards whether he should accept this offer or make another of his own. If a stalemate is reached in negotiation and the patient's decision remains unacceptable on biomedical or ethical grounds, then the therapeutic contract and alliance is broken. At that point referral to another physician should be offered. At any time, based on his explanatory model and value system, the patient himself may decide to abrogate the therapeutic alliance and seek care elsewhere. Rather than see this option as noncompliance or "doctor shopping," the physician must recognize it as an absolutely legitimate option for the patient — one that he should make the patient aware of and facilitate if the patient so chooses.

(8)   Each negotiation must involve ongoing *monitoring* of the agreement and of each party's participation. Not only should the physician see this as his role, but he should encourage the patient and family to monitor the ongoing status of the doctor-patient agreement as well. Such monitoring may necessitate renegotiation of the key clinical issues at a latter date.

We will now present several case examples of patient-physician conflict to illustrate actual clinical negotiations. We will take the reader through a detailed step-by-step negotiation in the first case and then present three brief case vignettes to further clarify the process.

Mrs. G was a 56-year-old Hispanic American with a past history of chronic kidney failure, status postrenal transplant in 1974, chronic anemia and hypertension who presented to the Orthopedic Clinic in June 1978 with pain in her left ankle after "twisting" it at work. She was initially diagnosed as having tendonitis of the left Achilles tendon and placed in a short leg cast for three weeks. Upon removal of the cast in clinic and weight bearing, a loud "crack" was heard by both patient and doctor. She had avulsed (broken off) a portion of her calcaneous (the bone under the sole of the foot) and this portion of the bone was pulled by its tendon two inches up into the ankle. The patient then had a painful lump of bone protruding from her left ankle. The orthopedist felt that Mrs. G had suffered osteoporosis (thinning and weakening of her bones) secondary to long-term treatment with prednisone (an immunosuppressant used to prevent rejection of her kidney transplant). The osteoporosis was responsible for the pathological fracture dislocation.

Mrs. G's leg was again casted with her physicians' deciding to manage the fracture conservatively. They felt the displaced portion of calcaneous would reattach securely, so that surgery would not be necessary. They hoped it would heal in this manner, because they felt the risks of surgery were too great due to continued treatment with prednisone and Imuran (immunosuppressant drugs that often cause poor healing but which are required for maintenance of her kidney transplant).

Mrs. G. again presented to the University Hospital in October. At this time she admitted that she was severely depressed and had suicidal ideation. The orthopedic surgeons hospitalized her because of the psychiatric problem and to review their management of the case. The patient was dissatisfied with her care and was quite angry with the orthopedists' recommended treatment. As a result of the depression, suicidal ideation and patient dissatisfaction with care, psychiatry was consulted.

We will now present our step-by-step clinical negotiation.

STEP I: Mrs. G., who was a traditionally oriented Hispanic woman, had the following explanatory model. She viewed the large bump on her ankle that was secondary to the displaced fracture as unsightly. It made her feel unattractive and was a severe blow to her self-image. She could not wear the type of shoes that she believed were suitable for her and, hence, felt "unladylike." In addition, she held that her family didn't appreciate the amount of pain she experienced and that consequently they failed to realize that she couldn't work or keep house the way she had prior to her injury. She admitted to being depressed, suffering insomnia and wishing that "God would take me." She stated that her doctors did not appreciate how upset she was because of her deformity and was angry at their decision not to operate. Also because this injury severely affected her ability to work she said she was worthless to her family.

STEP II: Mrs. G.'s illness problems included:

(1) Depression with the psychophysiological concomitants of insomnia, decreased energy, feelings of worthlessness, hopelessness, and suicidal ideation.

(2) Vocational problems created by her injury and resulting inability to do physical labor.

(3) Family problems secondary to members' expectation that she continue in her accustomed role in the household despite her injury.

(4) Body image disturbance caused by the lump on her ankle and her cast.

(5) Miscommunication and conflict with her physicians as a result of cultural and language differences. The patient wanted surgery to repair an injury that produced an unacceptable change in her body image and provoked serious psychosocial problems. The surgeons viewed conservative management as best and feared surgery might make the injury worse due to problems in healing resulting from the patient's medications.

STEP III: If evaluated in the traditional medical and psychiatric paradigm, the patient would be diagnosed as having a major depressive disorder secondary to her medical illness and the treatment would be antidepressants and/or psychotherapy. Utilizing the clinical social science concepts that we have presented, however, it was apparent that there were serious discrepancies and conflicts in the patient's and physician's explanatory models that were a direct result of personal and cultural factors. The orthopedic surgeons did not realize that Mrs. G. perceived the injury as an unacceptable threat to her body image that undermined her self-esteem and created difficult illness problems involving her family, marriage and vocation. The patient explained to the psychiatric consultant through an interpreter that traditional Hispanic women, such as she, are extremely concerned with physical beauty in order to please their husbands. Any sickness or injury causing cosmetic damage is likely to cause serious emotional problems, and had in fact done so in her case.

After eliciting Mrs. G.'s and her family's explanatory model, assessing the illness problems, and determining the orthopedic surgeons' model, we explained to the patient that in our view her calcaneous fracture and the resulting cosmetic deformity of her ankle had resulted in serious illness problems involving her family, vocation, marital life and body image and caused her to suffer a severe depression. We noted that though she believed only surgery would alleviate the pain and deformity in her ankle, her surgeons, who also wished to alleviate the pain and cosmetic disfiguration, believed that conservative management with rest and casting would be best. In addition, surgery could result in a worse injury because the patient was on immunosuppressant drugs that often cause poor healing. Besides clarifying the conflict to the patient between her desire for surgery and the surgeons' recommendation for further conservative measures, we explained in full the biomedical rationale for the proposed treatment plan.

In addition, we recommended to her treatment of the illness problems via psychotherapy with a Spanish-speaking social worker, who would deal with the specific vocational, marital, and family concerns troubling the patient, and a trial of tricyclic antidepressants for her severe depression.

The patient and her family, however, still requested surgery. Together with the surgeons, we then countered with a compromise plan to manage the patient's fracture for one more month using conservative management; if at the end of that time either the physical deformity or pain were intolerable, it would be surgically repaired. The patient and her family agreed to this compromise plan as well as the psychosocial interventions mentioned above.

Mrs. G.'s fracture healed well with the conservative management including rest, casting and eventually physical therapy. She had brief supportive psychotherapy that helped alleviate the family problems and her depression cleared one month after starting the antidepressants. Due to continued weakness and pain in her left Achilles tendon she has been unable to resume her vocation as a nurses aid and currently plans to enter a vocational rehabilitation program to train for an alternative position requiring less physical labor.

The following are further case examples of successful clinical negotiations. The first case is an example of the patient and physician having differing explanatory models and the second of a situation where the patient's model and illness problems were simply not elicited causing a major patient-physician conflict.

CASE 7: Mr. J. was a 33-year-old white male who came to his family physician with complaints of recurrent episodes of inability to concentrate, weakness, insomnia, anxiety and anhedonia that lasted from three to six months and are often accompanied by a dysphoric mood. His mother died of cancer when he was two and he was raised by an alcoholic father. He had had a poor work history with frequent job losses that he felt were secondary to the above "physical" problem. Mr. J. believed that all his symptoms were due to "hypoglycemia." He had read extensively on this subject and brought in pages of dietary information and charts of foods that he thought he could not eat. The charts were tremendously detailed accounts of his day-to-day diet and symptoms. He had been tested in the past with at least two full glucose tolerance tests which were only borderline abnormal. He felt desperate and wanted treatment for the hypoglycemia. It was felt that the patient had a major depressive disorder with an obsessive-compulsive personality style and that the appropriate treatment would be antidepressants and psychotherapy. However, the consulting physician was doubtful that he could convince the patient to accept this treatment plan because of his explanatory model that his symptoms were caused by an endocrine disorder. After eliciting the patient's explanatory model and illness problems the psychiatrist presented the following explanation: "Although it is possible that hypoglycemia may be a significant problem, you are managing that dietarily as well as possible. On the other hand, the symptoms you present are often best treated by an antidepressant. It may be that these recurring episodes that you suffer are actually depression and I believe an antidepressant is the treatment of choice." The patient was surprised at this diagnosis and recommendation and still insisted that hypoglycemia was the cause of his symptoms but agreed to a one-month trial of antidepressants provided the medical staff reassessed his putative hypoglycemia. The staff agreed to perform the appropriate blood tests if he went along with the trial medication. The patient responded dramatically to the antidepressants with a loss of virtually all his symptoms over a three to four-week period. A new negotiation was undertaken regarding psychotherapy.

This patient had a major depressive disorder but the dysphoric affect had been masked by his use of somatization (a defense or coping mechanism whereby dysphoria is experienced and expressed in somatic terms, i.e., headaches, backaches, hypoglycemia). In this case we were able to negotiate a compromise and develop an effective treatment strategy. In primary care, however, physicians are familiar with patients who somatize to an almost delusional extent and often seem not to experience psychological symptoms. It is essential to utilize the explanatory model technique here especially with ethnic patients to learn about these patients' beliefs about experiencing and expressing emotions. In many cultures and families there are strong sanctions and taboos against expressing emotions and in many countries and small communities psychological treatment is unavailable so that somatization becomes a culturally sanctioned coping mechanism for eliciting care for psychosocial problems. For many such somatizing patients intrapsychically oriented psychotherapy is inappropriate because it is antagonistic to their belief system (which often puts negative connotations on the experience and expression of emotions) but other psychological treatments like hypnosis, biofeedback, meditation, stress management, and supportive, problem-solving psychotherapy, especially when provided by the primary care physician, are well received and effective. Perhaps an equally important physician goal is to prevent iatrogenic harm which is quite common in these patients. Due to their use of somatization their psychosocial problems are often not recognized and inappropriate somatic treatments prescribed. As in the case described above, somatization often can be negotiated with the physician working within the patient's idiom for articulating distress. But in certain cases where either patients refuse to negotiate their illness status, perhaps due to the social gain they receive from it (i.e., financial compensation or emotional support from family), or doctors refuse to consider alternatives to somatic intervention, negotiation will not be feasible.

CASE 8: Mrs. T. was a 42-year-old female brought into the Harborview Medical Center with an overdose of a sedative hypnotic. Upon awakening she admitted that she had tried to kill herself. She had become depressed over the last year due to side effects of an intestinal bypass surgery that she had undergone for obesity and secondary hypertension. Mrs. T. had severe side effects including diarrhea, orthostatic hypotension, fecal incontinence, and flatulence. These side effects caused recurrent hospitalization, problems with her job due to absences, significant economic problems, and social embarrassment and withdrawal secondary to the diarrhea, flatulence, and occasional incontinence. She did lose 100 pounds and her blood pressure returned to normal. She decided, due to the illness problems, to have her bowel reanastomosed and visited five successive surgeons all of whom refused stating that her surgery was successful due to the weight loss and normalization of blood pressure and that her side effects were an expected physiologic result of the surgery. Mrs. T. became increasingly depressed and took the overdose. During her subsequent hospitalization she again demanded that her bowel be reanastomosed or she would again consider suicide. She was quite angry at the surgical team and her past surgeons who she viewed as taking an unempathic stand that was unresponsive to her needs. We established a negotiation process, elicited her explanatory model and illness problems and presented a compromise plan to conservatively treat her side effects for three months and treat her illness problems with psychotherapy, antidepressants and social work assistance. But if at the end of the three months the patient still had side effects that she was concerned about the surgeons would reanastomose her bowel. The patient agreed to this compromise plan and was subsequently followed by psychiatry and surgery. She continued to have intolerable symptoms and therefore her bowel was reanastomosed two months later. Subsequently, the patient has done well and has an excellent relationship with her surgeons (Katon and Kleinman (1980)).

At times negotiation will reach an impasse. Again it is the patient's responsibility to make the final choice of whether to accept the physician's proposed treatment. If an impasse is reached then the physician should offer referral.

CASE 9: Mr. Z. was a 30-year-old male who presented to the Seattle Veterans Administration Hospital Emergency Room for the fourth time in one and a half months complaining of anxiety and insomnia. He had a long-term history of problems with anxiety, abuse of alcohol, a poor work history, and unstable interpersonal relationships. He said Valium was the only thing that worked for his "nerves" and he requested a prescription. In his chart were several notes by physicians stating that the patient appeared to be having problems with dependency on Valium. He had been prescribed a total of 200 5 mg tablets over the last thirty days. The psychiatric consultant let Mr. Z. know that he was concerned about the amount of Valium that he was taking and that they could be habit-forming, especially in a person with a history of alcohol problems. The psychiatrist recommended that Mr. Z. be admitted to the Psychiatric Ward for detoxification and evaluation. The other option presented was for Mr. Z. to enter an outpatient therapy program for patients with drug abuse. The patient refused these options, stating the only problem he had was that he was out of Valium. The psychiatrist felt medically and ethically that the patient was abusing Valium and needed to be on an ongoing program to evaluate and treat the apparent addiction. He therefore refused the patient's request and referred him again to the Outpatient Program. The patient became angry and left abruptly. He returned a week later stating that he felt he did have a problem with drugs and agreed to admission at that time.

We have found a negotiation approach, like the one illustrated in these cases, to be especially effective when dealing with somatization of mental illness, maladaptive coping response to chronic or terminal disorders, transference-countertransference problems, patient-family or doctor-family conflicts in labeling illness, inappropriate use of the sick role, serious divergence in ethnic and biomedical conceptual orientations, and patient and physician conflicts due to the unusual psychosocial demands of special treatment environments. But we also regard this as the appropriate approach for clinical relationships generally.

We feel that negotiation should be an integral part of the primary care physician's work, a core clinical task. It certainly isn't necessary or feasible to go through all the negotiation steps each time. The physician can expand or contract the process as needed just as he does with his history taking or physical examination. It is essential, however, to be able to have the skill to conduct the negotiation process in its entirety when necessary. The fact that some negotiations do take up significant amounts of time is not an argument for exonerating the physician from the negotiation process, but surely is an argument for the necessity of macro-social structural change in the organization and financing of care accompanying the micro-clinical alterations presented in this paper.

REFERENCES

Balint, M.
    1957 The Doctor, His Patient and the Illness. New York: International Universities Press.
Berkman, L. F. and S. L. Syme
    1979 Social Networks, Host Resistance and Mortality: A Nine-Year Follow up of Alameda County residents. Amer. J. Epidemiol.
Blinder, B. J., D. M. Freeman, and A. J. Stunkard
    1970 Behavioral Therapy of Anorexia Nervosa: Effectiveness of Activity as a Reinforcer of Weight Gain. Amer. J. Psychiatry 126:1083–1089.
Blumhagen, D.
    1980 A Folk Illness with a Medical Name. Culture, Medicine and Psychiatry, in press.

Brown, G. W.
    1962 Influence of Family Life on the Course of Schizophrenia. Brit. J. Prev. Soc. Med.
          16:55–68.
Brown, G. W. and J. L. T. Birley
    1968 Crisis and Life Changes and the Onset of Schizophrenia. J. Health Soc. Behav.
          9:203–214.
Brown, G. W., M. N. Bhrolchain, and T. Harris
    1975 Social Class and Psychiatric Disturbance Among Women in an Urban Population.
          Sociology 9:225.
Bruch, H.
    1973 Obesity, Anorexia Nervosa and the Person Within. New York: Basic Books.
    1978 The Golden Cage: The Enigma of Anorexia Nervosa, Cambridge, Massachusetts:
          Harvard University Press.
Cay, E. L., et al.
    1975 Patient's Assessment of the Result of Surgery for Peptic Ulcer. Lancet 1:29–
          31.
Chrisman, N., and A. Kleinman
    1979 The Teaching of Clinically Relevant Anthropology at the University of Washing-
          ton. Paper presented at the American Association of Anthropology Meeting,
          Cincinnati, November 28, 1979.
Day, M., and E. Semrod
    1978 Schizophrenic Reactions. In The Harvard Guide to Modern Psychiatry. Armond
          M. Nicholi, Jr., ed. Cambridge, Massachusetts: The Belknap Press of The Harvard
          University Press.
Eisenberg, L.
    1977 Disease and Illness. Culture, Medicine and Psychiatry 1(1):9–24.
    1979 Interfaces Between Medicine and Psychiatry. Comprehensive Psychiatry 20:1–
          14.
Engel, G. L.
    1977 The Need for a New Medical Model: A Challenge for Biomedicine. Science 196:
          129–136.
    1979 The Biopsychosocial Model: Resolving the Conflict Between Medicine and Psy-
          chiatry. Resident and Staff Physician 25:70–74.
Greenson, R. R.
    1967 The Technique and Practice of Psychoanalysis, Vol. I. New York: International
          Universities Press, pp. 190–206.
Gunderson, J. G., et al.
    1974 Special Report: Schizophrenia 1973. Schizophrenia Bulletin 9:15–54.
Guralnik, D., ed.
    1968 Webster's New World Dictionary. New York: William Collins and World Publishing
          Company, Inc.
Harwood, A.
    In press Communicating About Disease: Clinical Implications of Divergent Concepts
          Among Patients and Physicians.
Henderson, S., D. B. Byrne, P. Duncan-Jones, et al.
    1978 Social Bonds in the Epidemiology of Neurosis: A Preliminary Communication.
          Br. J. Psychiatry 132:463.
Herceg-Baron, R., B. Prisoff, et al.
    1979 Pharmacotherapy and Psychotherapy in Acutely Depressed Patients: A Study
          of Attrition Patterns in a Clinical Trial. Comprehensive Psychiatry 20:315–
          325.
Holmes, T. and R. Rahe
    1967 The Social Readjustment Rating Scale. Psychosomatic Res. 11:213–218.

Horowitz, M., N. Wilner, and W. Alvarez
    1979 Impact of Event Scale: A Measure of Subjective Stress. Psychosomatic Medicine
          41:209–218.
Johnson, D. W., and F. P. Johnson
    1975 Joining Together: Group Therapy and Group Skills. Englewood Cliffs, New Jersey:
          Prentice Hall, pp. 171–202.
Katon, W., and A. M. Kleinman
    1980 A Biopsychosocial Approach to Surgical Evaluation and Outcome. Western J. of
          Medicine 133:9–14.
Kleinman, A. M.
    1975 Explanatory Models in Health Care Relationships. In National Council for Inter-
          national Health: Health of the Family. Washington, D. C.: National Council for
          International Health; pp. 159–172.
    1979 Patients and Healers in the Context of Culture: An Exploration of the Borderland
          Between Anthropology, Medicine and Psychiatry. Berkeley: University of Cali-
          fornia Press.
Kleinman, A. M., L. Eisenberg, and B. Good
    1978 Culture, Illness and Care. Annals of Inter. Med. 88:251–258.
Kleinman, A. M., and G. Smilkstein
    1979 Psychosocial Issues in Assessment in Primary Care. In Medical Behavioral Science:
          Basic Applications in Family Medicine. Rosen, G. M., Geyman, J. P., Layton,
          R. H. eds. pp. 95–108. New York: Appleton Century Crofts.
Lazare, A., et al.
    1978 Studies on a Negotiated Approach to Patienthood. In Gallagher, E. ed.: The
          Doctor-Patient Relationship in the Changing Health Scene, DHEW Publication
          No. (NIH) 78–183. Washington, D. C.: United States Government Printing
          Office; pp. 119–139.
Lipowski, Z.
    1969 Psychosocial Aspects of Disease. Annals Intern. Med. 71:1197–1206.
Ludwig, A. M., and E. Othmer
    1977 The Medical Basis of Psychiatry. Amer. J. Psychiatry 134:1087–1092.
Medalie, J. H. and U. Goldbourt
    1976 Angina Pectoris Among 10,000 Men. Amer. J. Med. 60:910–921.
Meissner, William W. and Armand M. Nicholi, Jr.
    1978 The Psychotherapies: Individual, Family, and Group. In The Harvard Guide to
          Modern Psychiatry. Armand M. Nicholi, Jr., ed. pp. 357–386. Cambridge: The
          Belknap Press of Harvard University Press.
Minuchin, S., B. L. Rosman, and L. Baker
    1978 Psychosomatic Families: Anorexia Nervosa in Context. Cambridge, Massachusetts:
          Harvard University Press.
Moore, D. C.
    1977 Amitriptyline in Anorexia Nervosa. Amer. J. Psychiatry 134(11):1303–1304.
Mosher, L. R., and S. J. Keith
    1979 Research on the Psychosocial Treatment of Schizophrenia. A Summary Report.
          Amer. J. Psychiatry 136:623–631.
Nader, L., and H. F. Todd, eds.
    1978 The Disputing Process. New York: Columbia University Press.
Needleman, H. L. and D. Wafer
    1976 Amitriptyline in Patients with Anorexia Nervosa. Lancet 2:580.
Nicholi, A. M., Jr.
    1978 The Therapist – Patient Relationship. In The Harvard Guide To Modern Psy-
          chiatry. Armond M. Nicholi, Jr., ed. Cambridge, Massachusetts: The Belknap
          Press of the Harvard University Press.

Nuckolls, K. B., J. Cassel, and B. H. Kaplan
   1972 Psychosocial Assets, Life Crisis and Prognosis of Pregnancy. Amer. J. Epidemiology 95:431–440.
Rush, A. J., A. T. Beck, M. Kovacs, et al.
   1977 Comparative Efficacy of Cognitive Therapy and Pharmacotherapy in the Treatment of Depressed Outpatients. Cognitive Therapy Res. 1:17–37.
Svarstad, B.
   1976 Physician-Patient Communications and Patient Conformity with Medical Advice. *In* The Growth of Bureaucratic Medicine. David Mechanic, ed. pp. 220–228. New York: Wiley Interscience Publications.
Vaughn, C. E., and J. P. Leff
   1976 The Influence of Family and Social Factors in the Course of Psychiatric Illness: A Comparison of Schizophrenic and Depressed Neurotic Patients. Br. J. Psychiatry 129:125–137.
Weissman, M. M.
   1979 The Efficacy of Drugs and Psychotherapy in the Treatment of Acute Depressive Episodes. Amer. J. of Psychiatry 136:555–562.

SOCIAL LABELING AND OTHER PATTERNS OF SOCIAL COMMUNICATION

13. THE SOCIAL LABELING PERSPECTIVE ON ILLNESS AND MEDICAL PRACTICE

Recent research has turned up some rather puzzling findings. For example, in California a child's "failure" on the school psychologist's IQ test does not insure a diagnosis of "mental retardation"; in fact, whether a child is diagnosed as mentally retarded and referred to special classes is more closely associated with whether he is Mexican-American or Black than with his score on an IQ test (Mercer 1973). Or, persons who think they have heart disease but in fact do not often alter their lives on the basis of their beliefs about themselves, not on the basis of presence or absence of symptoms (Eichorn and Anderson 1962). The psychiatric patients who feel that they are "back to normal" one month after their first hospitalization are no different, diagnostically, from the "still sick" group; instead, their better clinical outcome can be explained by the greater power certain hospitals give patients to re-negotiate their legal status, treatment plans and diagnoses with hospital staff (Waxler et al. 1979). Whether a hospitalized tuberculosis patient gets well quickly is partly explained by whether he has cooperated with the ward staff; those who cooperate stay sick longer, those who do not cooperate get well more quickly (Calden et al. 1960).

None of the above findings is easily explained by reference to medical text-books nor to the ways physicians have been taught to apply the biomedical model of disease. The patient's diagnosis, not his ethnic group, should determine his referral and treatment. Outcome for treated disease should be predictable from diagnosis and treatment, not from the bureaucratic organization of the treating hospital. Patients who cooperate with treatment are expected to do better and certainly not expected to do worse than non-cooperative patients.

All of these findings, however, can be explained by an alternate sociological theory, the theory of social labeling (Schur 1971; Scheff 1966; Gove 1975). For labeling theory who is to be called "ill" is determined by the individual's social position and society's norms rather than by universal and objectively defined signs and symptoms. Further, a person is labeled as "ill" in the course of social negotiations between himself, his doctor, his family, sometimes ward staff and others. The outcome of such social negotiations is influenced by each person's beliefs and training and also by the social and organizational contexts in which the negotiation occurs. Once labeled as "ill" the individual may find himself caught in the midst of a self-fulfilling prophecy. Depending upon his social position he may find that de-labeling is difficult, that continued illness is expected and therefore that his symptoms continue.

These examples contrast two perspectives on illness and treatment, the

L. Eisenberg and A. Kleinman (eds.), The Relevance of Social Science for Medicine, 283–306.

biomedical and social labeling perspectives. Each perspective uses a conceptual
model to organize an abundant array of small facts, to weigh, select, discard, and
integrate facts about disease, illness and treatment; neither model is coterminous
with the facts themselves. While both the biomedical and social labeling models
are used to analyze medical phenomena they do not compete directly with each
other in an attempt to better explain or predict these phenomena. Instead, the
biomedical model of disease is used by practitioners in their everyday work to
understand a client's symptoms and to make decisions about etiology, diagnosis,
prognosis and treatment. Balint (1957), for example, shows how the general
practitioner questions and listens, selecting from a patient's report certain facts
that "fit" his biomedical conception of disease, thus providing him with a
particular diagnosis and treatment plan. This model of disease underlies all that
doctors are taught in medical school.

The sociologist using a social labeling model to understand disease, illness and
medical practice stands outside the doctor-patient interview and asks how the
social context, the social roles and relationships, the application of the biomedical model of disease itself, influence what the doctor does and what happens
to the patient. A social labeling theorist looking at the general practitioner's
interview might ignore altogether the patient's report of physical symptoms but
attend, instead, to the relative power and control exerted by physician and
patient, and use these selected bits of data to predict whether the sick person
will remain "ill" or return to his normal routine.

AN INTRODUCTION TO SOCIAL LABELING

Mercer's study of mental retardation (1973) shows how the social labeling model
can be used to analyze diagnostic and treatment practices and thus the careers
of children who may or may not be called "retarded". The biomedical model,
followed by physicians, most teachers and school psychologists, assumes that
"mental retardation is a pathological condition" and that "although organic
involvement cannot be established in cases classified as undifferentiated, familial
or sociocultural, it is assumed that 'minimal brain dysfunction' exists but cannot
be detected because of the inadequacy of diagnostic tools". (Mercer 1973:7—8)
Intelligence tests are the usual diagnostic tools and special education and training
for those who can respond is the normal treatment. One might expect, then, that
the diagnosis of a mentally retarded child follows quite routine and universal
medico-psychological procedures.

Using social labeling theory as a guide Mercer traced this diagnostic process,
one in which children in a California community were referred for IQ testing,
evaluated, diagnosed and sent to special classes within the public school system.
While all children who were diagnosed as retarded did, indeed, have IQ scores
lower than 80, her investigation of the series of steps leading to this diagnosis
shows clearly that many children with equally low IQ scores were never so

diagnosed. In fact it is the social characteristics of the children, their families, the schools they go to, that are better predictors of who, out of the pool of all low IQ students, are to be treated as "retarded".

A brief description of this social labeling process will introduce some of the ways in which labeling theory examines all medical questions.[1] Think of the diagnosis of mental retardation as the end-point in a series of decisions; at each decision point it is possible for some low IQ children to be returned to the pool of "normal" children, thus never to be called "retarded". The very first sorting point is at school enrollment itself. Children enrolled in private schools (mostly Catholic parochial schools in this case) are immediately saved from the diagnosis of retardation, not because these children have higher IQ's (1.1% had IQ's less than 80), but because parochial schools do not have school psychologists, testing programs, nor procedures for referrals. Since, by law, a child must be tested before being sent to special classes, no child in the private school system is diagnosed as "retarded" nor "treated". Teachers perceive most of the low IQ students as simply poor in their academic work. Thus, the organizational structure of the parochial schools serves as a social context in which no diagnosis of retardation can occur.

Public schools, however, do have psychologists, special classes and formal procedures for making decisions about who is to be called "retarded". The first step in this procedure consists of "failing" or "keeping the child back" a grade. The elementary school teacher is the prime decision-maker and uses his/her norms as a basis for this decision; many children are initially labeled as retarded at this point because they are poor in social and academic skills. However it is the family background that profoundly distinguishes between children "held back" and children promoted. The former are much more likely to be Spanish-speaking Mexican-Americans of low socioeconomic status. At this very early stage in the sorting process, then, students from certain backgrounds have a much greater likelihood of being provisionally labeled as "retarded".

If a child is held back in school he may, next year, be referred by the school principal for psychological testing. This decision is not affected by the child's family background but it is influenced by an organizational characteristic of the school system. A school policy protects overburdened psychologists by imposing a quota on referrals for psychological testing; each school is allocated an equal number of psychologist-days, regardless of the size of the school. Thus, children tentatively labeled by teachers as retarded are much more likely to be sent on to the next labeling stage if they go to a small school. Children of equally low levels of academic and social performance escape the next diagnostic stage because school principals must limit the numbers of children they refer. Again, an organizational constraint has an impact on who is to be called retarded.

Referrals from the school principal do not necessarily insure that the child will actually be tested, however. Since psychological testing is a legal requirement for "treatment" (i.e., referral to special classes) it is apparent that the psychologist's decision to test or not is a crucial one for the child's career. While the child's family background has no bearing on the psychologist's decision, that is, he/she does not choose to test proportionately more Mexican-Americans or children from middle class families, the decision to test is highly related to the principal's reason for referral, mentioned in his/her referral statement. Those children presented as "possibly retarded" were tested 90% of the time. Thus, the psychologist chooses most often to "rubber stamp" the provisional label of mental retardation made by the principal and teacher. Children referred for academic difficulties, but in which no mention of retardation is made, are not as likely to be tested.

Of the children who are referred and actually tested by the psychologist, some "pass", that is have IQ scores greater than 80, while others "fail". "Once tested, a child's IQ becomes the most critical variable determining whether he retains the status of 'normal' student or moves closer to the status of 'mental retardate'" (Mercer 1973:114). The children who were referred for testing were similar to the whole population of the school district; those who "failed" were significantly more likely to be from poor and minority, Mexican-American or Black, homes. Failure of larger proportions of Mexican-Americans is probably not due to a lower level of intelligence in that group but is more reasonably explained by the middle class biases of intelligence tests which rest heavily on verbal skills. Many of the Mexican-American children come from Spanish-speaking homes but are taught and tested in English.

Diagnoses of "mental retardation" are applied by the school system to a selected sample of children, but that is not the end of selective processing. In fact, some children who are called retarded are never referred to special classes; these non-referred children are significantly more often from white or middle class families. The children who are selected for special classes have scores similar to the non-referred group but are significantly more likely to be Mexican-American, from poor families and to have been provisionally labeled as retarded by their classroom teachers. Further selection is apparent when Mercer examines which children actually appear in the special classes, the final decision point. Ten of the 81 referred children escaped the label of "retarded" by not going to these classes; these tended to be younger girls from Anglo families. Two remained in their original classrooms; one transferred to a parochial school where she was not considered retarded; seven moved out of the community. There is the hint here that middle class white families may be more able to resist labeling of their child by negotiating alternative arrangements.

Thus, Mercer has shown that while one might assume that the diagnosis of mental retardation is an objective judgement based on IQ scores derived from a standard intelligence test, the actual operation of this process is systematically influenced by a number of social and organizational factors that have nothing to do with the child's basic intelligence. One result of the selective labeling is examplified in the following segment of Mercer's Table 7 (1973:112):

		Characteristics of public school pop. (6–15 years. age) in %'s (N = 1565)	Characteristics of children in special classes for retarded in %'s (N = 71)
Sex:	Male	50.4	69.1
	Female	49.6	30.9
Ethnic group:	Anglo	81.0	32.1
	Mex-Amer.	11.0	45.3
	Black	7.9	22.6
Social status:	Poor housing	36.1	74.6

After examining Mercer's data, then, some might recommend that the California school system "tighten up", "systematize" and "make more objective" the procedures for identifying the "truly retarded" so that no child in that category slips through the net and remains "untreated". Implicit in this recommendation are the assumptions of the biomedical model of disease.

Social labeling theory makes quite different assumptions, however, some of which are implicit in our discussion of Mercer's findings. First, there is no universal definition of "illness". Whether an individual is to be called "ill" is relative to the society or organization in which he is found; poor academic/social performance in parochial schools or in lower class Mexican-American families is believed to be just that, not evidence of mental retardation. Organizational practices as well constrain the definition of illness; only if the society or organization has procedures for defining or labeling illness does the illness exist. Thus, illness is a social fact, one that cannot be separated from the processes through which it is socially identified and labeled. From this perspective there are no "truly retarded" children waiting to be discovered.

This then leads to the second principle, that whether symptoms, unusual behavior, poor performance are to be called "illness" is the result of a social negotiation process among interested parties. Clearly many people – teachers, students, families, psychologists – have contributed to the final label or lack of it and each has brought to that negotiation process his own assumptions about mental retardation as well as his own interests in the child, the process, or the diagnostic outcome. Social labeling theory focuses much of its attention on the relative power of "labelers" and "labeled" and assumes that the negotiation process and its outcome can often be predicted from the interests of those in power. The fact that it is children from middle class white families who are more likely to escape the label "retarded" is thus consistent with social labeling hypotheses.

Since labels of "illness" result from social negotiations in certain social and organizational contexts, the theory also assumes that "de-labeling" occurs within these contexts. That is, whether a person who has been called "ill" returns to "normal" is predictable from his social characteristics, the expectations that others have for him, the interests of all parties, and the nature of the treatment organization itself. For some, returning to "normal" is easily done; this may have been true for some of the young, white girls from middle class families in Mercer's sample. For others, the label of illness and involvement in the treatment process may so delimit the range of normal interactions and relationships that the individual has only one available role, as a "sick person". Our classes, schools, and homes for the mentally retarded which are organized to "treat" or "train" children for participation in normal society may have the unintended effect of prolonging "illness" or of leading to what labeling theory calls "secondary deviant roles". Some of the children who are labeled as retarded in the school system may have been given a label that sticks for life, and that has profound implications for jobs, marriage, and future social relationships.

SOME EVIDENCE FOR SOCIAL LABELING THEORY

Mental retardation is a "fringe" disease. It is quite easy to see how social factors might become involved in decision-making in the face of symptoms that are unclear and thus difficult to evaluate. But social labeling theory is used to analyse the selection, negotiation and treatment of all sorts of illnesses including those diseases that one might assume are objectively defined and routinely processed.[2] It assumes, then, that the process of becoming ill, being treated and getting well is a social process. It also allows for, and even predicts, that some patients who are treated within a medical system may, from the biomedical perspective, have no "true" disease (for example, the "crocks" whom physicians feel get in the way of treating the "truly ill") and that some "truly diseased" people never appear in any medical system (for example, the Indian woman who sees her pregnancy as a normal phenomenon, the busy mother who ignores her headaches, the man who attributes his shortness of breath to old age). For social labeling theory the "crock" and the old man who has difficulty breathing are not evidence that the medical system is not working well but instead are predictable in terms of how the social processes of identification, selection and negotiation actually work.

We will look here at three general stages of illness labeling. The first is the initial decision that something is wrong that should be called "illness". The second stage involves the negotiation among interested parties regarding what sort of illness it is and what should be done about it. Finally, the third stage is one in which the negotiated label (which, in reality, may change several times) influences social relationships and symptoms, and thus affects whether the labeled individual is able to "de-label" and return to normal. We have selected a few empirical studies relevant to each of the stages to provide concrete examples of the ways in which labeling theory examines the career of the ill person. These examples are not meant to provide a survey of empirical support for the theory since empirical evidence varies considerably, depending on the particular hypothesis; there is much more evidence for the initial selective labeling of ill people than for the later stages of labeling. Instead we use the examples to clarify the labeling hypotheses themselves.

SOME CONDITIONS UNDER WHICH "ILLNESS" IS IDENTIFIED AND LABELS OF ILLNESS ARE GIVEN

The first stage in social labeling of illness usually occurs when someone, often the individual himself, thinks that "something is wrong". Neither he nor his family may know what it is, even whether it is an illness; they may simply decide that things are not normal. There are, however, many social conditions under which the same individual feeling or behaving in the same way may never label himself nor be labeled by others as ill. Whether initial labeling occurs depends on the norms of the society in which he lives, his own social position within the society, and the characteristics of organizations with which he may be involved. We will look briefly at each of these three factors.

Cultural and Social Norms

Each society has its own peculiar definitions for the kinds of behaviors, dysfunctions, even feelings, that are to be called and treated as "illnesses". We see these culturally specific definitions of illness most clearly if we look across time within our culture or if we compare across cultures. For example, just recently in many places in the West the set of behaviors we call "alcoholism" has been legally shifted from the category of "crime" to the category of "illness", leading to new types of decisions about who is an "alcoholic" and to profound changes in the career of the labeled person. Definitions of other illnesses have also changed. Homosexuality is, formally, no longer an illness according to the American Psychiatric Association but "lack of sexual desire" now is, at least, as it is represented in textbooks describing specific etiologies and treatment strategies (Kaplan 1979). Further, in the West if a person does not go to work our first thought is that he might be "ill". This is not true in peasant Sri Lanka (Ceylon), for example, where "not working", while often deviant, is not necessarily a sign of illness. In Sri Lanka, too, the Western psychiatrist's cues for "depression" – withdrawal, lack of communication, lethargy – are seldom thought of as illness by the individual or his family (Waxler 1974a, b). One might also expect that in societies where diseases such as malaria, leprosy, hookworm, and schistosomiasis are highly prevalent they are less likely to be called "illness" than to be seen as "problems in daily living". For example, Indian mothers traditionally have not defined the high rate of infant death (often due to tetanus from the use of cowdung to treat the umbilical cord) as a problem of "illness" but instead have understood the repeated loss of their babies in religious terms. Thus, cultures vary in the extent to which a specific set of behaviors or feelings is judged to be deviant (e.g., "depression" in Sri Lanka is "normal"); cultures vary as well in terms of the type of deviance ("illness", "crime", "sin", etc.) the behavior is believed to represent.

Available Treatment Systems

Beliefs and norms within a specific culture allow for selective decisions about what phenomena are to be called "illnesses". But just as important in the labeling decision are the characteristics and capacities of available treatment organizations. Thus, whether an individual is to be called "ill" or "ill in a certain way" depends very clearly on the existence and kind of treatment and treatment systems that the society provides.

Hospital administrators have long had the uneasy feeling that the more beds they provide the more sick people there are to fill them. Recently Harris (1975) has shown that this is, indeed, probably true. Examining 56 counties in New York State he showed that increases in the number of hospital beds per 1000 population is associated with increases in the use of these beds, not because there was an initial demand or need, but because physicians respond to the new, and empty, beds by increasing admissions and lengthening patient stays. Thus, the availability of hospital services has a direct effect upon the norms of medical practice which, in turn, affects the number of individuals who will be labeled as "sick enough to be in a hospital". The fact of being so defined and treated may, according to labeling theory hypotheses, have important implications for the future of these hospitalized individuals.

We see just that in D'Arcy's analysis (1976) of changes in the health services in the Province of Saskatchewan during the period 1946–70. These changes led for a time to a startling increase in the numbers of older people labeled as "mentally ill". The high in 1950's for people over 70 was 600 per 100,000 people in Saskatchewan as compared with all-Canada rate for the same age group of 250 per 100,000.

The introduction of a program of free hospitalizations for mental illness interacting in the context of a rapidly increasing older age component in the population and the lack of facilities for the care of the aged had the effect of dramatically increasing the rate of mental illness . . . (D'Arcy 1976:5)

Free care for those old people who have no place to go was associated, then, with an enormous increase in psychiatric morbidity. A decrease in psychiatric hospitalization that was just as dramatic occurred in the early 1960's associated with changes in the delivery of health and welfare services, including

. . . increased old age allowance . . . the shift in the basis of allocating monies from a 'means test' to a 'needs' test, increased provincial funding for low cost housing . . . hostels, nursing homes . . . and the making of mental hospital admission discretionary (by the medical officer in charge of the hospital) (D'Arcy 1976:11).

Thus, by 1965 the psychiatric admission rates for patients over 70 years was down to 250 per 100,000. As D'Arcy suggests, changes in the availability of alternative social and health services clearly contribute to the "manufacture and obsolescence of madness". If the label of mental illness were benign and/or transitory one might view these changes as vagaries of the health bureaucracy but labeling theory hypothesizes that the label of mental illness in itself has significant and often negative effects on the social relationships of the labeled person. Thus, the increase in hospitalization rates has results that are not entirely benign.

Whether "trouble" is called "illness" is sometimes also dependent upon other characteristics of the practice of medicine, including whether an effective treatment is at hand to deal with it. For example, not until specific drugs were available to give to hyperactive children did "hyperkinesis" become a disease category that physicians and others attended to (Conrad 1978). Not until lithium became known as an effective agent for endogenous depression did manic-depressive psychosis come to be something other than an unusual disease, seldom seen in Western psychiatric hospitals (Kendell et al. 1971). Readily available treatments "create" diseases that might otherwise, and have in the past, not been called disease at all.

The decision to label some sort of "trouble" as "illness" is exceptionally common if the individual lives within the context of a "total institution" such as a prison or on a Navy ship. When all aspects of one's life occur within the boundaries of the prison walls the rate of labeled illness is four times the national average; that is, prisoners are four times as likely to make visits to the prison clinic requesting treatment. (Twaddle 1976). Characteristics of institutional life and the ways in which medical systems have been organized in response to them have the ultimate effect of producing large numbers of people labeled "ill". Some prisoners, called "skaters", label themselves as ill in order to use the clinic to meet friends; others appear often in the clinic due to the organizational policy that prescription drugs are given only one week at a time. Clinic physicians are also arbiters of who is allowed to purchase "civilian" shoes. Even when these unique characteristics are accounted for the rate of labeled illness is three times the national average.

These unique characteristics are important to social labeling theory. They appear clearly in the prison data but they illustrate a phenomenon that is more general. Whether an individual labels himself as "sick" occurs within and is affected by the norms of the society around him. Physicians following the biomedical model might say that some of these prisoners are not "really" sick; social labeling theory takes a different view, that all are labeled and processed as "ill" and that the very processing has important implications for the individual and the organization.[3]

What we have shown so far are some of the contextual factors that impinge on the labeling of illness. Cultural as well as treatment system variables have very clear and selective effects on whether the individual who feels or thinks that "something is wrong" is labeled as "ill".

The Characteristics of the Individual

Selective labeling is also contingent on characteristics of the individual himself, upon his position in the family and the society. For example, Campbell (1975) has shown that mothers are more likely to see their children as "ill" than themselves as "ill" even when the symptoms are identical. Two-thirds of a list of common symptoms (headaches, fever, toothache, sore throat, etc.) were judged by mothers to be "illnesses" in children while only one-half were believed to be illnesses if the mother had them. Further, mothers are twice as likely to call a doctor for a child's illness than for the same illness in themselves. Thus, the decision about whether "something is wrong" depends upon age and family position; the decision of mothers to normalize their own symptoms removes them from the set of labeled and treated patients.

Self-selection by the person who has symptoms is also often contingent, not on the symptoms or presence of "disease", but on the individual's social and economic background. The way in which social background impinges on these self-labeling decisions is apparent among physically handicapped individuals who drop out of a rehabilitation program before the prescribed regimen is completed (Ludwig and Adams 1968). Drop-outs are more likely to be men, white, in middle age groups, and to have had previous employment; those who complete the program are women, the very old and very young, blacks, and the unemployed. If the handicapped person has a job to return to he will redefine himself as "normal" and leave the rehabilitation program; this definition takes precedence over the physician's judgement that the individual has not yet returned to a normal physical state. It is those handicapped individuals who are in the relatively more powerful social positions (men, whites, but especially the employed) who can and do choose to think of themselves as "normal" rather than "sick" and who can and do act on this decision by dropping out of the treatment system.

LABELING AND DE-LABELING: A NEGOTIATED PROCESS

Cultural norms, the presence or absence of particular treatment systems and the social position of individuals within their social group are all variables significant in the initial decision about whether an individual is "ill" or not. If that decision is affirmative then the troubled individual often finds himself in a doctor's office or hospital emergency room. It is here that the "trouble" is transformed into a specific "illness" through a process of negotiation, often between professionals, family members and the sick person. The illness label, whether it is "pneumonia", "fatigue", "too much drinking", "just being ornery", is affected by the social positions and interests of all the parties involved.

Considerable research has focused on this negotiation stage, often following the biomedical perspective on disease. Many of these studies of physician-patient interactions look at communication and emotional and social class barriers that prevent the physician from obtaining diagnostic information, making a correct decision about treatment and getting the patient to follow, or comply with, his recommendations (Hauser 1979). Social labeling theory examines the same negotiations but follows quite different assumptions. It says that what the "trouble" is called is constructed within the interaction and is dependent, not on how accurately the physician can use interview and examination data to match the reported symptoms with a textbook description, but instead on social characteristics of the professionals and the patient and the social contexts in which they meet.

Characteristics of the Individual

What the trouble is to be called, and what is done about it is often predictable from the interests and relative social position of the troubled individual himself. For example, some individuals learn through experience with particular treatment systems how to state their case (regardless of their symptoms) in order to get what they want, either hospital admission or discharge. Those who want admission to a very selective psychiatric ward, for example, know that mention of suicidal tendencies is the key to admission since the law requires that; being "hospital-wise" tips the balance in the emergency room negotiations. A similar phenomenon occurs in a chronic care hospital (Roth and Eddy 1967) where the very small proportion of individuals who are informed about the variety of services are able to negotiate or to have others act on their behalf in order to be admitted to the most desirable "rehab" service. "Nearly always these knowledge-able individuals are chosen even though the physician may feel that little can be done to help them and may only take them to prevent their 'rotting away' on the less desirable wards" (1967:16).

The social and economic position of the potentially "ill" person along with that of his family or spokesmen may have a significant impact on the negotiation of the problem. This is often apparent in the negotiations around psychiatric hospitalization where the decision to label someone as "mentally ill" may have long-term negative effects. Some of these negotiations take place in commitment hearings where physicians, lawyers, prospective patients, sometimes family members, meet to consider whether the individual should be hospitalized against his will. One group of investigators systematically examined 81 hearings held in an Ohio state psychiatric hospital (Wenger and Fletcher 1969). In every one of these hearings the court-appointed referee (fulfilling the functions of a judge) rubber-stamped the recommendation made by the psychiatrist. Yet the psychiatrist's recommendation was not systematically based on the seriousness of the individual's symptoms nor the threat of his behavior to himself or others. Instead, recommendations were strongly related to the presence of a lawyer representing the individual's interests. If a lawyer were present not only was the hearing longer and less perfunctory but also the psychiatrist was significantly less likely to recommend hospitalization. Thus, only 26% of those with lawyers were involuntarily committed while 92% of those not legally represented were committed. This significant difference held true for individuals whose symptoms and behaviors met the legal criteria for admission as well as for those whose symptoms were less serious. While the lawyer's presence was a significant predictor of the recommended course, psychiatrists making the recommendations were not aware of that effect; one said, "Legal counsel has no effect on my decision . . . If the patient is sick, he's sick" (1969:71).

If we looked at these negotiation processes we would probably see a cluster of characteristics that are correlated with the "non-commitment" decision; the 18% of individuals who have lawyers are probably middle class with educational and economic resources that give them power. Even if they are not economically or socially "equal" to the examining physicians, the fact that they have a profes- sional speaking for them (since legal counsel is sometimes available free through Legal Aid) means that the label of illness (or lack of it) is negotiated between professionals of equal status. The investigators suggest that there exists "an uneasy peace which is sustained between the two professions, partly on the basis of the psychiatrists' unintended and unwitting trade-off of effective authority to the lawyers, in exchange for the privilege of ostensible authority in the carefully staged setting of the admission hearings" (1969:72). Thus, whether an individual is to be called "mentally ill" and to be involuntarily hospitalized is the result of a complex set of social relationships between several professionals and the prospective patient.

Characteristics of the Institution

The ways in which the institution operates has an important and selective effect on the negotiation of illness as well. Certain hospitals, dependent upon patient fees, may organize admission procedures in such a way as to produce the numbers of "ill" people that are required to keep the system going. For example, one private psychiatric hospital, in its brochure searching for "moonlighting" physi- cians to work at night, offers $ 125 per night *plus* $ 25 for each patient admitted. While we have no empirical evidence that the additional payment increases admissions, the incentive for admissions is an incentive to define individuals as "ill enough to need hospitalization".

More systematic investigation has been done linking the workings of treat- ment systems to the negotiation processes that result in someone being called "ill". In a study of 269 consecutive decisions for or against hospital admission to the psychiatric division of the Los Angeles County-U.S.C. Medical Center, it was discovered that the severity of the prospective patient's symptoms played no part in the outcome of negotiations (Mendel and Rapport 1969). However, the time of day and the day of the week that an individual appeared in the admissions office had a significant effect on the negotiation. Of those who appeared during regular working hours, 9—5, Monday through Friday, only 32% were admitted; of the others who showed up at night or on weekends, 51% were admitted, even though they were no different from the former group in severity of symptoms. A major factor in the increased admissions at night/weekends was the way the hospital organized its work-load, putting social workers and senior psychiatrists (who tend not to hospitalize) on duty during the day and residents on night duty. The resident on duty tended "to hospitalize patients to be 'safe' because he is unsure of his evaluation and is far less resourceful in planning and implementing an alternative to hospitalization" (1969:326). The resident's conservative stance interacts with the fact that individuals who request admission at odd hours are less likely to have or bring with them an interested family member who might provide an alternative to hospitalization. The way the hospital organization works, then, produces labeled illnesses that might not exist if, for example, social workers did night duty.

Similar institutional effects on negotiated illnesses appear in social agencies. For example, a person who becomes blind often voluntarily consults an agency for the blind and soon finds that "not all people who have been labeled 'blind' can follow a course entirely of their own choosing" (Scott 1969:73). Agency staff may negotiate an illness label with the individual that has little or nothing to do with the degree to which vision is impaired but is dependent instead on the ideology of the agency. A blind person who has residual vision (this is the most common form of blindness) is under strong pressure to think of himself as blind in the way which the agency happens to define it. For example, blind people who select one type of agency find that they are expected to "accommodate" to what the agency defines as a debilitating and life-long handicap. In these settings blind people are provided with extensive substitutes for sight, for example, tape record- ings in the elevators to announce the floors; cafeterias that serve food easily eaten by blind people; sheltered workshops geared to special handicaps of the blind rather than to training for regular jobs. The implicit assumption of these agencies is that blindness makes one incompetent and thus dependent (Scott 1969:85).

But some agencies take a different stand, that a blind person can be restored to quasi-normal life, provided he accepts the fact he is blind and receives training/ counseling. Blind individuals who appear in these agencies are encouraged to think of themselves as going through an emotional crisis in which personal independence and self-esteem has been lost with the loss of sight and in which reintegration of the personality involves pain. Stress, then, is on psychological rather than physical adaptation to poor vision. This "total psychological change" ideology contrasts with a third sort of ideology, represented by the Veterans' Administration, in which re-training of the blind is limited in time and the agency's expectation is that the individual will return to the normal community with the help of physical devices and some income maintenance.

The expectations of each type of agency for the blind are evident in the ways in which they negotiate with, or train, the blind person. Thus, one might expect that these varied negotiations produce blind persons whose lives follow quite different pathways. And this seems to be true. Compared with blind men treated in the V.A. program, blind civilians who receive services from other agencies "are less active in nonblindness-related clubs and organizations . . . they visit less; they have fewer sighted friends; they do not engage in social activities to the same degree; and they tend to be more isolated" (Scott 1969:116). Institutions such as agencies for the blind have a significant impact upon the kind of illness label that the sick person will take on and, in the long run, a significant impact on his social relationships.

Thus, what kind of illness an individual is believed to have, and what he and others expect of him is not a cut and dried affair dependent simply on the physician's diagnosis. Instead, illness labels are created in social negotiations between several parties, including professionals and the troubled individual, and they occur within institutional and social contexts that play an important part in the negotiation. Ideologies and organizational procedures as well as the relative power and interests of the negotiating parties contribute to the label of illness. Further, illness labels are often changed as the negotiation process continues. Thus, there is not only an on-going process of labeling, but also of re-labeling and de-labeling.

THE EFFECTS OF ILLNESS LABELS ON SOCIAL RELATIONSHIPS AND SYMPTOMS

Illness labels, we have seen, are given selectively, the result of negotiation between physician, patient and others, often in an institutional context. That these labels are not simply generated in a social exercise that is irrelevant to the individual's life situation is evident when we examine what happens to labeled individuals.

Someone who has been labeled as having cancer, who has been successfully treated, and who returns to work often finds that the label "sticks". Further, the label of "cancer" is a stigmatizing one (perhaps because of its equation with death) that often generates significant changes in the individual's social and work life. For example, in a recent study,

Many recovered patients complained of feeling isolated at work because their co-workers acted as though cancer was contagious . . . Over 80 percent of the blue-collar workers and 50 percent of the white-collar workers surveyed encountered some form of job discrimination relating to the fact that they had been successfully treated for cancer (New York Times 1979).

Discrimination with regard to promotions, work assignments, access to health insurance, etc., is common although illegal. Illness labels, therefore, are often difficult to discard, even when the disease has disappeared; it is the label itself that has impact on the individual's life.

An illness label may, as well, mean that the individual so labeled becomes enmeshed within certain institutions that sustain the label rather than encourage its discard. Certain illness organizations seem to have this function. For example, the Diabetes Clubs for adolescent diabetics, whose explicit function is to educate and support the patient so that he can take on a "normal" role, may, in reality, encourage the diabetic to spend more and more time in the company of others just like himself, thus sustaining the label of illness. Alcoholics Anonymous is a prime example of an institution that prolongs the illness label in its formal ideology (the requirement that individuals publicly confirm that they are "alcoholics") as well as in its function. A large percentage of AA members' social lives centers on the organization and other members, thus isolating them from normal relationships and further strengthening their role as "alcoholics".

Labels of "Illness" Affect Social Relationships

Whether and what kind of illness label one has, then, may have a profound effect upon one's social relationships, irrespective of whether the symptoms or the disease itself have disappeared. Others (and the labeled person) may continue to think of the individual as "a diabetic", "having cancer", "mentally ill" or "a heart patient"; further, organizational norms and functions may sustain the label and set limits on the role the individual can take.

The effect of a label on one's work is apparent in Eichorn and Anderson's (1962) comparison of farmers with labeled and unlabeled heart diseases. Two sets of farmers labeled themselves as having "heart disease", but only one set actually had, upon medical examination, any evidence of the disease. The group of farmers that mistakenly believed themselves to have diseased hearts, but in fact were well, received the label "through improper diagnosis or failure to understand the doctor's diagnosis" (Eichorn and Anderson 1962:242–243). The third and fourth sets of farmers did not label themselves as having heart disease but one group of them, upon examination, were found to have diseased hearts.

Comparison of the four sets provides for a test of the relative effects of disease and illness label on social role and findings show that both variables have some effect on the individual's life. Farmers with true heart disease, whether they were labeled or not, are more likely to cut down on the amount of work that they do; they reduce their hours of work, sell off some land, or take easier jobs in town. "Even though 'hidden cardiacs' did not believe they had heart disease they, like the true cardiacs, tended to report chest pains" (1962:246). Thus, the symptoms themselves, whether labeled as "heart disease" or not, may have had some effects on the farmers' decisions to cut down on work.

But labels have an effect on role, too, regardless of the presence of disease. If a farmer believes himself to have a diseased heart he will take more heart-related precautions than will the farmer who labels himself as "normal". Those who mistakenly labeled themselves or had been labeled as "heart diseased" chose to take naps, to use sun-shades on their tractors and to stop smoking just as did those who were "true cardiacs". The label itself – what the farmer or his family believes to be the case – has an important effect upon his behavior, even when he has no symptoms and no heart disease.

Another result of illness labeling may be longer or more frequent hospitalizations; once an individual is labeled as "ill" he is likely to be labeled again. For example, in the Los Angeles psychiatric service the one factor that residents, social workers and staff psychiatrists uniformly took into account in making a decision about hospital admission was whether the person had been admitted in the past, even though the decision-makers were unaware that they attended to this phenomenon (Mendel and Rapport 1969:325). In fact, sixty percent of previously hospitalized individuals were readmitted while only 11% of those not previously hospitalized were admitted, even though the two groups were almost identical in the severity of their symptoms. The implication of this tendency to re-label is important since in the course of re-hospitalizations the individual may become further and further removed from the normal world of work and his normal social relationships. Psychiatric patients who are removed from the labor market for considerable periods of time by virtue of their hospitalization have difficulty in finding jobs. Lack of work after discharge from psychiatric hospitalization is an excellent predictor of further re-hospitalizations, even when severity of symptoms is controlled for (Maisel 1967).

Some institutions, in fact, create and/or sustain lifelong roles for people labeled as "ill", roles that far outlast the disease itself. The Public Health Service leprosy hospitals, for example, accept the ideology that leprosy is socially stigmatized and thus provide patients with a small but isolated society in which they can remain for life. Houses, jobs, recreation, are all available on the grounds of the hospital. Thus, rather than discarding the label of "leper" once the disease is arrested ex-patients retain that label and are removed from society with the assistance of the institution whose goal is "cure" (Waxler 1979).

Similarly, some agencies for the blind offer broad services and encourage dependency such that some blind people become what Scott (1969) calls "professional blind men". These are blind individuals whose whole lives are organized around the fact of their blindness, and who are retained in the role partly as a result of their having been hired to work in such activities for the blind as sheltered workshops, home-teaching and counseling programs and residential schools.

Labels of Illness Affect Symptoms

To this point we have presented labeling theory as a conceptual model in which the label of illness is selectively applied to an individual, often on the basis of his social characteristics and the social context in which he lives, and in which labels are negotiated and re-negotiated, often within treatment institutions. The result of illness labeling is an alteration, temporary or permanent, in the individual's social relationships.

Nothing has been said about possible effects of labeling on the disease process or on symptoms themselves.[4] Yet this is probably the question of most interest to physicians. Practitioners are likely to ask, "Does the social labeling process impinge on the patient's illness and therefore on my job, the treatment of diseased individuals?"

The crucial question here is this: are labels of illness the result of disease or do they cause disease? Which comes first? The layman's assumption (and probably most physicians' as well) is that if one experiences symptoms then one labels oneself as ill. In this case labels are simply ways of conceptualizing a more basic biological process; they have no impact upon that process. Labeling theory hypothesizes just the opposite, that if one is labeled as "ill" this label has an effect upon disease; in this case we cannot conceive of the label simply as a cognitive phenomenon but must see it as having a direct impact on the illness itself.

Longitudinal studies of labels and disease and/or well-controlled analyses are required in order to sort out this "chicken-egg" phenomenon and few studies attempt to test these alternate hypotheses directly. However, there is considerable evidence that labels of illness and the expectations that others have of labeled individuals do have an impact on the disease process, particularly on prognosis. Often the mediating process is one in which the labeled person or the system around him comes to reject or to re-negotiate the label of illness and thus the individual drops the "sick role". He thinks of himself as "well", others treat him as "well" and expect him to be so and the organized, well-defined package of symptoms become diffuse, are not attended to, not rewarded, and may be redefined as "normal". Ultimately, as symptoms are socially redefined they disappear as significant biomedical phenomena as well.[5]

For example, acceptance of the label of "tuberculosis" as defined by a particular TB hospital is significantly associated with the rate of recovery from the disease itself. Calden et al. (1960) followed a cohort of newly admitted TB patients through the initial four months of hospitalization and classified them as having a relatively "fast" or "slow" recovery rate, relative to each patient's own initial condition. While very few of the medical/psychological variables were predictive of recovery rate, there was a "significant relationship between the patient's ward behavior and his rate of recovery" (1960:352). Patients who cooperated with the institutional regime – who accepted the label of "illness" – recovered slowly. Those who did not conform to the rules about bed rest and who were aggressive about getting what they wanted – that is, who rejected the label – recovered more quickly. It was the "good patient", the one who internalized the institution's label of illness, whose symptoms lasted longer.

A similar link between the label of illness and the retention of symptoms is apparent in psychiatric illness. Doherty (1975) looked at the acceptance and rejection of illness labels by psychiatric patients in the first four weeks of their hospitalization. In this hospital one of the major staff goals was to socialize patients to accept the fact that they were indeed "ill". The staff reasoned that not until one sees oneself as "ill" can the psychotherapeutic treatment orientation ("working out one's problems") be effective. Thus, one staff goal is to make sure that all patients label themselves as "mentally ill". In fact, some patients immediately so labeled themselves and retained that label of mental illness throughout the four-week period. Another group initially labeled themselves but quickly rejected the label and thought of themselves as "not mentally ill". A third group never did accept the label of illness. They denied that they were ill.

The three groups did not differ initially in overall psychopathology ratings by the staff; thus, whether one's symptoms were severely disturbing or only moderately so did not determine the initial label. But once the individual had

taken on (or not taken on) a particular illness label, that label predicted two
things: one, the extent to which the individual's global symptom level improved
and, two, the length of time he stayed in the hospital. It was only the group
of individuals who, at first, thought of themselves as "mentally ill" but then
rejected that label who improved significantly in terms of symptoms. Further,
this group (along with the "label deniers") stayed in the hospital a shorter period
of time. The crucial group, those patients who accepted the label of "mental
illness", were significantly less likely to improve and significantly more likely to
stay in the hospital longer.

A comparison of individuals labeled as "ill" in different cultures is another
way of examining the effects of labels on symptoms and prognosis. By varying
cultures we also often vary beliefs about illness, expectations for the labeled
person and modes of social processing. For example, in Sri Lanka (Ceylon)
mental illnesses are commonly believed to be supernaturally caused and easily
and quickly cured. Further, the availability of multiple types of treatments
(Western as well as Ayurvedic medicine, exorcism, several religion-based methods,
astrology, etc.) leave the power over the labeling and de-labeling processes and
the ill individual's life in his own and his family's hands. In contrast, in many
industrialized societies mental illnesses are believed to involve serious personality
change for which the individual is held responsible and which may last a lifetime.
Further, treatment agents work in large bureaucratically organized hospitals or
clinics that often take power and responsibility for de-labeling from the ill
person (Waxler 1977).

Social labeling theory predicts that these culturally based beliefs and expectations and the modes of social processing will produce illness outcomes congruent
with cultural expectations. Evidence suggests that this may be true for individuals
labeled as "schizophrenic" (Waxler 1979). A five year follow-up of diagnosed
schizophrenics living in Sri Lanka shows that social adjustment and clinical state
at the end of five years is remarkably good. The findings for Sri Lankan patients
are consistent with similar individuals in other traditional societies such as
Nigeria and India and consistently different from outcome for schizophrenia
in patients followed in industrial societies. For example, the proportion of
individuals labeled "schizophrenic" who have no further episodes of illness after
the first one ranges from 58% in Nigeria, 51% in India, 40% in Sri Lanka to 7%
in USSR and 6% in Denmark. These large and consistent differences suggest that
industrial societies process psychiatric patients such that large proportions are
alienated from their normal roles and continue to have symptoms. In contrast,
beliefs and practices in nonindustrial societies encourage short-term illness and
quick return to normality. Cultural differences in prognosis, then, may be the
result of culturally based labeling and de-labeling processes.

Physicians have always known that if they treat an individual as if he were
"ill" they may encourage illness rather than health. Administrators of old-style
state psychiatric hospitals saw new symptoms of withdrawal and regression
develop when patients were transferred to "chronic-care" wards (Wing and

Brown 1970). Our examples from tuberculosis and psychiatric patients in our own and other societies have shown that the everyday work of the treatment system, designed to foster recovery, may instead encourage the "sick role" and even sustain symptoms. There is evidence, then, that the labeling process is not simply a social phenomenon that is superimposed on the real work of diagnosing and treating biomedical phenomena but that labeling has an impact on disease and/or its symptoms. Labeling theory speaks of this phenomenon in terms such as "sick role" and "secondary deviance". The biomedical model refers to "iatrogenesis". The contribution that labeling theory makes to physicians' understanding of iatrogenesis is to broaden the range of iatrogenic variables and to specify just how the social processing of ill people contributes to the maintenance of or recovery from disease.

EFFECTS OF LABELING ON MEDICAL PRACTICE

We have shown how the social processing of people labeled as "ill" impinges on the lives of "ill" persons. Those who are selected into the domain of illness and medicine may find that the label of illness is not always benign nor temporary. Some illness labels are stigmatizing and some lead to social isolation. In some instances treatment systems are so structured that they unintentionally sustain labels and even symptoms.

These social labeling processes also have significant effects on the everyday practice of medicine. For example, the kinds of illnesses physicians and other health workers find they are called upon to treat are profoundly affected by the early stages of labeling. The large numbers of geriatric patients in Saskatchewan psychiatric hospitals (D'Arcy 1976) were admitted presumably because alternative services for old people were not available; the fact that they were selected into the hospital and given psychiatric diagnoses meant that physicians and others were obligated to treat them. Thus, physicians come to be specialists in geriatric psychiatry in response to the "new" illness. Similarly, medical practitioners have recently been called upon to treat such new problems as hyperkinesis, sexual desire disorders and alcoholism that now fall into the realm of "illness". Practitioners, then, often deal with illness or with ill people who are defined and selected by others (families or the individual himself) for reasons that have little to do with biomedical processes.

Labeling and social processing of sick persons, we have seen, sometimes even prolongs or creates symptoms that physicians are then asked to treat. Just as psychiatrists now must deal with the iatrogenic phenomenon of tardive dyskinesia they were also, in the past, called upon to treat symptoms of withdrawal and regression that resulted from prolonged psychiatric hospitalization on "back wards".

Selective labeling and social processing of ill people also impinges on the physician's practice in a somewhat more subtle way. These social processes provide most physicians with a very selected sample of patients, those who have been sorted into the "ill" category at several previous decision points. This pool of highly selected labeled individuals may serve as "data" for physicians' hunches about disease process and the effectiveness of treatment. Even the information from hospital or clinic records that we tend to think of as "hard" data can also be conceived as the product of social processing. Labeling theory suggests that facts such as diagnosis, length of stay, prognosis, may tell us much more about the social characteristics of selected patients and the workings of the treatment system than about a biomedical process. Highly selective diagnoses reported by physicians for medical insurance purposes are one example of this phenomenon.

But physicians and health workers do not stand entirely outside of the health system, prepared to treat or handle individuals who have been labeled as "ill" by family, self or society. They are active participants in the labeling and de-labeling processes; in fact, making decisions about who is to be called "ill" and who is "well" is central to a doctor's job. Labeling theory suggests that very often this labeling process is not entirely beneficial to the ill person and that medical personnel, in spite of their intentions, may process ill people in ways that prolong symptoms, socially isolate, or stigmatize. For example, psychiatrists working in a small ward in which demands for beds are very great and thus patient turnover rapid and length of stay short, find that they must continually argue that their patients are "still sick" if they are to retain patients long enough to gain their cooperation in taking medication and to make sure that their acute symptoms are controlled. This argument for "illness" is communicated to staff, family and often the patient himself and it may become a self-fulfilling prophecy (Howard, et al. 1979). Medical professionals' tendencies toward caution and conservatism may also often be a tendency to prolong the label of illness and thus to encourage the sick role, isolate individuals from normal social relationships and, perhaps, encourage secondary symptoms.

CONCLUSION

We have introduced some of the ways in which labeling theory is used to understand illness by looking at studies that examine specific segments of that process. Findings suggest that labels of illness are applied selectively, and that the physician's criteria for disease (symptoms, signs, severity, etc.) are only one of several factors that predict who is to be called "ill". Social characteristics of the individual (his family position, his socioeconomic status, etc.) or of his society (beliefs about illness, etc.) and the existence of and kind of treatment system available (how many beds, whether alternative services are present, etc.) are significant to the initial labeling decision. If the "trouble" is labeled as "illness" then the selected group of labeled individuals may appear in a treatment system where further negotiation and re-negotiation of the "illness" occurs. At this stage, too, whether an individual remains "ill" is associated with his background (his social position, how powerful he is, etc.) as well as with the organizational operation of medical practice and treatment systems (who selects, the pre-dominant ideology of the system, etc.). Finally, the selected group of labeled individuals may, as a result of social processing, find that they remain "ill" and that their symptoms are sustained. A selected group drops through this net and returns to "normal". The highly selected group of "ill" individuals appears in that category, not simply because they had the most severe or intransigent symptoms, but because they have been involved in a series of social processes that have led to their selection into the role of "ill person". Thus, whether an individual is called "ill" and remains "ill" is a social, not simply a biomedical, phenomenon.

In contrast, the biomedical model of disease assumes that whether a person is "ill" is an objective fact, whether and how he is to be treated is a technical decision and whether he "gets well" is related to the state of technical treatment and the patient's compliance with it. We have seen that this model does not always accurately predict the realities of illness careers and treatment system operations.

Labeling theory suggests that it is not simply that treatment systems and medical practices need "tinkering with" in order to get them to work more objectively and effectively but that the very selective way that individuals are defined as "ill" is inherent in our society's processing of all sorts of deviant people and fulfills more general social functions. For example, those who end up in prison are highly selected samples of the population of people who break the law. Police interrogation, court hearings and prison life then isolate the selected individuals from normal society and serve as training grounds for the "hardened criminal". In this system police, lawyers, judges, and court psychia-trists act as agents of social control, often removing and/or punishing selected individuals in ways that the society demands. Thus, formal law does not predict who will be labeled a "criminal".

Similar phenomena occur with regard to illness; physicians, social workers, even family members serve as agents of social control. They negotiate labels of illness that justify temporary (or sometimes permanent) isolation and abrogation of normal responsibilities on the part of the ill person. And they negotiate illness labels in a systematic way, based on our society's norms and beliefs, so that some individuals are more likely to be called "ill" and removed from society than are others. The biomedical theory of disease, then, does not always predict who is "ill". Some labeling theorists suggest that selective labeling of "illness" has little to do with disease itself but much more to do with the relative status, power and role of the individual. The illness labeling process, like the labeling of criminals, may, when seen in its broadest sense, simply be another way of removing society's unwanted.

NOTES

1. Mental retardation is, of course, not an illness that ordinary physicians often treat.

Instead, it has been handed over to psychologists and special teachers, probably because the most effective current "treatment" involves social/educational training rather than physical/medical "cure". However, the cause of mental retardation is explained in biomedical terms (as the result of minimal brain damage, etc.) and thus it falls within the biomedical theory of disease. We present Mercer's investigation of mental retardation because it is currently the most complete and systematic examination of the social labeling of a biomedical phenomenon.

2. Social labeling theory takes several forms. The most radical version questions the biomedical model of disease itself by stating that the labeling process "creates" the disease, that sick people are "sick" only because they have been so labeled. This leads very easily to a conclusion that physicians and other labelers are malevolent and motivated to cause trouble for people who would otherwise be well. If Mercer had followed this perspective she might have concluded that teachers and principals knowingly select Mexican-American and Blacks and call them retarded. Or that psychiatrists ignore real symptoms and selectively choose to recommend for long-term hospitalization and/or commitment only patients who are lower class or socially isolated.

A more conservative version of the theory, represented here, assumes that the labeling of illness usually begins when there are a set of diffuse or disorganized signs or symptoms, that is, when an individual evidences some sort of personal or behavioral deviation; whether these deviations are caused by genetic, biochemical, psychological, etc., factors is of no interest to the theory. Much of the time these signs and symptoms are ignored or explained away; only a small proportion are labeled and thus become grist for the medical negotiation process. In this version of the theory then there is no need to deny the presence of or significance of biomedical factors; these factors along with social characteristics of the individual and his social context contribute to the ways in which he is labeled or not labeled.

3. Waitzkin and Waterman (1974) suggest that the high rates of "sick call" in prisons may function to drain off tension that otherwise might take less controllable forms.

4. Some proponents of labeling theory would say that this question is irrelevant since "illness" is a social role and whether someone is called "diseased" is the result of a negotiation or decision in a social context. They say that "disease" is a concept of the biomedical model, a distinctly separate conceptual system.

5. Some authors call for an integration of the biomedical and social labeling perspectives when dealing with the hypothesis that predicts a causal effect of labels on symptoms or disease. Townsend (1978) discusses these relationships in some detail, pointing out that medicine's concern with psychosomatic illness, for example, already assumes that "role expectations mobilize organic systems of the body. . . . A person's biology *interacts* with his social experience; each influences the other" (1978:97).

Thus, the dichotomy between social processes and biomedical processes may be quite artificial and more a matter of relative emphasis than of competing explanations.

REFERENCES

Balint, M.
    1957 The Doctor, His Patient and The Illness. New York: International Universities Press.
Calden, G., W. Dupertuis, J. Hokanson, and W. Lewis
    1960 Psychosomatic Factors in the Rate of Recovery From Tuberculosis. Psychomatic Medicine 22:345–355.
Campbell, J. D.
    1975 Attribution of Illness: Another Double Standard. J. of Health and Social Behavior 16:114–126.

Conrad, P.
   1978 Identifying Hyperactive Children: The Medicalization of Deviant Behavior.
         Lexington, Mass.: D.C. Heath.
D'Arcy, C.
   1976 The Manufacture and Obsolescence of Madness: Age, Social Policy and Psychiatric
         Morbidity in a Prairie Province. Social Science and Medicine 10:5–13.
Doherty, E.
   1975 Labeling Effects in Psychiatric Hospitalization. Archives of General Psychiatry
         32:562–568.
Eichorn, R. and R. Anderson
   1962 Changes in Personal Adjustment to Perceived and Medically Established Heart
         Disease: A Panel Study. J. of Health and Human Behavior 3:242–249.
Gove, W., ed.
   1975 The Labeling of Deviance. New York: Wiley.
Harris, D.
   1975 An Elaboration of the Relationship Between General Hospital Bed Supply and
         General Hospital Utilization. J. of Health and Social Behavior 16:163–172.
Hauser, S. T.
   1979 Physician-Patient Relations. In Social Contexts of Health, Illness and Medical
         Care. E. G. Mishler, L. AmaraSingham, S. Hauser, R. Liem, S. Osherson and N. E.
         Waxler: Cambridge University Press.
Howard, L., S. Roses, N. Waxler, and J. Welsh
   1979 Environmental Constraints, Occupational Conflict, and Patient Definitions in
         Three Psychiatric Settings. Unpublished paper.
Kaplan, H. S.
   1979 Disorders of Sexual Desire. New York: Brunner/Mazel.
Kendell, R. E., J. Cooper, A. Gourley, and J. Copeland
   1971 Diagnostic Criteria of American and British Psychiatrists. Archives of General
         Psychiatry 25:123–130.
Ludwig, E. and S. Adams
   1968 Patient Cooperation in a Rehabilitation Center: Assumption of the Client Role.
         J. Health and Social Behavior 9:328–336.
Maisel, R.
   1967 The Ex-Mental Patient and Rehospitalization: Some Research Findings. Social
         Problems 15:18–24.
Mendel, W. and S. Rapport
   1969 Determinants of Decision for Psychiatric Hospitalization. Archives of General
         Psychiatry 20:321–328.
Mercer, Jane
   1973 Labelling the Mentally Retarded. Berkeley: University of California Press.
Roth, J. and E. Eddy
   1967 Rehabilitation for the Unwanted. New York: Atherton Press.
Scheff, T.
   1966 Being Mentally Ill. Chicago: Aldine.
Schur, E.
   1971 Labeling Deviant Behavior. New York: Harper and Row.
Scott, R.
   1969 The Making of Blind Men. New York: Russell Sage Foundation.
New York Times
   1979 August 26, 1979.
Townsend, J. M.
   1978 Cultural Conceptions and Mental Illness: A Comparison of Germany and America.
         Chicago: University of Chicago Press.

Twaddle, A. C.
  1976 Utilization of Medical Services by a Captive Population: An Analysis of Sick Call in a State Prison. J. of Health and Social Behavior 17:236–248.
Waitzkin, H. and B. Waterman
  1974 The Exploitation of Illness in Capitalist Society. Indianapolis: Bobbs-Merrill Co.
Waxler, Nancy E.
  1974a The Domain Called "Madness" in the Peasant Villages of Ceylon. Unpublished paper.
  1974b Culture and Mental Illness: A Social Labeling Perspective. J. of Nervous and Mental Disease 159:379–395.
  1977 Is Mental Illness Cured in Traditional Societies? A Theoretical Analysis. Culture, Medicine and Psychiatry 1:233–253.
  1979 Is Outcome for Schizophrenia Better in Nonindustrial Societies: The Case of Sri Lanka. J. of Nervous and Mental Disease 167:144–158.
  In press Learning to Be a Leper: A Case Study in the Social Construction of Disease. In Social Contexts of Health, Illness and Medical Care. E. G. Mishler, L. AmaraSingham, S. Hauser, R. Leim, S. Osherson, and N. E. Waxler: Cambridge University Press.
Waxler, Nancy E., L. Howard, S. Roses, and J. Welsh
  1979 Does Hospital Organization Facilitate De-Labeling? Unpublished paper.
Wenger, D. and C. R. Fletcher
  1969 The Effect of Legal Counsel on Admissions to a State Mental Hospital: A Confrontation of professions. Journal of Health and Social Behavior 10:66–72.
Wing, J. and G. Brown
  1970 Institutionalism and Schizophrenia. Cambridge, England: Cambridge University Press.

14. THE DOUBLE-BIND BETWEEN DIALYSIS PATIENTS AND THEIR HEALTH PRACTITIONERS

INTRODUCTION

One of the tasks of the social scientist in medicine is to provide models for analysis which are clear, elegant, and useful to clinicians. Such models provide rational, rather than empirical, guidelines for understanding phenomena, and impose economy on conjecture: models indicate the logically necessary features of an event or process. One model which has proved useful originated in the ethnographic study of the Iatmul people (Bateson 1958). This model has its most sophisticated formulation as a description of the antecedents of schizophrenia (Bateson et al. 1956), and has also been used as a descriptive construct with respect to psychotherapist-patient relations (Savage 1961), hypnotic trance induction (Haley 1958), identity confusion among twins (Rosenthal 1960), juvenile delinquency (Ferreira 1960), play, fantasy and courtship (Bateson 1955; Haley 1955), and disturbed behavior in experimental animals (Scheflen 1960). A great range of applications of the theory have been referenced by Watzlawick (1963): its original expression and elaborations may be found in Bateson's collected works, *Steps to an Ecology of Mind* (1972).

The model, usually called the double bind theory, is especially informative when applied to the dynamics of chronic illness. In the health care system there are a great number of persons who present for treatment but whose symptoms remain or proliferate after extensive medical care has been given. This population divides into two groups: those patients for whose symptoms medical professionals cannot find organic or psychogenic bases, and those patients whose symptoms are understood but for whom treatment is palliative at best or to no avail. Those in the first group are colloquially named "crocks", those in the second group are "chronics". The double bind model may be fruitfully applied to the problems generated by both groups: here, medically identified and sanctioned symptom persistence will be explored and the model applied to a chronic group of patients undergoing the treatment of hemodialysis. This patient group is notable because of the high incidence of psychiatric morbidity and suicide it sustains. Alternative explanations for illness behavior are first offered: the double bind model is briefly presented; the model is applied to clinical data obtained in a hemodialysis ward; and a brief discussion of case histories is given.

PARENT, CHILD OR PRACTITIONER, PATIENT

An influential view of sick persons appears to have originated with Talcott

L. Eisenberg and A. Kleinman (eds.), The Relevance of Social Science for Medicine, 307–329.

Parsons (1951, 1953, 1958; and Fox 1952). It has dominated much medical perception of patients, as will be shown. The essentials of his formulation are as follows:

That there are uniformities in the constitutions of all human groups at the organic level goes without saying, and hence that many of the problems of somatic medicine are independent of social and cultural variability (1958:168).

In spite of somatic factors, though, any individual's commitment to the values of his own society, including those pertinent to illness, is essentially moral, and variance with this morality is deviance. Illness is designated as illegitimate:

The stigmatizing of illness as undesirable, and the mobilization of considerable resources of a community to combat illness is a reaffirmation of the valuation of health and the counter-vailing influence against the temptation for illness, and hence the various components which go into its motivation, to grow and spread. (1958:177)

According to Parsons, there are four criteria which define the sick role and which transcend cultural boundaries. A particular culture may emphasize or be dominated by one or more of these criteria. The sick role consists of an exemption from other role obligations; it is an involuntary state and the sick person is not responsible for his illness; his illness is legitimized on a conditional basis; he is obliged to cooperate in altering his state and in evacuating the sick role.

Regarding the motivations for illness, Parsons says:

I may start by suggesting that all patterns of deviant behavior ... involve the primacy of elements of *regressive* motivational structure in the psychological sense. (1958:154)

With Fox, Parsons produces a metaphor based on the similarity they see between the sick person's incapacitated state and a child's immature state. Both are dependent and need the care of more adequate persons. "Thus in these two senses, illness is not unlike more or less complete reversion to childhood" (1952:235). The physician is analogous to parent, the hospital becomes a functional alternative to the family.

The level of generality intended by Parson's approach permits cross-cultural comparisons and a seminal means of categorizing the social consequences of illness. However, other writers have used the theory in a less than general manner:

The enforced state of dependency in illness can gratify strong needs to be taken care of, as the individual was cared for as a child (King 1963:112).
    ... the sick person's world becomes remarkably like that of an infant, and the behavior resulting from these aspects is necessarily infantile, too (Barker et al. 1953:321).
    In a small world like that of the provincial or the child, objectivity or the explanation of occurrences in terms of a wide context of relevant conditions is impossible ... [the sick person's] world is no longer plural, but singular and egocentric, like that of an infant (Barker et al. 1953:332).
    ... the state of convalescence is structurally and dynamically similar to adolescence. The behavior of the convalescent is analogous to that of the adolescent (Lederer 1958:256).

They do not realize that these "bids for attention" are much like the cries of a baby ... Most patients comply trustingly with the exigencies of treatment, but not all are "good children" (Roche Laboratories: 1968).

The characteristics alleged to accompany sick role regression are egocentricity, selfishness, exaggerated concern with trifling matters, domination, insecurity, intolerance, apathy and disinterest, dependency and hypochondriasis. On the surface the view of sick persons as children may appear sympathetic: children are the objects of gentle sentiments and affection in most cultures. But in fact the terms "regressed", "infantile", "dependent", are deprecatory and descriptive of psychopathology in this culture. This view of patients sanctions the delegation of control of large parts of their lives to others: the consequence of treating sick adults as children is destructive, as will be shown.

Hemodialysis patients are engaged in ongoing repetitive relations with health care professionals. They are exemplary of the population of patients we call "chronics", for whom modern medicine and technology have provided an illness-maintenance system rather than a health-maintenance system. Their interaction with the health care system is interminable, except by death or organ graft. They are immoral in the Parsonian sense; they may not evacuate the sick role. It is thus that we may see the cumulative effects of a health care professional attitude or prejudice in this group of patients. The literature on the problems accompanying hemodialysis is extensive and by its quantity testifies to the frustration experienced by all who are involved in it. The literature is imbued with an implicit view of the patient as infantile and regressed. A variety of causes are proposed for the high incidence of psychiatric morbidity and suicidal tendency in the dialysis patient population: patient predisposition, uremia and its concomitants, stress, body image distortion, anxiety, dependency, depression, deprivation, fear of loss, denial and the absence of denial are examples. The patients are characterized in the literature by their lassitude, organicity, psychosis or acute delirium, apathy, euphoria, acute and chronic anxiety, headaches, vomiting, depression, fatigue, insomnia, drive frustrations, fear of loss, denial, restlessness, irritability toward staff, family and employers, impatience, excessive demands, complaintiveness, anger, bizarre body image changes including phantom urination, philosophical passivity, and noncompliance. (Short and Wilson 1969; Blatt and Tsushina 1966; De-Nour 1969; Abram 1971; Abram 1974; Cummings 1970; Crammond et al. 1968; Norton 1969; Eisendrath et al. 1970; MacNamera 1967; Friedman et al. 1970)

The unfettered use of a Parsonian model leads directly to a punitive and manipulative medicine. On the other hand, its natural antithesis, humanism, has its own dangers and we will explore these next, before reviewing the deficits of both approaches and proposing an alternative.

VILLAIN VICTIM OR PRACTITIONER PATIENT

In contrast to the view of the sick person as regressed and helpless is the opinion that he is suppressed and deprived. As a victim of suppression, the patient contends first with his physician. The physician is both the product of a long personal history and of a standardized medical training. His training, once completed, entitles him to join a subcultural group characterized by homogeneity of attitudes and values. Homogeneity of medical training in the United States leads to a belief that adequate medical care can be given

... only under a certain type of social organization which, on examination, frequently turns out to be a close approximation to the patterns with which persons undertaking the program are most familiar (Saunders 1954:239).

The conditioning and patterning of the medical doctor renders him very different from most of his patients and

... of all the subcultural differences that may divide practitioner from patient in a given society, the subculture of the medical profession itself may well be the most critical (Wilson 1963:283).

All practitioners are professionals and all patients are amateurs (Wilson 1963:279).

Increasing specialization and the technological advances which demand it have seen the demise of the traditional general practitioner who once maintained a one-to-one relation with his patient: team care and unfamiliar rotating physicians typically confront the patient now and the encounter is depersonalized (Stevens 1971; Weaver 1968; Paul 1955). The interaction between doctor and patient is a matter of mutual role definition and the behavior of each is shaped by the other, but

The practitioner has a nearly exclusive monopoly of psychological and social leverage ... the practitioner has more to do with defining the patient's role than the patient has with defining the practitioner's (Wilson 1963:279).

That which the practitioner has, and the patient lacks, is information regarding the patient's diagnosis, prognosis, and treatment. The decision to share these data is the physician's and actual sharing is contingent on the mode and manner of communication, which is often flawed (Korsch and Negrete 1972). Communication may fail because of the level of abstraction used by the physician, the technical vocabulary or reference, or even the value assumptions which underlie his explications. In most instances the physician is operating on incomplete data and

... resorts to *a priori* assumptions and value orientations, many of which are shared with his colleagues. These make up the body of professional traditions (Ruesch 1963:74).

Whatever prejudices, motivations, or professional fashion trends comprise the body of professional traditions on which the physician relies, they are at best surmised or ignored by the patient. In effect, the patient relates as an individual to an institution.

With respect to the nature of hospitalization and its effect on the patient, much has been written in the sympathetic or humanistic vein. The hospital is likened to a prison:

Except for imprisonment, no other circumstance in our society requires one to surrender more of his personal liberty, prerogatives and identification (Wahl 1966:276).

Stress of hospitalization has been evaluated with behavioral and physiological measures (Tolson 1965). It is usually attributed to the patient's being separated from his loved ones and his customary lifestyle, to the increased social distance which prevails between himself and the doctors, to the hospital itself as an atmosphere of crisis and strain (King 1962; Simmons and Wolff 1954). Some studies have focused on the people with whom the patient relates while in the hospital: doctors, nurses, aides, orderlies, technicians, etc. These studies indicate that a hospital ward is a self-contained social system with medical personnel as the main actors. The patient plays a transient bit part. Members of the subgroups comprising the staff tend to interact mostly with others in their own specialty and ideologies between these groups tend to become more and more disparate (Wessen 1958). The channeling of interaction among personnel of various occupational levels is assumed to have dysfunctional influence on patient care (Croog 1963).

In addition to the anonymity and stress the hospitalized patient is alleged to experience are the consequences of the dualistic, hence competitive, social structure of the hospital (Smith 1958), the political and power interests of medical groups and factions (Stevens 1971), and the possibility that hospitals attract a relatively large number of "queer" people as employees (Smith 1958). Kiev points out that many of the symptoms manifested by hospitalized psychiatric patients are not characteristic of their actual disorder, but are "secondary symptoms grafted on" and result from their interrelations with hospital staff (Kiev 1970).

Recent literature, which will not be reviewed here, is marked by a growing accusatory and intemperate posture in those who criticize the institution of Western clinical medicine for its lack of personalized service and humanism. A sort of medical villainy is alleged to operate, with patients the hapless victims of resources controlled and relinquished only for the benefit of the professional caretakers. The implicit condescension in these purportedly humanistic critics toward patients is revealed in their depictions of patients as witless and incompetent to help themselves and as ignorant of options and passively manipulated by the system. In fact many of the assumptions about humanistic care have never been tested. That patients respond more readily to benign physician stereotypes – physicians who are warm, empathetic, compassionate, congenial – than to physicians who are brusque, terse, distant and competent, has not been shown, to my knowledge. While the functional design of hospitals results in separation from loved ones, social distance, arbitrary schedules, alien experiences, so do vacations which are designed to be recreational. That a detached, objective apprehension of patients is less curative than an involved, personalized apprehension has not been systematically or rigorously demonstrated. Sentimentality is the hallmark of the humanistic approach and like motherhood, the flag and apple pie, humanism presents itself as self-evidently good. In fact the non-obvious consequences of unexamined humanism and sentiment in medicine are degenerative.

Dialysis patients have presented larger interpersonal problems for health care professionals to consider than many other chronic groups, as indicated in the review of their characteristics above. Their care entails attendance to variables not usually included in treatment plans. The expansion of institutionalized care to include the impact of the treatment and disease on the patient's family, employment, economics, education, and life in general reflects a growing omnipotence in the medical profession's assumptions about chronic care. The "whole patient" concept is well illustrated in this expanding medical procedure and shown to be fallacious as well as damaging, as will be discussed below.

The literature reveals that patients are, in fact, sometimes seen as victims by their caretakers or observers. Nurses sometimes dream about hemodialysis (Foy 1970). Frequent topics in dialysis staff meetings are the "obnoxious behavior" of patients (Eisendrath et al. 1970). In a paper discussing patient withdrawal from dialysis programs as a clinical problem, it was noted that

Throughout the course of treatment, if the patient gained too much weight or failed to function up to staff expectations, the staff's exhortations, if not heeded by the patient, would be followed by anger, withdrawal, and explicitly expressed disinterest in the patient (McKegney and Lange 1971:271).

Nurses may feel overprotective and possessive of these patients and are jealous of other staff who work with them, are reluctant to relinquish control of the patient, and even resent patients assuming responsibility for themselves in certain areas (De-Nour and Czaczkes 1968). Social workers devote a large amount of time to these patients, arranging many aspects of the patients' lives to suit the demands of treatment. In one case a worker spent more than 150 hours on a patient's financial problems (MacNamera 1967) while in another similar case a patient purchased a new car while the social worker was on vacation, thus undoing all the work (Cramond et al. 1968).

One study documents that a change in the patient's perception of control does occur during the course of treatment. Goldstein and Reznikoff (1971), using Rotter's concept of locus of control, found that

According to this framework, individuals perceive the source of reinforcements on a continuum. Those with a purely internal locus of control perceive rewards and punishments occurring as essentially a direct consequence of their behavior . . . On the other end of the continuum are those individuals with external locus of control. They perceive events in their lives as occurring on a random or chance basis, independently of their actions (Goldstein and Reznikoff 1971:1205).

Hemodialysis patients evidenced a significantly greater degree of external control than did patients in another medical category. If perceiving that outcomes are unrelated to one's efforts is analogous to feeling a "victim", this study suggests that the conditions which operate to skew control radically, rendering some persons omnipotent and others helpless, may be present in hemodialysis contexts. However nothing in the literature recommends that we suppose villainy to be operating. In fact, the frustration and grief mutually expressed by professionals and patients in this difficult area of healing and ailing are poignant when so many best efforts are evinced but unsuccessful.

SYNTHESIS: THE DOUBLE BIND THEORY

The view of the patient as child and the view of the patient as victim are ultimately the same, in terms of their underlying structure. Both views assign a set of attributes or characteristics to one member in the patient-practitioner relation and then infer the attributes of the other. If the patient is like a child, it follows that the practitioner is analogous to parent. If a patient is a victim, there must be a victimizer: let organized American medicine be the villain. Both views adopt an extreme example of distribution of control, coercion, and authority, and neither deserves a finer analysis since they are stereotypic, trite, and they overlook the complex symbiosis and exchange that always obtain between individuals in relationships. Their prevalence, however, should give us serious pause. Such views were given recent impetus by popularized psychotherapy programs, for example, Transactional Analysis. Characterizations of patients as children and victims both implicitly recommend that a more egalitarian distribution of responsibility in such relationships would be corrective. Paradoxically both characterizations sanction and lead to more control rather than less by persons other than patients.

The double bind theory is known primarily for its formula for inducing context-dependent psychosis. The theory incorporates other concepts about relationships which are clear, elegant, and equally useful. A straightforward application of the theory has been given elsewhere (Alexander 1977). Here we want to explore the entire model subsumed by the name double bind and not only its more obvious paraphrase. We want to shift our focus now from entities, things, and people and their intrinsic attributes or dispositions, to the nature and structure of the relationships that obtain between them. We want to avoid reification of these relationships while at the same time categorizing them. And it is important to understand the precise definition of a paradox and not just its consequence in human affairs. It is important to distinguish the redundant paradox called double bind, a powerful pathogenic, from singular paradoxes, which can inspire creative response, and from contradictions, which are generative of oscillation and alternation rather than behavioral paralysis. In that interest, a review of concepts follows.

The theory assumes that all relationships have two and only two elementary forms. These are called symmetrical or complementary. A symmetrical relation is one in which the relating parties express or exchange the same kind of behavior.

Examples are boxing matches, debates, armament races, or all cases where "A is stimulated to do something because B has done the same thing; and where B does more of this because A did some of it . . . " (Bateson and Jackson 1964: 270). In a complementary relation, the relating parties express or exchange differing kinds of behavior.

This category of complementary interaction includes, for example, dominance and submission, exhibitionism and spectatorship, succoring and dependence, and so forth . . . a series of patterns where there is a mutual fitting between A's behavior and that of B (Bateson and Jackson 1964:270).

Complementary relations are antithetical to symmetrical relations and the predominance of one in a context precludes the effectiveness of the other.

Human relationships are complex, ongoing, qualified by feedback and context, and not amenable to simple analysis. To assign complementarity or symmetry, or some alternation between these two modes of interaction, to a relationship is to make a generalization about the quality of the relationship. For our purposes it is sufficient to use a generalization about the complementary nature of patient-practitioner relations, although far finer analysis is possible. The kinds of complementarity that predominate in the relationship between practitioner and patient are various: information-giving and information-receiving, teaching and learning, dominance and submission, succoring and dependence, intrusion and exposure, comfort and complaint, service and payment are a few. The kinds of symmetry that occur in these relationships are also various but infrequent, atypical, and always qualified by the overriding complement of healing and ailing.

Besides identifying the hierarchical or complementary structure of relationships, and the linear or symmetrical structure, the double bind theory relies on a conceptualization of communication which utilizes, in any given exchange, three levels of information *simultaneously*. Quite simply, these three levels of information include what is said (the verbal information), what is meant by what is said (usually expressed kinesically and nonverbally), and what is the case (situational information). For example, the patient says "I hurt" verbally; the patient's somatic state, posture, and facial expression confirm the presence of pain and render the verbal message "true"; and the patient is known to have a pain-producing lesion. Both the patient and the recipient of the patient's communication draw simultaneously on these three levels of information in order to complete a successful communicational exchange. In the example given, the total communication is congruent.

But communications are not always congruent. In the example given, the patient may be lying. One might as easily say "I love you" or "it is Wednesday" as "I hurt". In many cases nonsense results, but whenever one level of information simultaneously *negates* that which is *asserted* on another level, paradox results. In graphic terms, where "+" stands for assertion of a proposition and "−" stands for its denial or negation, all possible congruities and incongruities − paradoxes − are shown on the following matrix.

Verbal information $+ + + + - - - -$
Kinesic information $+ + - - + + - -$
Situational information $+ - + - + - + -$
                            1 2 3 4 5 6 7 8

Single or episodic occurrences of such paradoxes are common in our experience. A general example might be the professed efforts on the part of the United States in behalf of peace in the Viet Nam War, coupled with an escalation of heavy bombing. While not devastating to our beliefs in things as they are, such paradoxes produce distrust and skepticism. Another example is humor, which is the intended manipulation of levels of communication, in which case we laugh. But when whole complexes of ongoing interpersonal relations are marked by hypocrisy and paradox, we have pathogenesis.

Full double binds, or redundant "unresolvable sequences of experiences" (Bateson et al. 1956:174) are not common in our normal discourse with the world. Bateson specifies six criteria as conditions for the occurrence of the double bind (Bateson et al. 1956:175). These are paraphrased, simplified, and reordered below for their application to the context of chronic illness.

1. Two or more persons in an *ongoing complementary relationship*, wherein
2. one issues assertions which direct the behavior of the other and which implicitly or explicitly require compliance. These are called *primary injunctions* and are frequently, though not necessarily, verbal.
3. These assertions are simultaneously negated by *secondary injunctions* on another level of information. The secondary injunctions are usually, though not necessarily, conveyed through posture, tone of voice, kinesics, nonverbally. These also require compliance.
4. The recipient of these communications is directed by a *tertiary injunction* which prohibits escape from the relationship or corrective comment on it. This information is usually, though not necessarily, situational. A paraplegic may not cease dependency on others, an infant may not quit the relationship with parents.
5. The paradoxical communication pattern (2, 3 above) repeats in the relationship and comes to be *anticipated*, until
6. the person receiving the injunctions has *learned* to "perceive his universe in double bind patterns . . . almost any part of a double bind sequence may be sufficient to precipitate panic or rage." (Bateson et al. 1956:175)

In less rigorous terms, the theory tells us that if a person is routinely engaged in complementarity, and is repetitively punished for his response to directives (which are simultaneously negated and thus impossible to follow), he will lose trust. He will learn to anticipate punishment or disapproval and out of this pessimism will generate behaviors which appear to be unrelated to immediate stimuli. Psychosis is not the only possible outcome: various aberrant behaviors may result.

Paradox invokes an inappropriate response in the sense that no response can be appropriate when it issues from a directive which is simultaneously denied. But paradox needs to be distinguished from contradiction. Contradiction occurs when, in sequence, an assertion is made and then denied. The temporal factor distinguishes it from paradox and also permits adaptive response. For example we nurture our children when they are small but we switch to symmetry when they become adult, a sort of long term parental contradiction, appropriate to circumstance. Even less appropriate parental contradiction, as when a mother alternates frequently between nurturance and symmetry with her young child, can be negotiated by the child by oscillations, between passive-receptive behaviors and assertive behaviors. Contradictions demand oscillation in ongoing relations if the behaviors of A and B are going to "fit" or match: adaptations may be devised. Paradox produces behavioral paralysis and displacement activities, not oscillation.

DIALYSIS AND DOUBLE BINDS

Most people experience illness, and the social relations it entails, as a transient event. They either get well and regain their pre-illness roles, or they die. Palliation is a recent alternative, and hemodialysis is the epitome of illness maintenance. Chronicity, in this medical area, is not marked by episodic occurrences and remissions of symptoms, but by ramifying continuous sick role adaptations and treatments. The medical literature on hemodialysis, although only topically reviewed above, is an important sort of data in itself. Medical contributors from many different societies and cultures have described the problems incumbent on providing dialysis, yet the literature is pervaded by a homogeneity of descriptions of patient and staff behaviors. Israeli practitioners and patients share the problems of Marshall Islanders, Australians behave much like Africans in this context. While no suggestion is made here that cultural and communicational variables do not operate, or that the double bind model can replace all other explications for behavioral pathology in this circumstance, the use of the double bind theory does have nonobvious consequences in the development of plans for care.

The data presented below were obtained as part of a three-year participant observation or ethnographic study of an outpatient and home dialysis program in an urban general hospital. That the data are not idiosyncratic or confined to this particular hospital is confirmed by their similarity to that reported in the literature and found in other facilities by this and other investigators.

Hemodialysis patients are clearly involved in ongoing complementary relations with their practitioners. Their three-times-weekly, six or eight hours per treatment, schedules, require it. Whether treated as inpatients or outpatients in an institutional facility, or at home with the help of a spouse or family member, they are engaged in ongoing redundant complements. If we examine the kind of communication transacted by these patients and practitioners, we find that most of it is injunctive or directive of action on the part of the patient. Prescriptions for proper dietary and fluid intake, attention to asepsis, urine output, and treatment procedure, as well as for proper attitude, activity, affect and self-presentation, monopolize the communications. The multitudes of different directives to patients issuing from practitioners, family members, agencies and institutions, and from the demands of the illness, can be categorized as of three basic sorts. These constitute primary injunctions in a double bind formula:

(1) Be independent.
(2) Be normal.
(3) Be grateful.

The directive "be independent" follows from the very real need to delegate as much as possible of this complex treatment to patients themselves, since its institutional provision is very expensive and the resources scarce. While necessary, the effort is also ambivalent and sabotaged by the complex liability system traditional in medicine. Evidence of the ambivalence is well shown in the following excerpt from a medical staff meeting where A, B, and C are medical practitioners:

A. The patient should be intimately involved with his dialysis. This is why we don't allow patients to sleep during their treatments.
B. What about patients changing the light bulbs in their machines? We've always relied on the use of a technician . . . now I'm reconsidering, maybe patients should know more about the mechanical aspects of it.
C. I don't think patients should get involved in the mechanical part . . .
B. After the first dialysis, patients aren't allowed in bed at _____ (another dialysis facility). They dialyze in a chair, and they study or read.
A. I'm going to remove all the T.V.s from the Center. It should be a place of intensive training and sick people, not a place to sleep or watch T.V..
B. At least they should take their blood pressure sitting up . . .
A. There (another facility), they are allowed to take their time learning before they go home. Here, all the patients are supposed to learn at the same rate. There's sort of a feeling of urgency.
C. Most of them don't want to learn.
A. Effective now, a new policy, no T.V.s in the Center.

In this verbal exchange, patients are seen as malingering in the sense that they watch television or sleep rather than participate in their treatment. At the same time they are seen as "sick people". They are incompetent to change light bulbs in the machine and they don't want to learn, yet they are ultimately expected to learn to administer the entire treatment, and to learn at the same rate.

Teaching is systematic and determined with dialysis patients, instituted soon after they are admitted to the program. It is in the teaching-learning complement, embedded in the larger healing-ailing complement, that most aberrant behaviors and discrepancies were observed, although discrepancies occurred in other situations as well. Reading, graphic and lectured materials were presented to patients during their treatments. Routine procedures such as meter reading, blood pressure recording, heparin administration, etc., were taught and were intended to keep patients involved in their treatment. Sleeping was prohibited and reliance on other patients for help or information was discouraged. Patients were given the information they needed to properly complete some procedures, but much information was also withheld at the practitioners' discretion, being potentially disruptive of standardized and expedient procedure and subject to patient innovation. For example, the fact that many patients do not need a full six-hour treatment three-times weekly would never be professionally divulged, although many patients on home dialysis soon discovered this by experiment. Such information would jeopardize the economy that must underlie the administration of a service involving two treatment shifts, fifteen highly trained personnel, over fifty patients, and the resources of a busy general hospital.

The purpose of the training was ultimately to move the patient out of the expensive institutional frame and into his or her own home with treatment. Patients assigned a very different risk to their own treatment-maintenance than did practitioners. They could acknowledge their resistance to assuming control of their own care to some extent, usually however offering excuses such as "the landlord won't let me change the plumbing so we can install the machine," "my wife works and the kids have their own families and can't help with the treatment": these initial resistances were later replaced with frank admissions of terror and anxiety.

Patient: Every time the nurse comes in here, she asks me the same question. Everytime, I forget the answer. There's something wrong with my mind.

Patient: You see that patient over there? He always forgets about the saline. One time he's going to die. The only thing is, I get scared, I don't remember about the saline either.

Patient: I don't see how they can get away with this. It's *their* job. The money I pay them, and they want me to do the work.

Patient: Please, find out for me when they plan to make me go home. You don't think they'll make me go home next week, do you? I'm not ready yet. I don't know enough to go home yet.

Implicit in the directives to the patients that they learn the treatment are rejection and abandonment, from the patients' point of view, and a primary injunction that they be independent and not needful of professional care. "Be independent" is distinct from the possible variants of a directive to "do what I tell you to do". Compliance, conformity, cooperativeness, and doing what one is told are exceedingly different from trying to mobilize self-sufficiency and independence of decision in a complementary frame where the required resources for such action are controlled by others. In fact patients in this context cannot exercise independence, yet practitioners often interpret patient resistance as intended rather than inevitable. Some practitioner remarks in this respect are:

Practitioner: She's the worst of the lot. She's not stupid, she just doesn't give a damn.

Practitioner: You can assume that, anytime a patient says he doesn't understand something, that he's had it explained to him thoroughly.

Practitioner: He's just dense. If you take the little intelligence some of these people have, and take the rest away with uremia, you aren't left with much.

Practitioner: Sure, they're sick. Very sick. Every time they're supposed to do something, they're sick. You can sit around and listen to them complain. But if they do what they're supposed to, watch the diet and fluid, dialyze when they should, they'd be perfectly all right. I think they like being dependent.

The primary injunction to be independent is intrinsically paradoxical. One cannot be independent if one is made dependent on the directive to be so. It is also paradoxical in terms of extrinsic secondary injunctions which require conformity to the sick role in this society. Western institutional medicine reserves for itself the responsibility for the care of sick people who present themselves for care. In dialysis, it is typical to see a practitioner retake and rerecord the patient's bloodpressure, after the patient has independently taken and recorded it. Staff override patient preferences on lunch and dinner menus, on needle insertion sites ("But there's no flow there, I have to put it higher"), on saline, heparin, dialysate, medication administrations, on almost all aspects of the procedure.

They must. Within the rigid liability system that operates in medical facilities, negligence is not a trivial charge. It should be clear by now that there are no victims in a double bind. All participants are caught in mutually destructive behavior. That practitioners in the case at hand are guilty of negativism and accusation towards patients is a symptom of a problem of high order, not its cause.

Before proceeding to the other primary injunctions, "be normal" and "be grateful", we may pause to consider the tertiary, non-escape injunction that must be in effect for the six criteria of a double bind to be met. The infant may not cease dependency on parents, the paraplegic may not choose to be self-sufficient. What about hemodialysis patients?

Organ graft is a viable option for some, but kidney transplantation is also palliative. It is a temporary respite from dialysis, but it is not curative and it entertains its own risks, one viable risk being death. Death is also an alternative to dialysis. Patients who voluntarily withdraw from treatment are called "suicides", although patients denied treatment for any reason are not yet called "homicides". Transfer to another dialysis facility or to home treatment may or may not offer alternatives to problems associated with treatment at a given place. In most cases, it cannot, because as we hope to show, the problems of dialysis are in large part inherent in the structure of the relationships it requires. They are, in its largest sense and meaning, iatrogenic.

If transplant, death, or transfer do not serve as alternatives to patients, they may serve as potent threats. The temptation to a program to offer a patient who is difficult to maintain on dialysis a less than ideal cadaveric or related-donor kidney match is great. And whether real or not, patients express anxiety over the possibility of their expulsion from a program, of being "hated" by the practitioners who treat them, of receiving inferior medical treatment or being assigned dialysis times they cannot meet without tremendous inconvenience, of being gossiped about . . . the threat of punishment if they do not comply with the directives they encounter is very real to patients, even if their anxiety is unwarranted from a practitioner point of view. Patients may not easily escape from their perceived dilemma.

Because the dialysis procedure is ramifying in its impact on the patient's life, intruding on marital, sexual, employment, economic, and recreational domains, as well as physical and sensual domains, the practitioners in this specialty have felt it necessary to concern themselves with large areas of their patients' lives. A typical measure of rehabilitation in medicine is the patient's resumption of a pre-illness lifestyle and activity pattern. This measure of "health" has permeated the expectations of dialysis practitioners. It expresses itself in the primary injunction "be normal". It is negated simultaneously and secondarily by the frank reality of abnormality that must accompany this illness and its palliation. Dialysis patients cannot be normal. The dietary and fluid restrictions inhibit normal gratification and socializing, urine output can be a many-times-daily preoccupation, asepsis constrains physical activities, gross scarring on limbs caused by cannula are visible and evident. The literature on dialysis summarizes at great length the losses and deficits the patients experience. Moreover, the need to see normalcy of patient behavior is primarily a practitioner need, not a patient need. That practitioners desire to see their patients respond positively to the large manipulations they attempt is understandable: nonresumption of a normal lifestyle is a direct indication of practitioner failure to negotiate the "whole patient" concept. In order for patients to oblige this practitioner need, dialysis must be perceived as a compartmentalized event, a thing that occurs only three days a week. Paradoxically, practitioner interventions themselves, because they encompass so many aspects of patient life, increase the multiplicative effect of the treatment.

Failure to respond to the directive to be normal leads to the imposition of a third injunction of a primary nature. Patients should at least "be grateful". Hemodialysis is an expensive, intense, difficult service. Ostensibly its whole motivating principle is to treat people with end-stage renal disease. That such a large and involved enterprise should be mobilized to treat a relatively small group of sick persons is perhaps sufficient to explain practitioner expectations that patients should at least act "like they are being helped". When patients do not act like they are being helped, we usually see accelerated attempts on the part of practitioners to help more, or we see rejection of the patient and the emotional abandonment that is the ultimate paradox. Practitioners in the latter state of despair proclaim their helplessness to help, positing a patient domination and their own submission, while yet maintaining professional superiority and accountability.

These patients are not grateful for obvious reasons. The directive "be grateful" is possibly ironic. The obviously prestigious and financial functions of institutional medical service, and the personal and professional gains enjoyed by dominant practitioners, counter the directive on one level. The horrendous problems resulting from the disease and treatment counter it on another level. The chronic failure of patients in this situation to comply with the directives that they be independent and normal leads to pessimism, not to gratitude.

TWO CASES IN POINT

To illustrate the relatively innocuous but uneconomic process of contradictions in a practitioner-patient relation, as compared to the more complex pathology embedded in the relation when paradoxical, two case histories are briefly presented. The first relates a sequence of interactions between a patient from the South Pacific brought to the United States for acute treatment.

This forty-six year old woman was brought to the hospital unconscious, uremic, and diagnosed as in acute end-stage renal failure. No facilities existed to treat her in her area of Oceania. The patient's home government assumed the cost of her transport and care. While she remained comatose, the Renal Admissions Committee met to decide the conditions of treatment. Emergency dialysis was provided.

Clara stabilized on dialysis within two weeks. The staff was then confronted with the problem of whether to train the patient for home treatment, in which case she would have to remain in the United States, or to discontinue treatment. If Clara were to stay in the United States, it would be necessary to relocate her husband and three children as well. If she were returned to the South Pacific, she would die. It was decided to bring her family over and to train her for home treatment.

This required arranging for a home for Clara and her family. Clara spoke no English, her husband but a little. Fortunately some cousins of Clara's husband were located near the dialysis center and they moved in. Staff then concerned themselves with checking on, commenting on, the patient's living arrangements, which were crowded and inadequate according to staff standards. The patient and her husband apprehended this criticism and moved with the children into an expensive apartment. The staff reacted with dismay and sent the social worker to explain that the husband must get a source of income and that the apartment could not be included as a medical expense. The husband then, on counsel of his relatives, applied for public welfare. The social worker learned this would jeopardize their receipt of medical funds from their own country and told him he must get a job. The social worker arranged for job interviews for him. He got a job. However the job interfered with his learning back-up dialysis and translating the training for his wife. Thus training for home dialysis had to stop. The staff was again dismayed. A staff meeting included the following comments:

A. He hardly ever shows up for the treatments. He always has an excuse, either the job or the kids.
B. These people just cannot comprehend the United States. We just prolong misery by keeping them here, and we've disrupted everything. We should have sent them back.
A. If she'd died, everything would have gone on the same here. We can't take care of the whole world. We must do a good job with those we can reach.

Shortly after this meeting, Clara and her family returned to the South Pacific, where she died within three months. Staff reflected bitterly that her husband was accountable for her death, however indirectly.

In this case, we see the patient and spouse complying almost perfectly to demands imposed or implied by the caretakers, demands which over time were contradictory. Simply, they consisted of injunctions that treatment be accepted, that the family find housing, that the housing was inadequate, that the family find other housing, that the second housing was not acceptable unless the spouse find a job; the spouse found a job. The spouse must also attend the dialysis training, in order that the patient might be treated at home (in the apartment which required his employment). But the job precluded his participation in treatment. The climax of staff frustration was communicated to the patient and her spouse who, in keeping with their compliant pattern, merely did what they were told and went home. However unfortunate, this case is relatively simple and straightforward, marked by a sequence of contradictions and appropriate responses on the part of the patient and spouse. The second case is not so simple.

Ellen was a single twenty-year old woman, unemployed, living at home with her family. She had been undergoing hemodialysis for two years before receiving a cadaveric transplant. Those two years disclosed the following patient-practitioner interactional patterns.

Ellen was initially treated in the hospital for six months. During the time, family members were trained as back-ups, and she went home for treatment. After seven months at home, her parents refused ambiguously further care for her there. The hospital agreed to permit hospital dialysis on one condition, this condition made explicit to Ellen and her family. She would undergo treatment with minimal help from staff at the hospital. Needle insertion was specified as the only help she should expect. Otherwise she would monitor her own treatment, set up and clean up, and otherwise be independent. Patient and family agreed to the condition.

A pattern emerged almost immediately. Ellen would come on time for treatment, begin to set-up, largely ignoring staff and proceeding in a slow, methodical routine. The staff would have completed setting up and starting nine other patients before Ellen was ready for fistula needles. Often, they would have to wait for her. After discussion in staff meeting, the staff began to help out a little, so as to get her on and off the machine earlier.

Staff intervention in her treatment gradually increased. Expedience was the reason staff gave. As they increased their intervention, Ellen diminished her independent behavior. As she decreased her independent behavior, staff necessarily had to become more involved. After a time, Ellen's care and the explicit condition of her hospital dialysis were not discernibly different than the care of other patients. In addition, her attitude toward staff modified. She became somewhat critical of their methods, whereas originally she had tried to show her own competence. She began to come in late and overweight and was generally indifferent to social amenities. Staff discussed her case again, and arranged for vocational testing, hoping to induce Ellen to more independent behaviors if not on the machine, then off. The testing indicated she was of borderline mental ability. She was not normal.

This explained for the staff her slowness in self-dialysis and justified their interventions. It now became a question of whether she was legally competent to self-dialyze in the hospital. If up to this point Ellen had been indifferent to amenities, she now became hostile. Staff intensified caretaking, Ellen intensified dependent and critical responses, at one point striking a nurse. The content of her verbal exchanges were noted to be increasingly irrelevant and bizarre. The psychiatrist was asked to consult and found her to be having an acute psychotic reaction in response to stress. It is necessary to note, however, that the stress impinging on her was not significantly greater than on other patients, although staff persisted in feeling that she had taken advantage of a circumstance that they had arranged in good faith to help her and her family.

Ellen was then hospitalized, but eloped and was admitted one week later emergently, acutely ill. She was stabilized, treated with psychotherapy and antipsychotic medication and discharged to outpatient dialysis status again. Two weeks later two cadaveric kidneys became available and Ellen was one of four possible recipients. She received the transplant and after a recovery complicated by psychosis, went home. Another well-liked patient received the other graft but died. This indirectly intensified staff anger toward Ellen.

Three years after the transplant, Ellen was functioning well. There were no subsequent psychiatric episodes after discharge. However, Ellen summarizes her hospital dialysis experience this way: "Whatever you do, it's wrong." She wasn't grateful.

This brief case illustrates the progression of a double bind. Independent behavior was both demanded and precluded. Normalcy was qualified by vocational testing, which promoted greater patient dependency following intensified staff interventions. This provoked anger, the antithesis of gratitude, then more dependency, abnormalcy, ingratitude. Once begun, the cycles perpetuated themselves. The caretaking staff were concerned and motivated to do the right things for the patient and none of the cycles related to specific errors in judgment. Rather the whole situation and the total complement between Ellen and the practitioners constrained alternatives and accelerated a set of symptoms which then themselves renewed the pathologic relational cycles.

CONCLUSION AND CORRECTIVES

None of the problems presented here are easily resolved. They arise in the main from the very core of medical caretaking axioms and are merely premises derived correctly from an acute-care tradition now obsolete and inappropriate in the face of a large population of interminably ill people. Effective change requires compatible modifications on the level of perception and then in the structural bases of the care relationship. The changes must emanate from responsible attitude and action on the part of both patients and practitioners. Pathology has been defined here as a consequence of an overabundance of complementarity and control vested in caretakers. It is equally well defined as an excess of passivity and submission in patients. It should be obvious that the *unilateral* provision of symmetrical options as a corrective maneuver by health care professionals is in fact another *complementary* move and therefore not corrective. It is crucial that this be understood. Practitioners may not, on pain of further paradox, fully control or dictate the correctives.

A health care professional reading and understanding the text thus far will perceive a double bind emerging with the professional on the receiving end of conflicting injunctions. The injunctions are of the order, (1) you are accountable for a therapeutic outcome of your efforts, and (2) your efforts, if you are accountable, are not therapeutic. Fortunately the second assertion is not always true, nor is the first. But we may not ignore that serious pervading epistemological problems confront our medical and healing traditions.

It is suggested that the initial change must occur on the level of percepts. Practitioners and patients must expand their perception of illness systems to include the nature of relationships and not just the traits and attributes of the individuals engaged in them. Case conferences, staff meetings, patient forums and exchanges are all presently characterized by detailed itemizations of persons' proclivities, symptoms and character, rather than by consideration of the interactive structures that occur in clinical environments. We are conditioned socially, academically and professionally to view cause and effect, stimulus and response, activity and passivity as linear events rather than as reciprocals. Thus we perpetuate complementarity even where symmetry potentially exists. The required change in perception entails unlearning, which is more difficult than learning.

Another initial step in correcting perception is in the redefinition of the social sick role. This requires destigmatizing illness while not diminishing the fact of its intrusive and degenerative impact. A society which mobilizes huge medical enterprises to sustain and nurture its physically deficient persons cannot at the same time condemn these objects as immoral in their maintenance of the sick role. Nor can such a society afford to romanticize chronic illness, nor infantilize those who remain ill. A pragmatics of chronic illness will include a direct non-sentimental accounting of the optimal uses of illness, as well as the costs of illness maintenance.

There is a consistent de-emphasis of patient suffering by practitioners who engage with dialysis patients. Patient pessimism or expressions of hopelessness, anger, defiance, remorse, inadequacy, dependency and ingratitude are met with contest:

Patient: Can't you see that I'm dying?
Practitioner: Oh, now, you are in a bad mood today.

Patient: I don't think I can go on with this . . .
Practitioner: You just have to try harder.

Practitioner: What's the matter?
Patient: I'm sick of all this.
Practitioner: You complain about this kind of life?
You got a choice . . . like six foot under.

Practitioner: When the patients feel angry with what has happened to them, and turn their anger toward the staff, it's really hard to communicate with them. They feel like we are trying to kill them, when we are trying to help them. They are like children. You have to make them see that what we do, we do to help them.

At the same time, patient optimism is defined as denial. The denial is some-times seen as therapeutic, sometimes not. Patient optimism is tolerated until it affects their view of necessity of some area of the treatment regimen. Some patients might feel so much better on dialysis that they decide they need less of it, rather than more. This sort of optimism is not rewarded by practitioners, while optimism that leads to patient conformity with practitioner standards is consistently reinforced. Suffering is a universal human condition. It needs to be acknowledged and understood, even in a system designed to alleviate it.

While shifts in perception are preliminary to correction, the structure of the health care system itself must ultimately change to permit healthier outcomes. What can be done practically in this interest by practitioners?

A first move is to detach professional rewards from cure and control of patients and illnesses. Professionals in academic settings have long had access to the approval and critical feedback of colleagues and peers and their identity as professionals is not entirely contingent on their success as clinicians. But clinicians without strong effective peer affiliation tend to rely on patient response as the measuring stick for success or failure. In the circumstances we have discussed, this is anachronistic and forces the burden of proof on patients who cannot provide it. The serious development of professional liaisons and goals, and the support of these by institutions employing and serving health care practitioners, will be corrective. Reciprocally, the development of patient and consumer groups, which suffer the same loss of relevancy and immediacy of all group processes in terms of the needs of individuals, nevertheless provide patients alternative references and impose on the health care system a symmetrical, albeit sometimes combative, corrective.

A related second step in structural change lies in the depersonalization, the mechanization of the treatment system. The use of audio and videotape devices, graphic and printed materials, instead of individuals in the teaching and maintenance of treatment are anathema to current notions of humanistic care. We noted that reference to ideas promoted by the double bind thesis leads to nonobvious strategies in planning care. It follows from the views above that while much of the treatment must by definition remain complementary, it does not necessarily have to be conveyed by way of interpersonal relations. Minimizing the interpersonal transactions marked by injunction and control, while retaining efficacy, is the corrective intent. Neutralizing relations of their complementarity can also be done by rotating staff and limiting the one-to-one intimacies and mutual dependencies that tend to develop between individual practitioners and patients over time. Mobilizing patients into teaching, support and modelling roles also serves this purpose. This recruitment of patients has double benefits. It provides a controlled complementary communication route between patients who are primarily engaged in symmetry with one another, and it gives patients a constructive secondary use for their illness.

Yet this suggestion, like the one to follow, involves risks, expense, and loss of certainty. Minimizing the standardization imposed by the economics of health care institutions underlies each and every potential corrective. A third structural change would involve re-examination of the present tendency to send patients home for treatment, regardless of their idiosyncracies or unique preferences. Home dialysis promotes the usurpation by illness of a non-illness option, the home. It perpetuates the sick role of the patient as a primary identity in the eyes of important others and enlists them in treatment. At the same time, it can permit more patient control and innovation in treatment, leading to a more manageable illness program. Some home patients will admit in confidence that they radically modify the regimen but do not reveal their ingenuities on the records they submit to their practitioners. Patients thus differ in their response to the dictum that they must assume their own care. The care system, having commited itself to a very expensive maintenance enterprise for hemodialysis patients, cannot afford to render it insensitive to the individuality of those it serves.

A final recommendation for correction regards revision of the liability structure of health care. Until patients can be held truly accountable for the consequences of self-care, the imposition of self-sufficiency on them remains an hypocrisy. If in the course of self-treatment in a medical institution a patient makes a damaging or lethal error, it is yet the practitioners who are accountable. A currently litigious public and a predictably defensive health professional response increase the problem. The ambiguities surrounding liability and responsibility can suffice to entirely sabotage the assumption of self-care and accountability by patients. Involving legal agencies, third party carriers, administrators, practitioners and patients in ongoing discussion with an intent to generate clear explicit guidelines for liable behavior is obviously a necessary as well as notably absent corrective process.

The rapid advance of medical technology and reliance on institutional medicine by many sick people is resulting in a growing population of hard core chronically ill. Illness maintenance is becoming a major function of our medicine and it is critical that this reality become a proper subject matter for our study. The main message in this article is to the effect that hypocrisy, sham, and the sustained discrepancy in our premises about care and cure are ultimately the most powerful of pathogenics. One may live well with a disease, if its treatment does not require deceit or paradox. One may live equally well with the failure to cure, if one's objective is the maintenance of congruent, meaningful interpersonal communication. If both patients and practitioners maintain congruence as a communicational ethic, they share in the healthiest of symmetrical objectives.

REFERENCES

Abram, H. S.
    1974 The "Uncooperative" Hemodialysis Patient. *In* Living or Dying. N. B. Levy, ed. Springfield, Illinois: Charles C. Thomas.
Abram, H. S., G. Moore, and F. Westervelt, Jr.
    1971 Suicidal Behavior in Chronic Dialysis Patients. Amer. J. Psychiat. 127:1199–1203.
Alexander, L.
    1977 The Double-Bind Theory and Hemodialysis. Arch. Gen. Psychiat. 33:1353–1356.
Barker, R., et al.
    1953 Adjustment to Physical Handicap: A Survey of the Social Psychology of Physique and Disability. Social Science Research Council, Bulletin 55, revised. New York: Social Science Research Council.
Bateson, G.
    1955 A Theory of Play and Fantasy. Psychiat. Res. Rep. 2:39–51.
    1958 Naven. 2nd ed. Stanford: Stanford University Press.
    1972 Steps to an Ecology of Mind. San Francisco: Chandler Publishing Co.
Bateson, G. and D. D. Jackson
    1964 Some Varieties of Pathogenic Organization. *In* Disorders of Communication V.LXLII. Association for Research in Nervous and Mental Disorders Meeting, New York, 1962. Vol. 42, pp. 270–290. Baltimore: Williams and Wilkins Co.
Bateson, G., et al.
    1956 Toward a Theory of Schizophrenia. Behav. Sci. 1:251–264.

Blatt, B. and W. T. Tsushima
   1966 A Psychological Survey of Uremic Patients Being Considered for the Chronic
         Hemodialysis Program: Intellectual and Emotional Patterns in Uremic Patients.
         Nephron 3:206–208.
Cramond, W. A., et al.
   1968 Psychological Aspects of the Management of Chronic Renal Failure. Brit. Med. J.
         1:539–543.
Croog, S. H.
   1968 Interpersonal Relations in Medical Settings. In Handbook of Medical Sociology.
         H. E. Freeman, S. Levine, and L. G. Reeder, eds. New Jersey: Prentice-Hall,
         Inc.
Cummings, J. W.
   1970 Hemodialysis – Feelings, Facts, Fantasies. Amer. J. Nurs. (January), 70–82.
De-Nour, A. K.
   1969 Some Notes on the Psychological Significance of Urination. J. Nerv. Ment. Dis.
         148:615–623.
De-Nour, A. K. and J. W. Czaczkes
   1968 Emotional Problems and Reactions of the Medical Team in a Chronic Haemo-
         dialysis Unit. Lancet 2:987–991.
Eisendrath, R. M., et al.
   1970 Service Meetings in a Renal Transplant Unit: An Unused Adjunct to Patient Care.
         Psychiat. in Med. 1:53–58.
Ferreira, A. J.
   1960 The "Double-Bind" and Delinquent Behavior. Arch. Gen. Psychiat. 3:359–
         367.
Foy, A. L.
   1970 Dreams of Patients and Staff. Amer. J. Nurs. (January), 82–84.
Friedman, E. A., N. J. Goodwin, and L. Chandhry
   1970 Psychosocial Adjustment to Maintenance Dialysis. N. Y. State J. of Med. 70:629–
         637.
Goldstein, A. M. and M. Reznikoff
   1971 Suicide in Chronic Hemodialysis Patients from an External Locus of Control
         Framework. Amer. J. Psychiat. 127:1204–1207.
Haley, J.
   1955 Paradoxes in Play, Fantasy, and Psychotherapy. Psychiat. Res. Rep. 2:52–58.
   1958 An Interactional Explanation of Hypnosis. Am. J. Clin. Hyp. 1:41–57.
Kiev, A.
   1970 Commentary. In Anthropology and the Behavioral and Health Sciences. O. von
         Mering and L. Kasden, eds. Pittsburgh: University of Pittsburgh Press.
King, S. H.
   1962 Perceptions of Illness and Medical Practice. New York: Russell Sage Foundation.
   1963 Social Psychological Factors in Illness. In Handbook of Medical Sociology. H. E.
         Freeman, S. Levine, and L. G. Reeder, eds. New Jersey: Prentice-Hall.
Korsch, B. M. and V. F. Negrete
   1972 Doctor-Patient Communication. Sci. Amer. 227:66–74.
Lederer, H. D.
   1958 How the Sick View Their World. In Patients, Physicians and Illness. E. G. Jaco,
         ed. Glencoe, Illinois: The Free Press.
MacNamera, F. M.
   1967 Psychosocial Problems in a Renal Unit. Brit. J. Psychiat. 113:1231–1236.
McKegney, F. P. and P. Lange
   1971 The Decision to No Longer Live on Chronic Hemodialysis. Amer. J. Psychiat.
         128:267–274.

Norton, C. E.
    1969 Attitudes Toward Living and Dying in Patients on Chronic Hemodialysis. Annals
          N.Y. Acad. Sci. 164:720–728.
Parsons, T.
    1951 Illness and the Role of the Physician: A Sociological Perspective. Amer. J. Ortho-
          psychiat. 21:452–460.
    1953 Illness and the Role of the Physician. In Personality in Nature, Society and
          Culture. 2nd ed. C. Kluckoln and H. A. Murray, eds. New York: Knopf.
    1958 Definitions of Health and Illness in the Light of American Values and Social
          Structure. In Patients, Physicians and Illness. E. G. Jaco, ed. Glencoe, Illinois:
          The Free Press.
Parsons, T. and R. C. Fox
    1952 Illness, Therapy, and the American Family. J. of Soc. Iss. 8:31–44.
Paul, B. D., ed.
    1955 Review of Concepts and Contents. In Health, Culture and Community. New
          York: Russell Sage Foundation.
Roche Laboratories
    1968 Patterns of Tension # 15. Monograph. Hoffmann-LaRoche Inc.
Rosenthal, D.
    1960 Confusion of Identity and the Frequency of Schizophrenia in Twins. Arch. Gen.
          Psychiat. 3:297–304.
Ruesch, J.
    1963 The Healing Traditions: Some Assumptions Made by Physicians. In Man's Image
          in Medicine and Anthropology. I. Galdston, ed. New York: International Univer-
          sities Press.
Saunders, L.
    1954 Cultural Difference and Medical Care. New York: Russell Sage Foundation.
Savage, C.
    1961 Countertransference in the Therapy of Schizophrenics. Psychiatry 24:53–60.
Scheflen, A. E.
    1960 Regressive One-to-One Relationships. Psychiatry Q. 34:692–709.
Short, M. J. and W. P. Wilson
    1969 Roles of Denial in a Chronic Hemodialysis Unit. Arch. Gen. Psychiat. 20:433–
          437.
Simmons, L. and H. G. Wolff
    1954 Social Science in Medicine. New York: Russell Sage Foundation.
Smith, H. L.
    1958 Two Lines of Authority: The Hospital's Dilemma. In Patients, Physicians and
          Illness. E. G. Jaco, ed. Glencoe, Illinois: The Free Press.
Stevens, R.
    1971 American Medicine and the Public Interest. New Haven: Yale University Press.
Tolson, W. W., et al.
    1965 Urinary Catecholemine Responses Associated with Hospital Admission in Normal
          Human Subjects. J. Psychosom. Res. 8:365–372.
Wahl, C. W.
    1966 The Psychosomatic Emergency. Calif. Med. 105:276–280.
Watzlawick, P.
    1963 A Review of the Double Bind Theory. Family Process 2:132–153.
Weaver, Thomas
    1968 Medical Anthropology: Trends in Research and Medical Education. In Essays
          on Medical Anthropology, T. Weaver, ed. Southern Anthropological Society
          Proceedings # 1. Athens: University of Georgia Press.

Wessen, A. F.
    1958 Hospital Ideology and Communication Between Ward Personnel. *In* Patients, Physicians and Illness. E. G. Jaco, ed. Glencoe, Illinois: The Free Press.
Wilson, R. N.
    1963 Patient-Practitioner Relationships. *In* Handbook of Medical Sociology. H. E. Freeman, S. Levine, and L. G. Reeder, eds. New Jersey: Prentice-Hall.

SECTION 6

SOCIOPOLITICAL AND SOCIOECONOMIC ANALYSES

15. A MARXIST ANALYSIS OF THE HEALTH CARE SYSTEMS OF ADVANCED CAPITALIST SOCIETIES

The Marxist viewpoint questions whether major improvements in the health system can occur without fundamental changes in the broad social order. One thrust of the field — an assumption also accepted by many non-Marxists — is that the problems of the health system reflect the problems of our larger society and cannot be separated from those problems.

The health systems of the United States and other advanced capitalist countries contain a series of troubling contradictions. In part, these contradictions mirror those of the larger society. My own understanding of these issues gained clarity from my clinical work as a primary care doctor in California and Vermont. In the analysis that follows, I present some concrete illustrations from these and other clinical settings. One of the strengths of the Marxist viewpoint is its ability to explain difficult practical dilemmas in the day-to-day experiences of health workers. Drawing the connection between theory and practice, this approach also points to needed directions of change. I should add that by focusing on the health systems of capitalist countries, I do not mean to imply that socialist systems have no problems (I discuss some of these problems later in this chapter). Instead, my purposes are to describe some contradictions of capitalist health systems as clearly as possible, to point out the relevance of this analysis for health workers' clinical activities and commitments, and to offer suggestions for progressive medical-political action.

DIMINISHING RETURNS, ESCALATING COSTS

During the twentieth century this contradiction has arisen in the health systems of essentially all capitalist nations. These countries include those characterized by the "monopoly capital" form of economic system (Baran and Sweezy 1966; Edwards, Reich and Weisskopf 1978) — especially the United States — and also those with "mixed" capitalist systems in which some industries have been nationalized — for example, Great Britain.

In these countries, costs for health care have risen rapidly. On the other hand, increasing costs have not coincided with improved health. Instead, there is now much evidence of decreasing returns in the face of escalating costs for health care.

Figure 1, from the work of John Powles (1973), summarizes this contradiction. This figure shows the gradual declines in infant mortality and gradual increases in life expectancy that have occurred during the last century. There has been little apparent relationship between these trends and the specific advances of modern medicine. In the meantime, health expenditures have risen dramatically, especially since the end of World War II.

L. Eisenberg and A. Kleinman (eds.), The Relevance of Social Science for Medicine, 333–369.

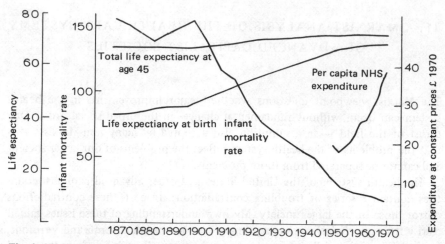

Fig. 1. Mortality trends over the last century, England and Wales, with recent expenditure trends. (Source: Modification of Powles (1973). Reproduced by permission of author and publisher.)

Modern medicine's *effectiveness* in improving health is very hard to prove. Recently a convergence has occurred in the work of several specialists in public health. This work shows that, with a few exceptions, the technical advances of modern medicine have not led to major improvements in measures of health, illness, life expectancy, or death (Powles 1973; Dubos 1959; Cochrane 1972; McKeown 1976, 1977; Illich 1976). Instead, the health of large populations seems much more closely related to broad changes in society, including socio-economic development, better sanitation, other environmental conditions, and nutrition.

These conclusions are most startling in the field of infectious diseases. When we think about problems that respond to medical treatment, infectious diseases seem most obvious. It has been shown that antibiotics have reduced deaths from a few infections – for example, pneumonia and meningitis (Haggerty 1972). But the major improvements in deaths and illness that have occurred for most other infections were *not* clearly related to the development of antibiotics or similar technical advances.

In a remarkable speech written as president of the Infectious Diseases Society of America, the physician Edward Kass searched for evidence that modern medicine had been effective in reducing the impact of infection (Kass 1971). He traced death rates back over a century for several diseases thought responsive to antibiotics (tuberculosis, diphtheria, and scarlet fever) or immunization (whooping cough and measles).

Figures 2–6 show Kass's results. For each disease studied, he found that the major declines in mortality *preceded*, rather than followed, the diagnostic tests and specific treatments developed by modern medicine. This observation held true for diseases caused by bacteria for which antibiotics had been discovered, and by viruses, for which immunization had been introduced.

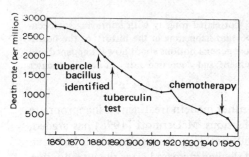

Fig. 2. Mean annual death rate from respiratory tuberculosis, England and Wales.

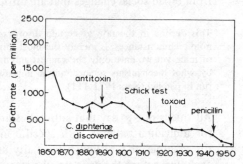

Fig. 3. Mean annual death rate from diphtheria in children under 15 years of age, England and Wales.

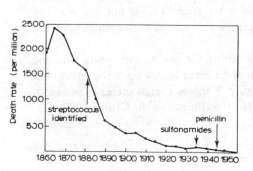

Fig. 4. Mean annual death rate from scarlet fever in children under 15 years of age, England and Wales

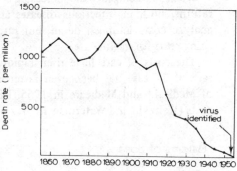

Fig. 5. Mean annual death rate from measles in children under 15 years of age, England and Wales.

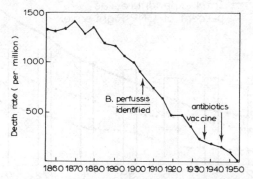

Fig. 6. Mean annual death rate from whooping cough in children under 15 years of age, England and Wales

(Source: Kass (1971). Reproduced by permission of author and publisher.)

Kass concluded that, contrary to current belief, improvements in infectious diseases generally did not result from advances of modern medicine, but rather from broad social changes that are difficult to pinpoint:

This decline in the rate of certain disorders, correlated roughly with improving socioeconomic circumstances, is merely the most important happening in the history of the health of man, yet we have only the vaguest and most general notions about how it happened and by what mechanisms socioeconomic improvement and decreased rates of certain diseases run in parallel (Kass 1971:111).

All this is not to say that antibiotics or other modern treatment is inappropriate for individual patients with specific infections. McDermott (1978) has argued, for example, that although mortality and morbidity from tuberculosis had been declining before the drug era, the rate of decline increased after the introduction of specific drug therapy. The point is that the most impressive improvements in these diseases have not occurred because of modern medicine.

We need to consider the increasing costs of medical care in light of diminishing returns, both in infectious diseases and other areas. This is not the place to analyze costs in much detail, but rather to outline some components of the rising costs for health care.

The costs of care have risen rapidly during the last twenty years, and the rate of increase has been even faster in the United States since the enactment of Medicaid and Medicare in 1965. Figure 7 shows overall increases in health costs (Waitzkin and Waterman 1974:9–10; U.S. Bureau of the Census 1977:93):

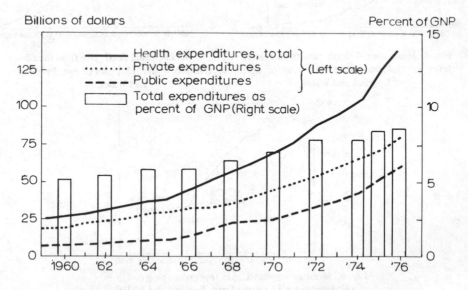

Fig. 7. National health expenditures, United States, 1960–1966. (Source: U.S. Bureau of the Census (1977:93).)

Clearly, part of this rise in costs comes from general inflationary trends in the economy. However, two specific sources of increased health costs are worth noting.

The first source is doctors, who consistently have maintained the highest level of income among the professions (Table 1).

TABLE 1
Median annual income by profession, 1975

Professions	Income ($)*
Physicians	47 520
Attorneys	24 996
Engineers	21 888
Professors	17 899
Accountants	16 200
Teachers	10 272

* Net income, indicates income after deduction of expenses related to professional activities. (Sources: U.S. Bureau of the Census 1977:102, 411; U.S. Department of Labor 1977:12.)

It is also important to realize that doctors' incomes have risen much more quickly than those of non-professional health workers (Figure 8) (Waitzkin and Waterman 1974:10; U.S. Bureau of the Census 1977:102; U.S. Department of Labor 1977:12; Navarro 1975a).

The price that doctors charge for their services is not subject to ordinary supply and demand. Access to the profession — which determines supply — is limited at two points: admission to medical school and licensure to practice (Fuchs 1974; Waitzkin and Waterman 1974:11–12). Because the supply of doctors is limited, the price of services can rise without the usual constraints of competition. Also, doctors directly affect the demand for their services. Patients generally rely on their doctors' advice in deciding the frequency of appointments. Doctors also raise the demand for their colleagues' services by advising referrals and consultations, which patients usually feel bound to pursue. This is a source of what medical economists call "derived demand", that is, demand directly created by the producers of services. Derived demand also tends to drive costs up.

A second important source of high costs is the so-called "medical industrial complex" (Ehrenreich and Ehrenreich 1970:29–39, 95–123). Increasingly, illness has brought profits to large U.S. corporations. The most obvious example of profit from illness is the pharmaceutical industry, whose drug sales total over $ 8 billion per year and increase at about 9% annually. The drug industry spends approximately 25% of its income from sales on advertising and promotion, including gifts to doctors and medical students that are intended to influence physicians' prescribing habits. Year after year, the pharmaceutical industry's profits rank among the highest of all U.S. companies (Silverman and Lee 1974).

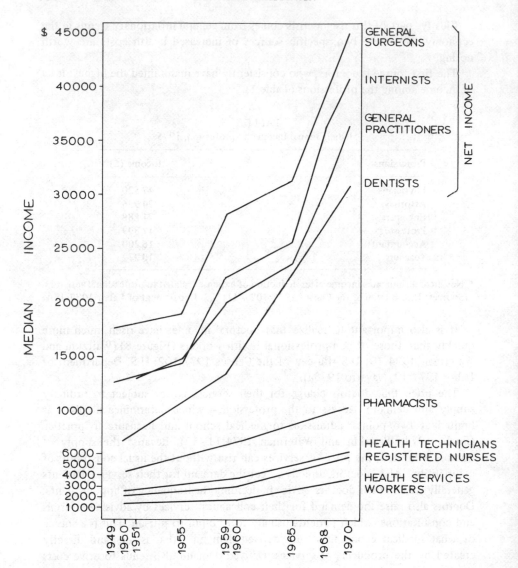

Fig. 8. The rise in income of selected personnel in the delivery of health services in the United States. Only self-employed physicians in solo practice and under 65 years of age are included. (Source: Navarro (1975a). Reproduced by permission of author and publisher.)

Other rapidly growing industries include firms producing hospital supplies and equipment, whose profits climbed 15 to 25% after Medicare and Medicaid took effect in 1965, and the private nursing home corporations, that have expanded quickly since federal funds for elderly patients became available (Ehrenreich and Ehrenreich 1970:113–117; Bodenheimer, Cummings and Harding 1972). Hospitals are the major buyers of drugs, equipment, and supplies. Profits enjoyed by the medical industrial complex in large part account for the problem of rapidly increasing hospital costs.

Rising costs during the past three decades have come partly from other sources in the health sector, as well as general trends that have affected the economy as a whole. Two undeniable components of increasing costs, however, are the profits going to health professionals and private corporations.

To sum up, we have witnessed declining mortality rates of most diseases that were common in the mid-nineteenth century. These improvements have not been clearly related to the specific technical advances of modern medicine and certainly have not been linked to rapid increases in health expenditures during the past three decades. Infectious diseases, which we often think are most amenable to medical intervention, responded mostly to broad sanitary and environmental changes and better nutrition that had little to do with medicine itself. As A. L. Cochrane, an eminent public health expert, has concluded, the twentieth century has been a "straightforward story of the ineffectiveness of medical therapy historically", as contrasted to the "layman's uncritical belief in the ability of the medical professional at least to help if not to cure" (Cochrane 1972:8).

As health care has become more expensive, the contradiction has become clearer that greater expenditures have not yielded more effective health care. Indeed, the returns have diminished as costs have increased.

CURING, CARING

The contradiction of diminishing returns in the face of escalating costs is tied to a more fundamental contradiction. During the twentieth century the goals of medicine shifted from caring to curing (Powles 1973; Illich 1976). The emphasis moved away from nurturent support for a person under physical and emotional stress. Instead, the curing of specific physical abnormalities, through technical means if possible, became the main goal.

The diagnostic search for a physical lesion, and the therapeutic search for a technical cure, perhaps made sense for a limited number of illnesses that were prevalent at the turn of the century. Examples included certain infections like pneumonia and meningitis, with which modern medicine could deal effectively. In addition, certain surgical procedures — such as operations for congenital heart disease and hip replacement — have produced undeniable benefits for patients with specific diseases.

Ironically, the diseases for which the "engineering" or "curing" approach are more suitable have nearly vanished from the scene of advanced capitalist nations. For example, major life-threatening infections occur much less often, relative to the past. On the other hand, we now are seeing an "epidemic" of chronic diseases (high blood pressure; chronic heart, lung, and kidney disease; and cancer), as well as accidents and violent deaths from homicide and suicide (Powles 1973). Most of these problems are diseases with no known cure, or are manifestations of social rather than medical conditions. The commonest causes of illness and death are no longer diseases caused by specific lesions or treated by specific remedies. They are "diseases of civilization"; it is doubtful that their occurrence will change drastically while our society remains what it is.

Whether struggling to change society is an appropriate part of progressive health work is discussed later in this chapter. Meanwhile, it is important to realize that the curing or engineering approach is not the most appropriate for most current medical problems. Of course, no one would advocate withholding antibiotics from a person with pneumonia, or argue against the limited application of technologic medicine when it is clearly necessary. But in most situations involving chronic diseases or manifestations of social stress, the *caring* function of health work needs recognition.

There is probably no better example of the overuse of the engineering approach, and the underuse of the caring approach, than the diagnosis and treatment of heart attacks. Heart attacks (myocardial infarctions) occur when part of the heart dies because it cannot get enough blood through the coronary arteries that bring blood to the heart. Most people who have heart attacks have developed other disturbances that have affected the coronary arteries prior to the heart attack itself. These disturbances include atherosclerosis and hypertension that usually build up over many years before a person has a heart attack. Even more important, atherosclerosis and hypertension are commoner in industrialized than unindustrialized societies. Many studies indicate that these problems are closely related to social stress, especially stress that people experience in their jobs or in economic hardship (Eyer 1975; Engel 1976; Jenkins 1976; Friedman and Rosenman 1974).

Until recently there has been very little attention to reducing social stress as one way to prevent heart attacks. Even now, most of the emphasis is placed on individual stress, and techniques like meditation and biofeedback by which individuals can try to lower the stress they experience (Benson 1975). These suggestions either ignore the structural sources of stress that come from the modern industrial system, or else they assume that changes in society needed to reduce social stress significantly would be so fundamental that they are not practical goals. In short, the *prevention* of heart attacks has received relatively little attention. What attention it has received focuses on individual changes that will not affect the societal origins of heart disease.

We have spent enormous amounts of money and energy in dealing with heart attacks after they occur. During the last two decades, coronary care units (CCUs) have become the accepted place for treating patients with heart attacks. CCUs are intensive care units, where patients are hospitalized for several days, have their heart rhythms monitored continuously, and receive medications through intravenous lines.

The justification for CCUs is apparently straightforward. One fairly common cause of death after a heart attack is an arrhythmia resulting from death of a portion of heart muscle. Abrupt changes in rhythm can lead to instant death. If the heart rhythm is monitored continuously, personnel in the CCU can discover a rhythm abnormality immediately and treat it, either by drugs or by electric shock applied to the chest. After several days in a CCU, the likelihood of rhythm disturbance decreases, and the patient can recuperate in an ordinary hospital ward.

Some heart attack victims have survived because rhythm abnormalities were caught and treated in CCUs. On the other hand, many patients have suffered life-threatening infections and abnormalities in blood levels of potassium and sodium because of medications and fluids given by vein. Numerous patients have shown worsening physical conditions associated with the emotional stresses they experience in a CCU, for example, observing another patient's death (Engel 1976). These complications of CCUs, like any other form of treatment, temper one's enthusiasm, since they must be balanced against whatever benefits are seen.

CCUs reflect the development of a high technology, capital-intensive innovation whose effectiveness has been assumed but never proven. Despite this lack of demonstrated impact, the effectiveness of CCUs has been widely accepted by the medical profession and has been promoted by the mass media.

CCUs are very expensive. During the past twenty years, CCUs have proliferated at medical centers and community hospitals throughout the U.S. and other countries. The initial cost of each CCU bed, which includes capital needed for monitoring devices and other equipment, is about $ 15,000 beyond the usual cost of a hospital bed. The cost for one day of CCU care is about twice that for ordinary hospital care (Hofvendahl 1971). There are different cost discrepancies between CCU and ward care in nonteaching hospitals (where CCUs are about 25% more costly) and teaching hospitals (where CCUs are about 75% more costly) (Bloom and Peterson 1973). The costs of coronary care also are increasing over time. A study of heart attacks in a single hospital from 1939 to 1969 showed escalating use of drugs (especially for sedation), chemical tests, bacteriology, radiology, and electrocardiograms, in the face of no demonstrable improvement in mortality (Martin et al. 1974).

How could the effectiveness of CCUs be tested? The standard approach in testing the effectiveness of any treatment is the *random control trial*. Here, patients are randomly assigned to two groups – a treatment group and a control group that does not receive treatment. Before and after treatment, the condition of patients in both groups is measured and compared. The treatment is effective only if patients in the treatment group show improvements that are greater than for patients in the control group.

Astonishingly, the medical profession accepted CCUs as the recommended treatment for heart attacks without any control studies showing effectiveness. In short, we have made high expenditures for coronary care, and subjected innumerable people to CCUs, without evidence that CCU treatment is better than no treatment at all. Recent random control trials that have been done in Great Britain led to a surprising result. In these courageous studies, the researchers randomly assigned heart attack patients to hospital or to home care (if provisions in the home were adequate). The findings showed either no difference or slightly better outcomes, in terms of mortality, for the group randomly assigned to home treatment (Mather et al. 1971, 1976; Hill et al. 1978). Although this research needs repeating, the preliminary conclusion is that the *engineering approach to heart attacks is no better, and possibly somewhat worse, than simple rest at home.* One other question that this finding suggests is this: Are we achieving more from our emphasis on *curing* and the engineering approach, than we would from a consistent effort to *care* for clients and to change the stressful social conditions that predispose people to heart attacks?

To summarize, a massive irrationality seems to have occurred. Enormous expenditures of valuable resources have been devoted to a treatment whose effectiveness has been assumed but not proven. What is the dynamic of our social system that fosters this irrationality?

The development of CCUs and similar technologic forms of treatment, whose effectiveness is dubious at best, makes sense only when analyzed from the structural features of capitalism. That is, although CCUs appear irrational given our health care needs, they become quite rational when seen from the needs of the capitalist system, especially since they support the expansion of monopoly capital and private profitability in the health sector (Waitzkin 1978b). This analysis does not imply that the doctors who pioneered CCUs and pushed for their expansion were motivated by profit considerations alone. Powerful ideologic forces influenced health professionals to believe that technologic solutions to heart disease were appropriate. Also, the dramatic salvage of occasional patients served to persuade coronary-care personnel that they were saving lives and that it was improper to withhold the presumed benefits of CCUs from heart attack victims. The contradiction between curing and caring in capitalist health systems mirrors the broad political and economic structures of society. It is doubtful that we can resolve the contradiction between curing and caring without basic change in the political and economic order.

CONCENTRATION, MALDISTRIBUTION

A third contradiction of the health system is that of concentration and maldistribution. Although various barriers limit the supply of health workers, there is great maldistribution of those workers who *are* available. Health facilities also are highly concentrated in certain parts of the country, while other areas remain underserved.

First, there is maldistribution based on geography — what might be called "horizontal" maldistribution. Rural areas like Appalachia and the Great Plains states, as well as urban districts with mainly black or Spanish-speaking populations, experience extreme shortages of health workers. On the other hand, more affluent parts of cities and suburbs, especially on the East Coast and West Coast, have large concentrations of medical personnel.

Table 2 gives a state-by-state breakdown in the distribution of active physicians.

The variation is enormous. There is a heavy concentration of doctors per population in such places as Washington, D.C., New York, and Massachusetts; other states like Mississippi, Alabama, and South Dakota have a startling relative lack of health workers.

TABLE 2

Number of active physicians and physician/population ratios, by geographic region division, and state: December 31, 1970

Region, division, and state	Number of active physicians	Resident population July 1, 1970 (in 1000's)	Number of physicians per 100,000 population
All locations	323,200	209,539	154
UNITED STATES	317,200	203,805	156
NORTHEAST	95,730	49,150	195
New England	22,530	11,873	190
Connecticut	5,730	3,039	189
Maine	1,240	995	125
Massachusetts	12,120	5,699	213
New Hampshire	1,010	742	136
Rhode Island	1,600	951	169
Vermont	820	447	184
Middle Atlantic	73,210	37,272	196
New Jersey	10,900	7,195	152
New York	43,080	18,260	236
Pennsylvania	19,270	11,817	163
SOUTH	83,750	62,990	133
South Atlantic	45,690	30,773	149
Delaware	780	550	141
District of Columbia	3,950	753	525
Florida	9,980	6,845	146
Georgia	5,360	4,602	117
Maryland	9,150	3,937	232
North Carolina	5,790	5,091	114
South Carolina	2,520	2,596	97
Virginia	6,240	4,653	134
West Virginia	1,930	1,746	111
East South Central	13,460	12,823	105
Alabama	3,200	3,451	93
Kentucky	3,440	3,224	107
Mississippi	1,970	2,216	89
Tennessee	4,850	3,932	123

(*Continued*)

Table 2 (continued)

Region, division and state	Number of active physicians	Resident population July 1, 1970 (in 1000's)	Number of Physicians per 100,000 population
SOUTH (continued)			
West South Central	24,590	19,396	132
Arkansas	1,830	1,926	95
Louisiana	4,600	3,644	126
Oklahoma	3,140	2,572	122
Texas	15,030	11,254	134
NORTH CENTRAL	76,500	56,730	135
East North Central	54,430	40,368	135
Illinois	15,770	11,137	142
Indiana	5,360	5,208	103
Michigan	12,810	8,901	144
Ohio	15,060	10,688	141
Wisconsin	5,430	4,433	123
West North Central	22,070	16,367	135
Iowa	3,260	2,830	115
Kansas	2,901	2,248	129
Minnesota	5,860	3,822	153
Missouri	7,020	4,693	150
Nebraska	1,760	1,490	118
North Dakota	630	618	102
South Dakota	630	666	95
WEST	61,330	34,930	177
Mountain	12,550	8,345	150
Arizona	2,860	1,792	160
Colorado	4,380	2,225	197
Idaho	700	717	97
Montana	770	697	111
Nevada	570	493	116
New Mexico	1,420	1,018	139
Utah	1,500	1,069	141
Wyoming	350	334	103
Pacific	48,780	26,589	183
Alaska	320	305	106
California	38,780	19,994	194
Hawaii	1,170	774	151
Oregon	3,105	2,102	148
Washington	5,400	3,414	158
Puerto Rico	2,480	–	–
Outlying areas	3,420	–	–

Sources: Hang, Roback and Martin 1971.

Note: Figures may not add to totals and subtotals due to independent rounding.

Note added in proof: During the two years this book has been in press, the data in Tables 2 and 3 have become more outdated, but the relationships still hold.

Even states that seem to have good doctor-population ratios contain severe *internal* maldistribution. For example, Vermont is a small state that seems to have an adequate number of health workers, as compared to other states. The most recent data show a ratio of 184 doctors per 100,000 population; this figure is well above the national ratio of 156 per 100,000. However, when the state-wide figure is broken down by counties, one finds enormous discrepancies (Tables 2 and 3). Most of Vermont's doctors are concentrated in a single county (Chittenden), where the state medical school and the largest city (Burlington) are located. In more rural countries there are severe shortages of health workers, and the statewide figures mask these shortages. Several counties have extremely poor doctor-population ratios, some worse than the state average of Mississippi.

TABLE 3

Number of active physicians, by county, in Vermont: December 31, 1971

County	Number of Active physicians	Resident Population December 31, 1971 (estimate)	Number of physicians per 100,000 population
Addison	20	25,100	80
Bennington	50	30,700	163
Caledonia	26	22,100	118
Chittenden	441	105,900	292
Essex	3	5,500	55
Franklin	30	33,500	90
Grand Isle	1	3,600	28
Lamoille	16	13,800	116
Orange	20	18,000	111
Orleans	15	20,100	75
Rutland	78	55,300	141
Washington	71	49,200	144
Windham	61	35,700	171
Windsor	54	44,900	120

Source: U.S. Public Health Service.

Secondly, besides the horizontal maldistribution based on geography, there is a "vertical" maldistribution based on income. Low-income patients cannot buy health care and medications as easily as higher-income patients. In addition, poor people more often have to use emergency room and outpatient departments of public hospitals for their care. Here they frequently face bureaucracy, impersonality, and lack of continuity because of rotating interns and residents who can follow their patients only for brief periods of time. To some extent, this situation has improved since the passage of Medicaid and Medicare legislation in 1965. But many private practitioners refuse to accept Medicaid or Medicare patients because of paperwork and delays in payment. In general, it is still more difficult for poor or lower-middle income people to get access to adequate health care than it is for the wealthy (Kosa et al. 1975; Strauss 1972; Koos 1967; Miller and Roby 1970; Wilensky 1975:98–104).

The forces that have led to concentration and maldistribution are complex. Regarding *health institutions*, finance capital has become more and more concentrated in a smaller number of medical centers and corporations. This concentration of capital in the health sector has paralleled similar trends in other sectors of the economy. "Monopoly capital" is the general term that describes this phenomenon; it is a major impediment to change in the health system (Waitzkin 1978a).

For *health workers*, maldistribution comes largely from the nature of professional education. Doctors, nurses, and other health workers receive their training in medical schools and teaching hospitals that emphasize advanced technology and specialization. This training encourages people to use diagnostic tests and treatments that require extensive laboratory and X-ray facilities, drugs and radiation therapy, and other advanced techniques. These facilities usually are available only in urban areas. Practitioners' education leads to a "trained incapacity" (Merton 1968:251) – involving a dependency on technology that itself is highly concentrated.

Health workers learn to respond to clinical situations by choosing tests and treatments that are possible in medical centers but are very difficult where technology is not present. As a result, health workers gravitate to medical centers. Technologically oriented training, of course, is not the only cause of maldistribution. For example, recreational and cultural facilities that people with advanced education usually value are more difficult to find in some rural and urban areas. These factors have created continuing difficulties even in socialist countries that have tried to correct maldistribution through a national health service which assigns health workers, for varying periods of time, to underserved regions. In advanced capitalist societies, however, monopoly capital and technologic training have been prime causes of the concentration of both facilities and health workers.

Maldistribution is not just a theoretical problem. While it is difficult to show the effectiveness of advanced medical technology like CCUs, many people in the U.S. do not have access to even the simplest forms of care. Because of maldistribution, there are still individuals who suffer death or permanent disability every year. The three case presentations that follow involve patients who used the clinics of the United Farm Workers Union (UFW) in California. The Union set up this system of clinics because of maldistribution and farmworkers' inadequate access to health services.

A Girl with Acute Glomerulonephritis

O. O. is an 11 year-old Chicana girl. Her family are migrant workers and were living temporarily in a shanty camp-without running water. The patient and her family are Spanish-speaking and know very little English. About a week before she came to the clinic, she scraped both feet on a rock in a fall. She and her parents washed the wounds with water from a well and bandaged them with a makeshift bandage. Four days later, both her feet became painful, hot, red, and swollen (symptoms of inflammation with infection). Two days after that, her ankles, fingers, and eyelids became puffy (symptoms of fluid retention), and she began to feel very sleepy. Her family brought her to a Union organizer, who drove them 75 miles to the clinic in Salinas – the closest medical facility the family could afford.

At the clinic, physical exam showed a sleepy girl in no acute distress, with a slight fever and elevated blood pressure. There was no heart murmur. Lesions with pus were present on both feet and were surrounded by areas that were tender, hot, red, and swollen. Her ankles, fingers, and eyelids were edematous.

Abnormal lab work included a urinalysis containing protein and red blood cell casts, elevated blood urea nitrogen and creatinine, and depressed creatinine clearance (all consistent with kidney disease); a markedly elevated antistreptolysin 0 titer and elevated erythrocyte sedimentation rate and depressed complement. Bacterial culture of the wounds showed beta-hemolytic Group A streptococcus.

The diagnosis was acute glomerulonephritis that was a complication from a streptococcal skin infection.

The patient's wounds were cleaned and dressed with an antibiotic ointment. A course of penicillin, rest, and a nutritive diet were started. After two weeks, the patient felt better. After three weeks, she could resume her usual activities. At six months, her creatinine, blood urea nitrogen, and creatinine clearance were consistent with kidney function about 60 per cent of normal.

In criticism/self-criticism session at the clinic, it was felt there was little the Union could have done to prevent the complication of the skin infection, because of the family's physical isolation and unavailability of health workers in the local area.

A Boy with Congenital Heart Disease

B.C. is a 5 year-old Chicano boy whose grandmother brought him to the UFW clinic because of poor appetite. The child had been delivered at home and had not been seen by a doctor previously. No one in the family speaks English.

Physical exam revealed a very small boy, with height and weight below the 3rd percentile. The child's fingernail beds and lips were slightly cyanotic; the fingernails showed clubbing. Examination of the heart showed a harsh grade V/VI systolic ejection murmer. Electrocardiogram showed right ventricular hypertrophy.

The tentative diagnosis was pulmonic stenosis with possible septal defect and possible pulmonary hypertension.

The child was referred to a university medical center. Catheterization confirmed the above diagnoses at a severe level. He underwent surgery to correct the pulmonic stenosis and septal defect. Most expenses were paid by the Crippled Children's Service. The surgeons believed that residual pulmonary hypertension would remain postoperatively.

This child faced the probability of permanent functional deficit from heart and lung disease. If he had had access to a health worker by age 3, the defect probably could have been corrected without permanent serious deficit.

A Teenager with Polio

A. G. is a 14 year-old boy, born in California, whose family are migrant farm workers. The boy had no immunizations or contact with health workers until age 9, when he developed a fever and subsequent nearly complete paralysis of both arms and the right leg. Details of contacts with other ill individuals at the time are sketchy. He is followed at the clinic for vague abdominal symptoms that are thought to be psychosomatic, probably deriving from upset that he cannot follow his peers into farm labor.

The incidence of polio has dropped markedly since the introduction of vaccines but has not yet been eradicated from the U.S., because of incomplete immunization.

All three of these young people are victims in our society. The girl with glomerulonephritis would not have suffered permanent kidney impairment if services that the family could afford were available close to home. The boy with congenital heart disease could have lived a normal life if he had been examined by age three — usually a routine for wealthier families in the U.S. Polio would not have crippled the teenager if the polio vaccine had reached him, but there are still many children in the U.S. who do not receive complete immunization because of maldistribution.

Some critics, notably Ivan Illich (1976), have argued against proposals to correct maldistribution, since these measures supposedly would distribute the *bad* effects of modern medicine more widely. This argument would make sense if all people currently had access to even the most basic forms of care and prevention. A minimum baseline of services is necessary. To argue against this minimum will mean further cutbacks in services for the poor; in a class society, the rich always will be able to buy the care they need (Waitzkin 1976; 1978c).

In summary, the U.S. produces many health workers and contains numerous capital-intensive health facilities. But both workers and facilities are concentrated in limited areas, or are available mainly to higher-income clients. Many people do not have access even to the simplest kinds of care that could prevent needless suffering and disability.

FREEDOM, EQUALITY

This classic contradiction pervades U.S. society, including its health system. One reason why many people enter the professions is that they cherish the ability to be one's own boss. This preference resonates with the general American ethos of individual "freedom" and voluntarism. Many health workers do not want to be told where to practice, how much to charge, how to improve what they are doing, or how to respond to organized consumer groups. Similarly, it is argued that clients should have freedom of choice.

Yet freedom of choice is heavily class linked. Here is what Marx and Engels (1848) said about the relation between class and freedom:

The abolition of [class society] is called by the bourgeois abolition of individuality and freedom! . . . By freedom is meant, under the present bourgeois conditions of production, free trade, free selling and buying.

In short, freedom is greatest for those who control property and wealth. This conclusion is no less true for health care than for other goods and services. Poor people never have had as much freedom as the wealthy to choose their sources of health care. More often than not, they have had to rely on the fragmented and depersonalized services of public hospitals and outpatient departments. Recently many public facilities have closed because of financial cutbacks resulting from the current economic crisis (Blake and Bodenheimer 1975). Freedom of choice is, for the most part, a theoretical freedom. It is an important ideology in U.S. society. But the reality of freedom is that some groups have enjoyed its fruits much more than others.

Equality also is a theoretical goal in the U.S., but a goal that does not square with reality (Waitzkin and Waterman 1974; Anderson 1972; Wilensky 1975; Lewis, Mechanic, and Fein 1976). I already have outlined the severe maldistribution of health workers and facilities, based on both geography and income differences. There is a growing concern that citizens should have equal access to health care — in short, that health care is a fundamental right, analogous to the right of public education.

But equality in health care will not happen just by talking about it. Major reorganizational changes in the health system must occur if equality is to become more than a rhetorical goal. These changes would necessarily limit the freedom that at least two groups — health workers and the industries that profit from illness — now enjoy.

Health workers would be less free to practice where, how, and when they choose. Other countries have tried several mechanisms to reduce financial and distributional impediments to equality (Waitzkin 1978a). Health workers may receive payments directly from some arm of government for services to low-income patients, or alternatively the government reimburses patients for payments they make to health workers. This financial structure is a system of national health insurance (NHI), which the U.S. still has not enacted. In countries with socialist or "mixed" capitalist-socialist economic systems, health workers generally are employees of a national health service (NHS), obtain a salary from government revenues, and receive either no or nominal fees from individual patients. These financial arrangements reduce health workers' freedom to set an independent price for their services. Health care ceases to be a commodity to be paid for like other goods and services. It is recognized that the "free market" structure necessarily stands in the way of equal health care. Alternative financing mechanisms rely on government intervention. They also decrease health workers' freedom to work strictly in a free-market mode.

Other measures also are necessary to reduce maldistribution. If health workers are entirely free to work where they choose, maldistribution will persist. Some countries have used financial incentives, through higher salaries, to influence health workers to serve in rural areas and urban districts with shortages. This technique remains essentially *voluntary*. Despite financial incentives, since health workers may choose to practice in areas of surplus, there is no way to assure redistribution according to need. As a result, maldistribution tends to persist to a greater or lesser degree.

Another method to overcome geographical inequalities involves *compulsory* measures, which require health workers to serve, for at least a specific period of time, in needy areas of the country. Some nations combine compulsory policies with training a corps of para-professional health workers. These workers perform most functions of doctors but refer people with difficult problems to urban centers. Compulsory assignment of health workers to needy areas has been the only technique that has relieved maldistribution problems. The problem of maldistribution has not disappeared in countries that use compulsory assignment of health workers. In the Soviet Union, for example, bureaucratic irregularities permit some doctors to avoid compulsory service in rural areas. China recently has begun a reevaluation of the "barefoot doctors," because their more limited training has left gaps in technical services for certain regions of the country. On the other hand, Cuba successfully has reduced maldistribution through a national health service that restricts the number of doctors licensed to practice in specific geographical areas. This approach — involving restrictions on practice opportunities in overserved areas in addition to temporary periods of compulsory service in underserved areas — has been advocated as a potential solution to the problem of maldistribution. These changes do not occur easily. Their implementation always depends on basic social changes. These policies include a strong emphasis on the importance of collective goals, even if these goals imply, for periods of time, the subordination of individual preferences.

The contradiction between freedom and equality, however, goes beyond the individual level. Measures to reduce inequality affect the free choice of individual health workers, but they apply even more strongly to industries that profit from ill health. A basic principle in countries that have tried to deal systematically with inequality is that *illness should not be exploited for profit*. Both financial and geographical inequalities are intimately linked to private profit making.

Earlier in this chapter, I discussed the escalating costs of health care during the last three decades. Profit making by insurance companies, pharmaceutical firms, medical equipment manufacturers, the nursing home industry, and many other enterprises accounts for a significant part (though of course not the only part) of these increasing costs. Corporate profit is a continuing drain of financial resources in the health system. How can a society seek equality in health services and still permit private profiteering? How can we complain that financial resources are limited, while we allow an enormous drain of money into the medical-industrial complex?

The goal of equality contradicts the goal of free enterprise in the health sector. Under capitalism, the sick are subject to exploitation for corporate profit. Countries seeking to increase equality have severely restricted the freedom to profit from illness. Both socialist and "mixed" systems have either eliminated or strictly controlled the proliferation of competing pharmaceutical companies, insurance corporations, health equipment industries, proprietary hospitals, and nursing homes. In most cases, hospitals, other institutions caring for the sick, and industries manufacturing health products are either owned or controlled by the state. This kind of change cannot occur in isolation from other fundamental changes in the society. But equality in health care will remain a rhetorical goal as long as freedom of profit making from illness persists.

CAPITALISM'S HEALTH, CAPITALIST DISEASES

Even more basic than the exploitation of illness is capitalism's role in causing and maintaining disease. Currently we are facing an "epidemic" of cancer, heart disease, and chronic illness (Powles 1973). Until recently, many have explained these problems largely as manifestations of better health care. That is, since modern medicine has controlled infection, the major killer of the past, the new problems we face result from increased life expectancy. By this explanation, most current health problems are "degenerative" conditions. They often are associated with aging and are "unmasked" by more effective treatment of diseases that previously killed people younger.

Earlier, I reviewed the historical evidence for this explanation. The conclusion was that improved mortality and morbidity probably did *not* result from the specific advances of modern medicine, as opposed to better sanitation and nutrition. So we are left with the question whether diseases that currently are increasing reflect — rather than "unmasking" — the problems and contradictions of modern society.

Whenever considering this question, it is important to distinguish between capitalism and industrialization (Navarro 1975b). There is no question that industrialization itself is associated with increases in some illnesses, especially occupational diseases, that are linked to the nature of industrial work. These illness-generating conditions exist in industrialized societies, whether capitalist or socialist. However, it is again important to focus on the issue of profit and the organization of production in capitalist industry. How do the constraints of capitalist production reduce the incentive to correct the conditions that generate illness? How does the nature of the capitalist labor force prevent workers from taking a stronger stand against these conditions? Why are governmental controls in this area so weak? It is worthwhile to study these questions in relation to specific diseases that result, at least in part, from the capitalist mode of production.

Farmworkers' Back

Chronic, disabling back injury is the commonest occupational disease that farmworkers endure in the U.S. This disease has nothing to do with industrialization; it occurs in agricultural work that historically has had little mechanization and that has depended almost entirely on manual labor. Here is a typical case history of a patient followed at a UFW clinic.

J.C. is a 32 year-old Chicano father of five. He began working as a farm laborer at age 14. He generally worked eight to ten hours a day in stoop labor with an arched back in such crops as lettuce. For about ten years he used the "short hoe" required of many farmworkers in the Western states. Several years ago, while bending at work, he suddenly felt a sharp pain in his back with radiation down the back of his left leg.

Physical exam at that time showed tenderness over the L4–L5 intervertebral space of the back, decreased reflexes and sensation of the left lower extremity, and positive straight-leg-raising test on the left. X-rays and myelogram showed advanced degenerative arthritis of the entire lower spine and a herniated nucleus pulposus at the L4—L5 level.

Severe pain on bending persisted after back surgery. The patient knows no English, cannot find a job outside farm labor, and is applying for permanent disability benefits.

The short hoe has a short wooden handle — about one foot in length. To use the short hoe, a person must work in a stooped posture, bent forward at the waist, so that the hoe can reach the ground. The short hoe has no intrinsic advantage over the long-handled hoe, which a farmworker can use in an erect posture. The only reason for the short hoe is supervision. If the foreman sees that everybody in a crew is bent over, he can be more sure that everybody is working. With long-handled hoes, since people can stand with straight backs, supervision becomes somewhat more difficult. It is harder for a small number of supervisors to be sure that a large number of workers are really working.

Farmworkers' back is an entirely preventable disease. It occurs in an un-industrialized, agricultural sector of the economy that is highly oriented to profit. The short hoe's human toll is crippling back disease for thousands of farmworkers. The main injuries are slipped disks and degenerative arthritis of the spine. These problems occur in young workers who do stoop labor. The physical effects are irreversible. Since migrant workers most often lack educational opportunities and frequently know little English, farmworkers' back usually means permanent economic disability.

There is nothing new about this disease. Medical specialists have testified about the short hoe's devastating effects for several decades. Yet farm owners (especially the "agribusiness" corporations that have gained control of many agricultural enterprises) consistently have refused to stop the short hoe's use. Farmowners generally give no reason for this policy, except that long-handled hoes would require higher costs of supervision. (A few companies also argue that the wood for longer handles increases costs! When analyzed, the costs of longer handles are minimal.) The profit motive and the nature of agricultural production lead directly to this illness-generating labor practice.

Until recently farmworkers were unorganized. A "reserve army" of migrant workers were available to replace individuals crippled by farmworkers' back or objecting to the conditions of work. Powerlessness resulted from lack of organization. Individual farmworkers had no alternative to the crippling effects of the short hoe, because resistance meant loss of work.

Since the mid-1960s the UFW has organized farmworkers throughout the West, Southwest, and Southeast. Like other unions, the UFW has fought for basic improvements in wages and benefits. Beyond these economic goals, however, the UFW has focused on the conditions of work. The UFW has launched organizing and publicity campaigns concerning the short hoe, dangerous insecticides and chemicals, and other occupational health issues.

After many years, the California legislature responded. It passed a law banning the short hoe in the state. When agribusiness interests did not succeed in stopping legislation, several companies turned to the courts. One court issued an injunction against the new law; the ruling accepted the companies' claims that conversion to the long-handled hoe would lead to excessive costs. This injunction later was reversed. But even after legislation, California farmworkers — as well as workers in other states without such laws — continued to use and suffer from the short hoe. Other states have not passed legislation banning the short hoe. The contradiction between the health of capitalist agriculture and the illness of farmworkers' back persists.

Plastic Workers' Liver Cancer

Plastic is everywhere in modern society. It wraps our food, upholsters our furniture, transports our water in pipes, amuses our children as toys, entertains us as phonograph records, and attracts our attention as signs. During the past three decades, plastic production and consumption in the U.S. and other countries have spiraled upward.

The basic component of plastic is polyvinyl chloride. Through chemical reactions polyvinyl chloride (a solid) is manufactured from vinyl chloride (a gas). Beginning in 1938, a series of scientific reports have appeared, showing toxic damage of the liver and other organs in animals exposed to vinyl chloride in laboratory experiments. Studies conducted under several different conditions verified these findings. Although many scientists and officials in the plastic industry knew about these results, they did not change the utilization of vinyl chloride in the manufacturing process.

In 1974 three workers in a plastic factory in Louisville, Kentucky, developed angiosarcoma of the liver — an otherwise very rare cancer. During the next two years investigators found that more than 26 other cases of angiosarcoma were linked to occupational exposure to vinyl chloride. These people with cancer attracted worldwide attention. New studies showed an association between vinyl chloride exposure and cancer in organs besides the liver; they also found increasing rates of many types of cancer among people exposed to the chemical. One researcher summarizes in this way the discovery of vinyl chloride's cancer-producing effects: "It is probable that we are just beginning to see a larger epidemic" (Peters 1976:653).

Production of vinyl chloride in the U.S. has increased since 1939 at an average annual rate of 12%. Despite definite, unambiguous evidence that vinyl chloride causes cancer of the liver and other organs, the plastic industry has resisted attempts to reduce occupational exposure. The production process itself has several steps. During one step, the cleaning stage when workers crawl into the reactors where polyvinyl chloride is formed, the concentration of vinyl chloride may exceed 1000 parts per million (ppm). In experiments with rodents, investigators have found liver damage at exposures of 50 ppm. Although the minimum toxic level for humans is unknown, occupational health officials recommended engineering changes that would assure exposure levels of 1 ppm or less. The plastic industry's response was that a reduction to 1 ppm would raise the cost of polyvinyl chloride by 50%. As a compromise, in 1970, the U.S. Occupational

Safety and Health Administration set a standard that allowed exposure levels up to 25 ppm. The plastic industry challenged even this intermediate level by court appeals, which have delayed but not stopped the new regulations. Currently, although the safe level remains unclear, the industry continues to oppose exposure levels that are 25 times greater than experts' recommendations.

The profit issue, which is the industry's main concern, is not the only impediment to effective controls. Since implementation of safer standards is costly and time-consuming, it is likely that many plants producing polyvinyl chloride would close, either permanently or temporarily. If plants were closed until safe production procedures or substitutes for polyvinyl chloride were developed, it is estimated that about two million workers would lose their jobs (Boden 1976).

This is labor's classic dilemma in occupational diseases. Workers frequently face the contradiction between job safety and continued employment. Workmen's compensation laws provide financial benefits only *after* a worker has suffered injury or disability from the work process. There are no adequate provisions for financial assistance during changes in the production process that would *prevent* the development of occupational diseases. Workers' desire for a safe workplace thus is an ambivalent desire. The threat of unemployment is always present in any struggle to reduce occupational hazards (Stellman and Daum 1973; Berman 1978).

The question is: Your job or your life? Historically, organized labor has favored occupational safety legislation and tighter regulations. But when workers confront job loss, they often have accepted compromises that they recognize are inadequate.

As the dangers of vinyl chloride have become clear, plastic workers' unions have supported the recommendation of 1 ppm. But political and economic realities have restrained the unions' activism. In general, unions have not opposed the compromise regulation of 25 ppm. Since the society gives no assurance of alternative employment during industry's transition to safer standards, the unions have little choice. To keep their jobs, workers must accept the risk of cancer.

Or do they? Some socialist countries, unencumbered by private profit, have taken drastic measures to prevent occupational disease (Nee and Peck 1976). Also, later in this chapter, I describe the simplicity of solutions, even in the U.S., that are possible when workers own their factories. First, however, it is important to understand how diseases of capitalism can spread beyond the workplace, to affect entire communities and larger populations.

Brain Disease from Mercury Poisoning

In 1907 a chemical company built a factory in Minamata, Japan. Minamata is a small seacoast community whose economy for centuries had been based on fishing (cf. Smith and Smith 1975). Over the years, the factory grew and became part of a large petro-chemical conglomerate, the Chisso Corporation. Because the factory dumped its waste products into Minamata Bay, fish began to die or to avoid the area. In 1925 Chisso started to give payments to local fishermen who complained. In 1932 Chisso began to produce acetaldehyde, a chemical used in the manufacture of drugs, perfumes, plastics, and many other products. Organic mercury is a catalyst in acetaldehyde production.

Beginning in 1952, cats in Minamata began to die after developing convulsions, bizarre behavior, and paralysis. Between 1956 and 1957, 52 children and adults started to have similar neurologic disorders; 21 people died. Outside investigators reported that the cause of the disease probably was heavy-metal poisoning carried to humans and cats who ate fish from Minamata Bay.

In 1959 a scientist working for Chisso fed material from an acetaldehyde waste pipe to a cat in his laboratory. Soon the cat showed the typical signs of Minamata Disease. The scientist reported this finding to the Chisso management. The management suppressed the finding and ordered the scientist not to conduct more experiments concerning Minamata Disease. The scientist, perhaps concerned about his continued employment, remained silent (the results of his experiment came to light during trials that took place in the late 1960s). The company publicly announced there was no scientific proof that Minamata Disease was related to Chisso manufacturing processes. The company installed a purification device in 1959. Nevertheless, Chissa continued to dump waste products containing mercury into Minamata Bay until 1968, when it switched to catalysts that were technically more efficient than mercury.

During the late 1960s and early 1970s, over three thousand patients brought legal suit against Chisso for financial compensation and medical expenses. Residents also held demonstrations, sit-ins, and other protests at the Minamata plant. Company guards, together with unionized workers at the plant, physically attacked the protestors several times; there were many injuries, some serious. In 1973 the Central Pollution Board decided that Chisso would pay medically "verified" patients $ 68,000 for "heavy" cases, and $ 60,000 for "lighter" cases. As of early 1975, 798 patients had been verified, and approximately 2800 other applicants were waiting for decisions. Many of these patients were children with *congenital* Minamata Disease, whose mothers had eaten mercury-containing fish during pregnancy. Meanwhile, the provincial government announced that fish outside Minamata Bay, marked by buoys, were safe to eat. This decision ignored the fact that fish throughout the Shiranui Sea, of which Minamata Bay is a part, can swim past buoys. Researchers in Japan estimate that as many as ten thousand people, who are currently or were previously eating fish from the Shiranui Sea, may eventually fall ill with Minamata Disease.

The structure of capitalist production is responsible for such tragedies of environmental poisoning. For more than a decade, Chisso management suppressed evidence of the company's responsibility for Minamata Disease. Management recognized the financial burden it would face if it accepted responsibility. Indemnity payments would drastically affect profits. There were no mechanisms by which Japanese society as a whole would compensate the victims or pay their medical expenses. Moreover, in this situation, workers at Chisso had structural interests that overlapped with management's. Major payments to Minamata victims, or a less efficient production process without mercury catalysis, by reducing profitability, ultimately would threaten workers' jobs. During the protests and suits, these economic realities forced unionized workers at Chisso to side with managers and against their injured neighbors. If profit were not the guiding motivation of industry, and if the society guaranteed people's material subsistence, prevention and protection from industrial poisoning would not encounter such fundamental resistance.

The implications of Minamata Disease go far beyond Japan and mercury. During the 1960s a paper company in northern Ontario, Canada, dumped mercury-containing wastes into the English—Wabagoon River (Smith and Smith 1975:140—143). This region of Canada is fairly isolated. The people who live there are mainly Native Americans and the operators of popular tourist camps. Several citizens, concerned about the mercury problem, obtained tests that showed toxic levels in the river fish. Government officials have investigated the situation. The paper company has reduced but not eliminated mercury in its waste discharges. Although it is estimated that river fish will contain toxic mercury levels for about 70 years, the government has not stopped the company's mercury dumps. Nor has the government banned fishing — apparently responding to pressures from the tourist industry that caters to visiting sports fishermen. Inaction persists, despite the fact that several people living in the region have developed classic symptoms of Minamata Disease and have shown high mercury levels in tests of blood and hair.

Outbreaks of mercury and other heavy-metal poisoning occur periodically in many parts of the U.S. and other countries (Center for Disease Control 1976; Pierce et al. 1972). In the early phases of the Minamata epidemic, investigators found that Chisso was pouring into the sea more than fifty chemicals that can cause disease in humans. Later research showed that thallium, manganese, and selesium — all present in high concentration in Chisso's effluents — were not the cause, and that mercury was. Other industries have discharged these elements and related compounds (including lead, hydro-carbons, asbestos, and occasional radioactive "spills"). Environmental poisons have caused temporary epidemics of acute illness. Their chronic effects, especially in the development of cancer, only recently are receiving more attention. The social, economic, and political issues involved in many geographic areas, and in relation to many specific poisons, resemble those of Minamata. Some socialist countries have tolerated industrial pollution for varying periods of time. On the other hand, China and Cuba have made remarkable progress in reducing hazards of pneumoconiosis in mining and bagassosis in sugar production (Nee and Peck 1976; Occupational Health Delegation to Cuba 1979). While the structure of capitalist production remains what it is, however, we can expect more of the same devastation that the people of Minimata have faced.

Asbestos Workers' Lung Disease and Cancer

Asbestos is one of several compounds that cause occupational lung disease. Industries that expose workers to asbestos include manufacturers of insulation (pipes, heatproof screens, etc.), construction, shipyards, and textile makers. The disease asbestosis occurs in the following way. Industrial dusts containing asbestos settle in the small airways of the lungs, form dust deposits, and inflammation. The inflammation leads to fibrosis in the cell layers between airways and small blood vessels. As a result of fibrosis, it becomes more and more difficult for a person to get adequate oxygen from the lungs into the bloodstream. Workers in many industries develop similar chronic lung disease from exposure to other types of dust:

- aluminosis ("bauxite lung") from aluminum in smelting, explosives, paints, and fireworks manufacturing;
- baritosis from barium sulfate in mining;
- beryllium disease from beryllium in aircraft manufacturing, metallurgy, and rocket fuels;
- byssinosis ("brown lung") from cotton, flax, and hemp dust in textile manufacturing;
- coal workers' pneumoconiosis ("black lung") from coal dust in mining, coal trimming, and the graphite industry;
- kaolinosis from hydrated aluminum silicates in china making;
- platinum asthma from platinum salts in electronics and chemical industries;
- siderosis from iron oxides in welding and iron ore mining;
- silicosis from silica in mining, pottery, sandblasting, foundries, quarries, and masonry;
- stannosis from tin oxide in smelting; and
- talcosis from hydrated magnesium silicates in the rubber industry.

Although many of these diseases produce chronic disability and early death from lung pathology alone, asbestos has the added danger of cancer. Since 1935 the medical literature has contained reports of lung cancer associated with asbestosis. The industry's response followed the predictable pattern of denial and suppression of information (Kotelchuck 1974; Lynch and Smith 1935; Holleb and Angrist 1942; Selikoff et al. 1965, 1972). For many years major asbestos companies in the U.S. and Canada publicly claimed the evidence that asbestos caused cancer was not convincing enough to reduce exposure levels. Several companies also gave financial support to researchers whose published studies showed no relation between asbestos and cancer. Retrospectively all these studies used inadequate methods. For example, industry-sponsored research studied young people who had worked in asbestos production for short periods of time. This research generally ignored the "latent period" between exposure and development of disease.

During the 1960s several investigators not receiving industry support for the first time were able to study workers who had longer periods of exposure. These definitive studies showed a clearcut association between asbestos exposure and cancer (including mesothelioma, an otherwise rare cancer of the chest or abdominal cavity). Fifty years after the initial reports of asbestosis, and forty years after the observed association between asbestos and cancer, only now are we seeing attempts to reduce workers' exposure to safe levels.

Again, as in other occupational health problems, it is not only industry's profits that stand in the way of change. The prospect of unemployment inhibits unions of asbestos workers from taking a strong stand on working conditions. Many asbestos workers already have lost their jobs during production cutbacks resulting from environmental protection regulations. The threat of job loss, and the changes that can occur when workers take control of their factories, are clear from the story of the Vermont Asbestos Company (VAC).

For many years, the GAF Corporation of New York (a multinational corporation controlling numerous industrial subsidiaries) had owned and operated an asbestos mine in northern Vermont. About 300 people worked at the mine, which served as the main employer for families in two small towns. In 1974, the U.S. Environmental Protection Agency and the Vermont Occupational Safety and Health Agency asked the mine to install dust-control devices and procedures to lower asbestos exposure to acceptable levels. The estimated cost of these changes was about $1 million. Rather than spend this money, GAF decided to close the mine.

Facing massive unemployment, workers at the mine began to think about an unusual alternative — owning and running the mine themselves. At first the price, $5 million, seemed impossible. Still, several workers approached the Vermont Governor's office to see if they could get the state to underwrite the risk of loans from local banks. The governor's office agreed. Workers then obtained the necessary loans, bought the mine, and began operating it themselves. Profit no longer went to New York, but instead to workers and their families who held shares in the company. Productivity increased enormously. Within a year, VAC paid off all outstanding loans. In 1½ years it was making such a profit that the board (composed jointly of manual and managerial workers, all of whom held shares in the company) decided to create a new industry, making construction material from asbestos waste products. The new plant, creating about 70 jobs, will be located in the county of Vermont with the highest current rate of umemployment.

Many problems remain at VAC, particularly concerning the distinction between managerial and non-managerial workers. One problem that workers have corrected, however, is hazardous asbestos exposure levels. Within one year of taking control, workers have installed the dust-control devices that bring asbestos levels below current safety standards. They have met all the requirements of federal and state regulatory agencies. The contradiction between profit and health evaporates when "profit" goes entirely to workers. (Since the company's revenues no longer go to outside capitalists who own the means of production, they are hardly profits in the traditional sense.) Workers' monetary rewards mean nothing if they face disability, cancer, and early death. The value of safety in the workplace is never clearer than when workers own the workplace. VAC's success in solving its occupational health problems sets an example for other workers. It also clarifies the question whether we can prevent capitalism's diseases while capitalism persists in its present form.

HEALTH PRAXIS

Marxist analysis conveys another basic message: analysis is not enough. "Praxis," as proposed throughout the history of Marxist scholarship, is the disciplined uniting of thought and practice, study and action (Gramsci 1971). It is important to consider political strategy, especially as it concerns the health system of the United States.

Contradictions of Patching

Health workers concerned about progressive social change face difficult dilemmas in their day-to-day work. Clients' problems often have roots in the social system. Examples abound: drug addicts and alcoholics who prefer numbness to the pain of unemployment and inadequate housing; persons with occupational diseases that require treatment but will worsen upon return to illness-generating work conditions; people with stress-related cardiovascular disease; elderly or disabled people who need periodic medical certification to obtain welfare benefits that are barely adequate; prisoners who develop illness because of prison conditions. Health workers usually feel obliged to respond to the expressed needs of these and many similar clients.

In doing so, however, health workers engage in "patching." On the individual level, patching usually permits clients to keep functioning in a social system that is often the source of the problem. At the societal level, the cumulative effect of these interchanges is the patching of a social system whose patterns of oppression frequently cause disease and personal unhappiness. The medical model that teaches health workers to serve individual patients deflects attention from this difficult and frightening dilemma.

The contradictions of patching have no simple resolution. Clearly health workers cannot deny services to clients, even when these services permit clients' continued participation in illness-generating social structures. On the other hand, it is important to draw this connection between social issues and personal troubles (Mills 1959). Health praxis should link clinical activities to efforts aimed directly at basic sociopolitical change. Marxist analysis has clarified some fruitful directions of political strategy.

"Reformist" Versus "Nonreformist" Reform

When oppressive social conditions exist, reforms to improve them seem reasonable. However, the history of reform in capitalist countries has shown that reforms most often follow social protest, make incremental improvements that do not change overall patterns of oppression, and face cutbacks when protest recedes. Health praxis includes a careful study of reform proposals and the advocacy of reforms that will have a progressive impact.

A distinction developed by Gorz (1973) clarifies this problem. "Reformist reforms" provide small material improvements while leaving intact current political and economic structures. These reforms may reduce discontent for periods of time, while helping to preserve the system in its present form:

A reformist reform is one which subordinates objectives to the criteria of rationality and practicability of a given system and policy . . . . [It] rejects those objectives and demands – however deep the need for them – which are incompatible with the preservation of the system.

"Nonreformist reforms" achieve true and lasting changes in the present system's structures of power and finance. Rather than obscuring sources of exploitation by small incremental improvements, nonreformist reforms expose and highlight structural inequities. Such reforms ultimately increase frustration and political tension in a society; they do not seek to reduce these sources of political energy. As Gorz puts it:

. . . although we should not reject intermediary reforms . . . , it is with the strict proviso that they are to be regarded as a means and not an end, as dynamic phases in a progressive struggle, not as stopping places.

From this viewpoint health workers can try to discern which current health reform proposals are reformist and which are nonreformist. They also can take active advocacy roles, supporting the latter and opposing the former. Although the distinction is seldom easy, it has received detailed analysis with reference to specific proposals (Waitzkin and Waterman 1974; Kotelchuck 1976; Alford 1975; Navarro 1974).

Reformist reforms would not change the overall structure of the health system in any basic way. For example, national health insurance chiefly would create changes in financing, rather than in the organization of the health system. This reform may reduce the financial crises of some patients; it would help assure payment for health professionals and hospitals. On the other hand, national health insurance will do very little to control profit for medical industries or to correct problems of maldistributed health facilities and personnel. Its incremental approach and reliance on private market processes would protect the same economic and professional interests that currently dominate the health system.

Other examples of reformist reforms are health maintenance organizations, prepaid group practice, medical foundations, and professional standards review organizations. With rare exceptions that are organized as consumer cooperatives, these innovations preserve professional dominance in health care (Freidson 1976). There have been few incentives to improve existing patterns of maldistributed services. Moreover, large private corporations have entered this field rapidly, sponsoring profit-making health maintenance organizations and marketing technologic aids for peer review (Salmon 1975).

Until recently, support for a national health service in the United States has been rare. For several years, however, Marxist analysts have worked with members of Congress in drafting preliminary proposals for a national health service (Dellums et al. 1978). These proposals, if enacted, would be progressive in several ways. They promise to place stringent limitations on private profit in the health sector. Most large health institutions gradually would come under state ownership. Centralized health planning would combine with policy input from local councils to foster responsiveness and limit professional dominance. Financing by progressive taxation is designed explicitly to benefit low-income patients. Periods of required practice in underserved areas would address the problem of maldistribution. The eventual development of a national drug and medical equipment formulary promises to curtail monopoly capital in the health sector. Provisions for occupational health and safety would aim toward reducing illness-generating conditions in the workplace and environment.

Although these proposals face dim political prospects, support is growing. For instance, the Governing Council of the American Public Health Association has passed two resolutions supporting the concept of a national health service that would be community based and financed by progressive taxation (Governing Council 1977). This reform contains contradictions that probably would generate frustration and pressure for change. In particular, these proposals would permit the continuation of private practice and, therefore, the inequities of the private-public dichotomy. Yet because a national health service provides a model for a more responsively organized system, advocacy of this reform seems a key part of health praxis (Sidel and Sidel 1977). In this context, it is worthwhile considering some problems and strengths that have emerged in socialist health systems, as well as directions of progressive medical-political action in the United States.

The Problem of Bureaucracy Must be Surmounted

Any attempt to construct a coordinated public health system would involve the formation of a bureaucracy organized on a national level. The dehumanizing and alienating manifestations of bureaucracy have made themselves felt in many socialist countries which have tried to establish effective health care systems (Weinerman 1969; Waterman 1971). As a result, patients often must face cumbersome procedures which inhibit their ability to obtain the health care they seek. Bureaucratic obstacles to adequate health care arise primarily at two points: overcentralization of policy making and inefficient referral networks.

Centralized planning can produce health systems which are rational on paper but ineffective in reality. Each region of a nation experiences unique health problems, which relate to such variables as the dominant economic enterprise, terrain and transportation, degree of urbanization, and so forth. Rural areas which are organized around agriculture, for example, show an incidence of occupational diseases and difficulties of access to medical facilities which differ markedly from those of urban districts with predominantly industrial enterprise. Several Eastern European countries have constructed health systems which, in practice, fail to take into account such local variations. As a result, particularly in rural areas, patients encounter severe inconveniences in obtaining needed services, despite national policies which make health care theoretically available to all citizens (Waterman 1971). Clearly, a centralized bureaucracy will have difficulties in planning adequately for the diverse needs of an entire population.

A second bureaucratic problem arising in nationally organized health systems concerns the availability of general practitioners, as opposed to specialists. To cite the Yugoslavian example, local health centers are staffed predominantly by general practitioners, who must see a large number of patients each day (Waterman 1971; cf. Weinerman 1969). Specialists are available in provincial areas but spend most of their time at large provincial hospitals. Patients with non-emergent conditions who require specialty attention must wait long periods of time and travel long distances to obtain care at these hospitals. Because the separation of general versus specialty services is fairly rigid, difficulties arise at both the local and provincial levels. For patients whose conditions fall within the competence of general practitioners at local health centers, medical care tends to be brief and perfunctory. For problems requiring specialists, patients face inconvenient delay and geographic inaccessibility; their care at the provincial hospitals tends to be impersonal. In short, in countries where health services are organized mainly along bureaucratic lines, the balance of general and specialty services tends to be poorly matched to the specific health needs of local patient populations.

The problem of bureaucracy emerges in any attempt to formulate a framework for a nonexploitative health system. Its solution does not lie in the simple assertion that bureaucratic forms be minimized. Some mechanism must evolve through which planning — particularly involving the allocation of resources and personnel — can occur on a national level. Such a mechanism would inevitably involve some degree of bureaucratic organization. It is a fallacy to believe, as some have argued, that bureaucracy itself necessarily leads to an alienating, cumbersome health system (Halberstam 1971). As illustrated by health systems in Eastern Europe, bureaucracy exerts its worst effects when it interferes with the day-to-day activities of specific localities, rather than limiting itself to the setting of national goals. From this view, the problem of bureaucracy becomes an issue of central versus local control.

National Goals, Local Control

The role of a centralized bureaucracy in a nonexploitative health system need not be complex. In fact, its functions would be predominantly economic. First, a nation must determine on a federal level the priority which health care is to receive within a spectrum of national goals. This decision, basically evaluative, leads directly to budgetary implications. For example, the relatively small proportion of the national budget devoted to health activities in the United States reflects the evaluative priorities of central decision makers. Continued support of the military and related industries reflects policy preferences of the nation's leadership. Redirection of priorities at a national level is a necessary precondition for a humane health system. In brief, *national goals* must be redirected, to recognize the importance of the population's health and welfare needs. With a redirection of national goals, fundamental changes would ensue in the central budgetary processes. Presumably, resources which now are allocated to capital-intensive, defense-related industries would become available in the health sector.

Following these awesome modifications in national priorities, a central bureaucracy's formal functions might be fairly simple, at least in theory. The major goal of such a national organization would be to insure each citizen's right to health care. With a suitable budget, therefore, the bureaucracy's principal tasks would pertain to the distribution of resources. Money made available by a structure of progressive taxation would be distributed to local health institutions according to a formula based on local health needs. A variety of specific formulae might be imagined. One reasonable suggestion is that funds distributed to specific health centers or hospitals be determined by the number of patients using those institutions, and that communities with greater prior needs (i.e., higher rates of illness, lower average income, and so forth) receive somewhat greater initial funding (Bodenheimer, Cummings, and Harding 1972:120–121). The crucial point is that the scope of central bureaucratic activities would be quite limited. Once national priorities were realigned, a centralized bureaucracy would not play a major role in health policy. Nor would it control the day-to-day activities of local health facilities. The bureaucracy's major task, which theoretically could be accomplished with a relatively small number of personnel, would be the distribution of funds from a central collecting point to the health centers and hospitals which actually provide care.

Local control over health policy would circumvent the problems of a more extensive federal bureaucracy whose uniform procedures tend not to accommodate the variable needs of different groups and localities. Although local control is a problematic topic, its broad directions may be outlined based on the examples of countries in which it has proven effective – particularly Cuba and the People's Republic of China.

Because they are best acquainted with local health needs and working conditions, consumers and health workers would unite to form coalitions responsible for the policies of specific hospitals or health centers. Optimally, as in the case of Cuba and China, councils of workers and consumers would be elected through democratic procedures. On the local level, these councils would control health centers or hospitals – hiring personnel, constructing budgets, determining the type and scope of services provided, and so forth. To coordinate services on a regional level, each local council would elect representatives to a regional council. The regional council would make decisions about hospital expansion and new construction, the establishment and location of technically advanced and specialized facilities (radiation therapy, transplantation teams, etc.), and other matters which affect the availability of services throughout the region. The restriction of medical expansion would comprise one important goal of the regional council. From this view, tendencies of individual hospitals to expand by establishing duplications of nearby specialty facilities would be sharply curtailed.

The specific details of consumer-worker control need not be rigidly defined. In fact, effective local governance would depend in part on flexibility in establishing decision-making structures appropriate to the needs of different localities. For example, local health councils could contain variable proportions of consumers' and workers' representatives. In communities with significant ethnic or racial minorities, special arrangements might be made to encourage representation from these minorities. Moreover, special groupings could provide the basis for particularistic health facilities, such as women's clinics or health centers for migrant workers. In these cases, the composition of local health councils could be modified to take into account the unique needs of the clinics' clientele. Several health care projects in the United States currently try to follow principles of consumer-worker control (Rudd 1975; Douglas and Scott 1975, 1978; La Clinica de la Raza 1978).

There are several obvious problems inherent in this projected scheme. Perhaps the most significant is the expansionary tendency of all bureaucracies. Although the initial intention might be a limited bureaucracy whose principal function pertains to the distribution of economic resources, encroachment by bureaucrats into the policy affairs of local health councils would be an omnipresent problem requiring constant scrutiny. Also, the widely recognized tendency toward oligarchy might limit the true effectiveness of local control. In most democratic organizations, a leadership emerges which often grows distant from the constituency it represents. Furthermore, especially in relationships with the professional providers of medical services, local health councils could become objects of cooptation, providing legitimation for decisions which actually would continue to be made by a professional elite. These potential problems, however, do not undermine the basic premise of consumer-worker control as a desirable goal. In countries which have assigned high priority to the health and welfare needs of the population, local control has proven an obtainable reality.

Health Care and Political Struggle

Fundamental social change, however, comes not from legislation but from direct political action. Currently, coalitions of community residents and health workers are trying to gain control over the governing bodies of health institutions that affect them (Mullan 1976; Waitzkin 1970, 1977; Waitzkin and Sharratt 1977). Unionization activity and minority group organizing in health institutions are exerting pressure to modify previous patterns of stratification (Badgley and Wolfe 1971; Wolfe 1975; Bridges 1974; Rudd 1975; Chamberlin and Radebaugh 1976).

Gaining control of the state through a revolutionary party remains a central strategic problem for activists struggling for the advent of socialism (Lenin 1973). Party building now is taking place throughout the United States. Advocates of a "vanguard party" believe that historically all successful revolutions have resulted from the efforts of a small vanguard who hold consistent ideology and attract mass support during periods of political and economic upheaval. Activists adopting the vanguard approach frequently take jobs as lower-echelon health workers; they recruit members during unionization efforts and oppose cutbacks in jobs and health services. Supporters of a "mass party" argue that mass organizing must precede rather than follow the development of a coherent ideology; therefore, political energies should go toward building alliances that embrace a spectrum of anticapitalist views. Mass party organizers work toward community-worker control over local health programs, occupational health and safety, women's health issues, minority recruitment into medicine, and electoral campaigns for improved health services (Source Collective 1974).

Recognizing the impact of medical ideology has motivated attempts to demystify current ideologic patterns and develop alternatives. This work often involves opposition to the social control function of medicine in such areas as drug addiction, genetic screening, contraception and sterilization abuse, psychosurgery, and women's health care. A network of alternative health programs has emerged that tries to develop self-care and nonhierarchical, anticapitalist forms of practice; these ventures then would provide models of progressive health work when future political change permits their wider acceptance (Marieskind and Ehrenreich 1975; Levin 1976; Douglas and Scott 1975, 1978; Resnick 1976; Sweezy and Magdoff 1976).

A common criticism of the Marxist perspective is that it presents many problems with few solutions. Recent advances in this field, however, have clarified some useful directions of political strategy. This struggle will be a protracted one and will involve action on many fronts. The present holds little room for complaisance or misguided optimism. Our future health system, as well as the social order of which it will be a part, depends largely on the praxis we choose now.

REFERENCES

Alford, R. R.
  1975 Health Care Politics. Chicago: University of Chicago Press.
Anderson, Odin
  1972 Can There Be Equity? New York: Wiley.
Badgley, R. F., and S. Wolfe
  1971 Doctors' Strike. Toronto: Macmillan.
Baran, Paul A., and Paul M. Sweezy
  1966 Monopoly Capital. New York: Monthly Review Press.
Benson, Herbert
  1975 The Relaxation Response. New York: Morrow.
Berman, Daniel
  1978 Death on the Job. New York: Monthly Review Press.
Blake, Elinor, and Thomas Bodenheimer
  1975 Closing the Doors on the Poor. San Francisco: Health Policy Advisory Center.
Bloom, B. S., and O. L. Peterson
  1973 End Results, Cost and Productivity of Coronary-Care Units. New England Journal of Medicine 288:72–78.

Boden, Leslie I.
    1976 Vinyl Chloride: Can the Worker Be Protected? — Economics. New England
        Journal of Medicine 294:655—656.
Bodenheimer, Tom, Steve Cummings, and Elizabeth Harding
    1972 Billions for Band-aids. San Francisco: Medical Committee for Human Rights.
Bridges, K. R.
    1974 Third World Students. Harvard Medical Alumni Bulletin 49 (September—October):
        23—25.
Center for Disease Control
    1976 Organic Mercury Exposure — Washington. Morbidity and Mortality Weekly
        Report 25:133.
Chamberlin, R. W., and J. F. Radebaugh
    1976 Delivery of Primary Care — Union Style. New England Journal of Medicine
        294:641—645.
Cochrane, A. L.
    1972 Effectiveness and Efficiency: Random Reflections on Health Care. London:
        Nuffield Hospital Trust.
Dellums, Ronald V., et al.
    1978 Health Service Act, H. R. 11879. Washington: U.S. House of Representatives.
Douglas, C., and J. Scott
    1975 Toward an Alternative Health Care System. Win Magazine 11 (August 7): 14—19.
    1978 Alternative Health Care in a Rural Community. Win Magazine 14 (July 27, August
        3): 20—24.
Dubos, René
    1959 The Mirage of Health. New York: Harper.
Edwards, R. C., M. Reich, and T. E. Weisskopf, eds.
    1978 The Capitalist System. Englewood Cliffs, New Jersey: Prentice-Hall.
Ehrenreich, Barbara, and John Ehrenreich
    1970 The American Health Empire. New York: Vintage.
Engel, George L.
    1976 Psychologic Factors in Instantaneous Cardiac Death. New England Journal of
        Medicine 294:664—665.
Eyer, Joseph
    1975 Hypertension as a Disease of Modern Society. International Journal of Health
        Services 5:539—558.
Freidson, E.
    1976 Doctoring Together: A Study of Professional Social Control. New York: Elsevier.
Friedman, Meyer, and Ray H. Rosenman
    1974 Type A Behavior and Your Heart. New York: Knopf.
Fuchs, Victor
    1974 Who Shall Live? Health, Economics, and Social Choice. New York: Basic Books.
Gorz, A.
    1973 Socialism and Revolution. Garden City, New York: Anchor.
Governing Council, American Public Health Association
    1977 Resolutions and Policy Statements: Committee for a National Health Service.
        American Journal of Public Health 67:84—87.
Gramsci, Antonio
    1971 Selections from the Prison Notebooks. New York: International.
Haggerty, Robert J.
    1972 The Boundaries of Health Care. Pharos 35:106—111.
Halberstam, M. J.
    1971 Liberal Thought, Radical Theory and Medical Practice. New England Journal of
        Medicine 284:1180—1185.

Hill, J. D., J. R. Hampton, and J. R. A. Mitchell
  1978 A Randomised Trial of Home-Versus-Hospital Management for Patients with
       Suspected Myocardial Infarction. Lancet 1:837–841.
Hofvendahl, S.
  1971 Influence of Treatment in a Coronary Care Unit on Prognosis in Acute Myocardial
       Infarction: A Controlled Study in 271 Cases. Acta Medica Scandinavica Supple-
       ment 519:1–78.
Holleb, H. B., and A. Angrist
  1942 Bronchiogenic Carcinoma in Association with Pulmonary Asbestosis. American
       Journal of Pathology 18:123–131.
Illich, Ivan
  1976 Medical Nemesis. New York: Pantheon.
Jenkins, C. David
  1976 Psychologic and Social Risk Factors for Coronary Disease. New England Journal
       of Medicine 294:987–994, 1033–1038.
Kass, Edward H.
  1971 Infectious Diseases and Social Change. Journal of Infectious Disease 123:110–
       114.
Koos, Earl
  1967 The Health of Regionville. New York: Hafner.
Kosa, John, et al., eds.
  1975 Poverty and Health. Cambridge: Harvard University Press.
Kotelchuck, David
  1974 Asbestos Research. Health/PAC Bulletin 61:1–6, 20–27.
Kotelchuck, David, ed.
  1976 Prognosis Negative. New York: Vintage.
La Clinica de la Raza
  1978 Personnel Policy. Oakland: Private printing.
Lenin, V. I.
  1973 The State and Revolution. Peking: Foreign Language Press, pp. 5–25, 99–
       122.
Levin, L. S.
  1976 Self-care: An International Perspective. Social Policy 7:70–75.
Lewis, C. E., D. Mechanic, and R. Fein
  1976 A Right to Health. New York: Wiley.
Lynch, K. M., and W. A. Smith
  1935 Pulmonary Asbestosis. American Journal of Cancer 24:56–64.
McDermott, Walsh
  1978 Medicine: The Public Good and One's Own. Perspectives in Biology and Medicine
       21:167–187.
McKeown, Thomas
  1976 The Role of Medicine: Dream, Mirage, or Nemesis? London: Nuffield Provincial
       Hospitals Trust.
  1977 The Modern Rise of Population. New York: Academic Press.
Marieskind, H. I., and B. Ehrenreich
  1975 Toward Socialist Medicine: The Women's Health Movement. Social Policy 6:
       34–42.
Martin, S. P., et al.
  1974 Inputs into Coronary Care during 30 Years: A Cost Effectiveness Study. Annals
       of Internal Medicine 81:289–293.
Marx, Karl, and Frederick Engels
  1959 The Communist Manifesto. In Marx and Engels, Basic Writings on Politics and
  (1848) Philosophy. Garden City: Anchor.

Mather, H. G., et al.
  1971 Acute Myocardial Infarction: Home and Hospital Treatment. British Medical
       Journal 2:334–337.
  1976 Myocardial Infarction: A Comparison Between Home and Hospital Care for
       Patients. British Medical Journal 1:925–929.
Merton, Robert K.
  1968 Social Theory and Social Structure. New York: Free Press.
Miller, S. M., and Pamela Roby
  1970 The Future of Inequality. New York: Basic Books.
Mills, C. W.
  1959 The Sociological Imagination. New York: Grove.
Mullan, Fitzhugh
  1976 White Coat, Clenched Fist. New York: Macmillan.
Navarro, Vincente
  1972 Health, Health Services and Health Planning in Cuba. International Journal of
       Health Services 2:397–432.
  1974 A Critique of the Present and Proposed Strategies for Redistributing Resources in
       the Health Sector and a Discussion of Alternatives. Medical Care 12:721–742,
       1974.
  1975a Social Policy Issues: An Explanation of the Composition, Nature, and Functions
       of the Present Health Sector of the United States. Bulletin of the New York
       Academy of Medicine 51:199–234.
  1975b The Industrialization of Fetishism or the Fetishism of Industrialization: A Critique
       of Ivan Illich. Social Science & Medicine 9:351–363.
Nee, V., and J. Peck, eds.
  1976 China's Uninterrupted Revolution. New York: Pantheon.
Occupational Health Delegation to Cuba
  1979 Final Report. Mimeograph, Boston.
Peters, John M.
  1976 Vinyl Chloride: Can the Worker Be Protected? – Perspectives. New England
       Journal of Medicine 294:653.
Pierce, P. E., et al.
  1972 Alkyl Mercury Poisoning in Humans: Report of an Outbreak. Journal of the
       American Medical Association 220:1439–1442.
Powles, John
  1973 On the Limitations of Modern Medicine. Science, Medicine and Man 1:1–30.
Resnick, J. L.
  1976 The Emerging Physician: From Political Activist to Professional Vanguard. In
       Professions for the People. Gerstl and Jacobs, eds. Cambridge: Schenkman.
Rudd, P.
  1975 The United Farm Workers Clinic in Delano, Calif.: A Study of the Rural Poor.
       Public Health Reports 90:331–339.
Salmon, J. W.
  1975 Health Maintenance Organization Strategy: A Corporate Takeover of Health
       Services. International Journal of Health Services 5:609–624.
Selikoff, I. J., et al.
  1965 Relation Between Exposure to Asbestos and Mesothelioma. New England Journal
       of Medicine 272:560–565.
  1972 Carcinogenicity of Amosite Asbestos. Archives of Environmental Health 25:
       183–186.
Sidel, V. W., and R. Sidel
  1977 A Healthy State. New York: Pantheon.

Silverman, Milton, and Philip R. Lee
   1974   Pills, Profits, and Politics. Berkeley: University of California Press.
Smith, Eugene W., and Aileen Smith
   1975   Minamata. New York: Holt, Rinehart and Winston.
Source Collective
   1974   Organizing for Health Care. Boston: Beacon.
Stellman, Jeanne M., and Susan M. Daum
   1973   Work Is Dangerous to Your Health. New York: Vintage.
Strauss, Anselm
   1972   Medical Ghettoes. In Where Medicine Fails. Anselm Strauss, ed. New Brunswick,
          N.J.: Trans-Action Books.
Sweezy, P. M., and H. Magdoff
   1976   More on the New Reformism. Monthly Review 28(November):5–13.
U.S. Bureau of the Census
   1977   Statistical Abstracts of the United States, 1977. Washington: Government Printing
          Office.
U.S. Department of Labor
   1977   National Survey of Professional, Administrative, Technical, and Clerical Pay.
          Washington: Government Printing Office (Bulletin 1980).
Waitzkin, Howard
   1970   Expansion of Medical Institutions into Urban Residential Areas. New England
          Journal of Medicine 282:1003–1007.
   1976   Medicine and Society: The New Reductionism. Contemporary Sociology 5:
          401–405.
   1977   What To Do When Your Local Medical Center Tries to Tear Down Your Home.
          Science for the People 9(March–April):22–23, 28–39.
   1978a A Marxist View of Medical Care. Annals of Internal Medicine 89:264–278.
   1978b How Capitalism Cares for our Coronaries: A Preliminary Exercise in Political
          Economy. In The Doctor-Patient Relationship in the Changing Health Scene.
          E. Gallagher, ed. DHEW Publication No. (NIH) 78–183. Washington: Govern-
          ment Printing Office.
   1978c Regressive Policy Implications of the 'Medicalization' and 'Self-help' Concepts.
          In Colloque International de Sociologie Medicale. Paris: Centre National de la
          Recherche Scientifique. Editions CNRS.
Waitzkin, Howard, and John Sharratt
   1977   Controlling Medical Expansion. Society 14(January–February):30–35.
Waitzkin, Howard, and Barbara Waterman
   1974   The Exploitation of Illness in Capitalist Society. Indianapolis: Bobbs-Merrill.
Waterman, Barbara
   1971   Impressions of the Yugoslavian Health System. Unpublished paper, Department
          of Social Relations, Harvard University.
Weinerman, E. R.
   1969   Social Medicine in Eastern Europe. Cambridge: Harvard University Press.
Wilensky, Harold
   1975   The Welfare State and Equality. Berkeley: University of California Press.
Wolfe, Samuel
   1975   Worker Conflicts in the Health Field. International Journal of Health Services
          5:5–8.

16. IMPORTANCE OF THE ECONOMY TO THE NATION'S HEALTH*

OVERVIEW

It has frequently been observed that the average life span is longer in countries at higher levels of economic development and in subpopulations at higher socioeconomic levels within countries. The hypothesis of this paper is that development of the economy continues to be central to the health of human populations. Underlying this hypothesis is the argument that the economy provides the basic material resources required for survival, including nutrition and management of the physical environment. The economy provides, as well, the sources of investment in the development and dissemination of empirical knowledge relating to human health and survival. It follows that the greater availability of the material and organizational sources of survival is a result of long-term economic growth.

The secular tendency for increased average life span concomitant with economic development is based on *heightened adaptive capacity* which results, in turn, from the availability of increasingly greater resources. It is further argued that this increased adaptive capacity related to economic growth has been sufficiently powerful to more than counterbalance the well-known health risks associated with technological development, affluence and urbanization. The latter include environmental contamination, crowding, hypernutrition and obesity, overuse of stimulants, such as tobacco, and of sedatives, such as alcohol, and the decline in muscular exertion and related cardiovascular fitness.

Nonetheless, the fundamental benefits to human health of economic development must be seen as partially offset by the stresses resulting from the disruptions to social life associated with the "cyclic" aspects of economic activity. These cycles, referred to as economic instabilities, are experienced as alternating periods of recession and rapid growth. In social-psychological terms, these are the periods of major stress for society — periods of economic loss and of adjustment to sharp social changes associated with industrial reorganization.

The combination of features of long-term economic development, rapid economic growth and recession provides a basis for understanding the major trends in morbidity and mortality. Given this conceptual framework, it becomes possible to estimate the impact of multiple factors on the health of populations. Toward this end, a quantitative model of the impact of the economy on mortality has been developed and tested successfully with United States data. In the present paper, this general model is further tested using British data over a span of four decades with results approximating the United States-based experience for the same time span. The general economic model of epidemiologic history is

371

L. Eisenberg and A. Kleinman (eds.), The Relevance of Social Science for Medicine, 371–398.

then discussed with respect to the contributions of medical science resulting
from investments in research that depend on economic development.

BACKGROUND

Since at least the middle of the nineteenth century in England and Wales, one
can observe a secular decline in mortality rates associated with long-term improvements in economic conditions. Long-term economic growth has entailed
both a very greatly improved standard of living and considerably reduced economic instability and insecurity, as reflected in the diminished amplitudes of
economic fluctuations. These two features of economic growth have played a
central role in the secular decline in mortality rates.

For the same time period, probably the single most consistent finding in the
epidemiological and demographic literature concerns the inverse relation between
socioeconomic status and mortality rates. In general, the higher the income,
occupational and educational levels of a population, the lower its mortality rate
(Antonovsky 1967; Kitagawa and Hauser 1973; Titmuss 1953; Girard et al.
1960; Febvay 1957; Benjamin 1965; Mechanic 1978). Nor are the socioeconomic
differentials in mortality confined to deaths caused by infectious diseases, which
have been associated with poor nutrition and sanitation and with overall poverty.
In the modern era for industrialized nations, infectious diseases no longer represent a substantial risk to mortality, and mortality due to many of the principal
chronic diseases constitutes the greatest source of the socioeconomic differential
(Kitagawa and Hauser 1973).

The relation between social status and mortality has been most regularly and
thoroughly studied on the basis of British data since at least 1851. The stability
of this relation does not appear to have changed either in Britain, or in such
other industrialized countries as the United States and France (Girard et al.
1960; Febvay 1957; Benjamin 1965; Morris and Heady 1955). In fact, there is
considerable evidence that in both the United States and Britain the socioeconomic differentials in mortality rates have increased since the Second World War
rather than decreased (Kitagawa 1977). This has been especially perplexing in
the latter case since Britain introduced a nationally available and high quality
health service in 1948. The evidence is inconclusive as to whether lower socioeconomic groups in Britain have had equal access to the Health Service. Nonetheless, it is probable that differential utilization of health care is not solely
responsible for the basic inverse relation between socioeconomic status and
mortality rates (Rein 1969; Townsend 1974; Roemer 1976).

At least three large research literatures point to factors other than health care
which could reasonably account for socioeconomic differentials in mortality.
The first of these literatures, one concerned with the epidemiology of both acute
and chronic illnesses, identifies intemperate life habits as pathogenic. Such habits
include the immoderate use of alcohol and tobacco, overeating and lack of
exercise (Morris 1979).

A second literature, which correlates broad demographic phenomena with mortality rates, indicates that the disruption of basic social patterns involving family and community is a risk factor to mortality (Benyoussef et al. 1974; Tyroler and Cassel 1964; Levine and Scotch 1970; Scotch 1960; Scotch 1963; Syme et al. 1965; Smith 1967; Cassel 1967; Marks 1967; Kitagawa 1972; Gove 1974). Such disruptions include migration, urbanization, and disturbances in family life brought about by divorce, separation, and widowhood.

A third literature, which deals with psychosocial stresses as they influence the probability of illness, has until lately concentrated on studies of the impact of specific deleterious events on health problems. These events include those involving loss (associated with depression), unemployment, retirement, work stress under conditions of financial and employment insecurity, and anxiety over extended periods, which has been related to hypertension (Friedman 1961; Cobb et al. 1966; Ferman 1964; Friedman et al. 1958; Pepitone 1967; Russek 1965; Palmore 1969; Sales 1971; Gross 1970; Haynes et al. 1977). Recently, research introduced by Holmes and Rahe, following the pioneering concepts of Meyer and Selye, has indicated that the cumulative influence of various stressful events over a considerable time span constitutes a substantial risk to illness for a large proportion of the otherwise healthy population (Selye 1956; Levi 1972; Cassel 1970; Holmes et al. 1974; Rahe et al. 1964; Thorell and Rahe 1974; Rahe and Romo 1974; Rabkin 1976; Rahe 1969; Wolff 1968; Paykel 1974).

It is the hypothesis of this paper that the comparatively high economic instability and insecurity of lower socioeconomic groups increase the likelihood of (1) immoderate and unstable life habits, (2) disruption of basic social networks, and (3) major life stresses. As a result, it is probable that the greater economic instability and insecurity of lower socioeconomic groups is a major source of their higher mortality rates.

A test of the general hypothesis, as elaborated, would at least require the establishment of a positive relation between economic instability and insecurity, on the one hand, and mortality rates on the other. It is possible to study the potential connection between these phenomena through an examination of the trends and fluctuations in mortality as compared with those in national economic indicators. It follows that indicators of economic instability and insecurity, such as unemployment and unusually rapid economic growth rates, should be associated, over time, with higher mortality rates. In addition, the smooth, long-term exponential trend in economic growth should be inversely correlated with mortality rate trends.

There is now a good deal of research experience in testing precisely this hypothesis, based on United States data. That experience has resulted in the development of a basic explanatory model of the relation between mortality and national economic conditions.

ECONOMIC FLUCTUATIONS AND LIFE STRESS

Two classic sequences of economic loss associated with life stress and, subsequently, with morbidity and mortality can be identified. The first of these concerns "cyclic" unemployment and related economic losses. This sequence involves populations in a long-term condition of continuous economic instability and insecurity which approach crisis levels during economic recessions. Particularly at risk are individuals employed in industries whose fortunes depend on cyclic changes in the level of national economic activity. The "cyclic industries" include, typically, consumer durable goods, e.g., household equipment and automobiles; clothing and related accessories; contract construction and housing; recreation; and other goods and services which are not vital to the purchasing populations and can be deferred until the recessional period has passed.

Semi-skilled and unskilled workers in nearly all industries constitute a second, and very large, population vulnerable to cyclic recessions. They are among the first employees to be released during recessions and among the last to be rehired in expansionary periods. Populations subject to cyclic unemployment show increased mortality largely following recessions, with mortality initially increased two to three years after the first recession which has initiated a process of morbidity.

The second classic sequence is associated with "structural" unemployment, or displacement, and related losses of income. This type of economic loss is produced by changes in the overall structure of the national economy. The primary cause of such structural change is technological innovation which brings about a decline in the work force of a particular industry, either through automation or the replacement of one industry by another — e.g., the replacement of natural fibers and chemical substances by synthetics. Another important source of structural economic loss is relocation of industry within a country, or a shift in investment to outside a country where an industry had traditionally flourished.

In this sequence, the morbidity process will also be initiated during recession, when the probability of displacement becomes relatively high for workers whose presence represents only marginal gain to a firm. For such workers, the main alternative source of employment is probably in another industry — and almost certainly at a job status and income level that are significantly below those previously held. This second classic sequence is thus the main source of downward social mobility as it has been experienced historically and in modern times. The sequence, involving radical change in the individual's social environment, includes the "industrial revolution" and migrations of farm populations to manufacturing centers; it is the basis of the lengthy process of urbanization of the world's population. It is similarly the basis for the post-War decline in manufacturing employment and the concomitant increases in employment in the services and, subsequently, in the communications industries.

In the sequence of downward social mobility, much as in the classic cyclic sequence of continuous economic instability, the illness process (especially for chronic disease) begins with the economic losses of the recession and, within two to three years, the likelihood of mortality is greatly increased — particularly if another source of stress appears. For the downwardly mobile, the next major source of stress usually occurs during their reintegration into the economy, which takes place most probably during the rapid economic growth following the recession in which economic loss was sustained. For these individuals, therefore, the probability of mortality increases during the rapid economic growth period.

The downward mobility sequence can also lead to a situation in which those who are not successfully reintegrated are thrust into the population which is only intermittently employed. Others may leave the labor force entirely, as in the case of the involuntarily retired. In these cases, mortality may be associated with recessions that occur considerably later than the period of initial economic loss.

Finally, on occasion, the rapid economic growth period will involve loss of employment, or lack of re-employment, of individuals whose work skills are no longer consistent with the pace of industrial development. The potential for job lossess suggested by the introduction of the micro-processor, as pointed out by Draper et al. (1979), is an example of this situation. Such persons will often be unable to become economically reintegrated either during the initial rapid growth period or, particularly, during the following recession. This last population group is at especially high risk to morbidity and even mortality prior to its encountering the second period of rapid growth and the renewed possibility of reintegration.

DEVELOPMENT OF THE BASIC MODEL

The basic model originated with the findings that the rate of first admissions to mental hospitals in New York State was inversely related to the rate of employment during 1914–1967 and to an index of business cycles for 1841–1909 (Brenner et al. 1968; Brenner 1973b). A subsequent study, using data for the entire United States, indicated that a variety of national indicators of acute pathological disturbances, including suicide and homicide, showed increases within a year of heightened unemployment rates (Brenner 1971b).

With psychopathologic indicators of morbidity and mortality showing relatively rapid reactions to increased unemployment, the research was focused next on the examination of mortality rate trends for the psychophysiologically involved chronic diseases, especially the cardiovascular group. Special attention was given to spectral and graphic analysis of the relation between coronary heart disease mortality, by age and sex, and the United States unemployment rate. Based on the earlier study of psychopathology, it was expected that, initially, increases in cardiovascular morbidity would follow increased unemployment within a few months (Kasl et al. 1972), but mortality increases would begin to appear only after a considerable lag since there is often an interval of several years between the incidence of morbidity and that of mortality in the chronic diseases.

Increased cardiovascular mortality was observed to occur at a lag of two to three years following increased unemployment for most age groups and both sexes (Brenner 1971a). While one criterion used in this investigation of the lagged relations was plausibility, as an editorial in *The Lancet* (1979) has indicated, the higher correlations were also found at lags of two or three years rather than at zero or a one-year lag. Only recently, I learned that the same relation, with a nearly identical lag structure, was found by Morris and Titmuss in 1944, using British data on rheumatic heart disease mortality (Morris and Titmuss 1944).

The findings on the impact of recession on cardiovascular mortality, which represents 60 to 70 percent of total mortality in industrialized societies, raised the question of whether the secular decline in the total mortality rate might be inversely related to the long-term economic growth trend. It was reasoned that since economic loss, via recession, leads to increased mortality, long-term sustained and stable growth, which minimizes loss, should lead to lower mortality. Evidence for this position came from findings that the infant mortality rate, long regarded as one of the most sensitive indices of national economic development, also showed increases within one or two years following economic recessions in the United States (Brenner 1975). It was further observed that the magnitude of recession — and thus the incidence of severe economic loss — had become progressively smaller and less devastating. If only on that account, it was assumed, the mortality rate should decline — but at a decreasing rate because of the simultaneous aging of the population.

Initial tests of equations incorporating indices of both long-term economic growth and recession began with mortality related to alcohol consumption, including cirrhosis of the liver (Brenner 1975). These tests were followed by a large-scale study, prepared for the Congressional Research Service and the Joint Economic Committee of the United States Congress, on the impact of national economic changes on pathology rates, including mortality for certain major causes (U.S. Congress, Joint Economic Committee 1976). The Congressional study employed a multivariate model which incorporated an indicator of economic growth, the rate of unemployment and the inflation rate. An additional innovation was the use of the polynomial distributed lag method, which permitted a test of the assumption that there probably was no single discrete lag between economic change and mortality rates for the entire population. Instead, it seemed realistic to assume that, within a five-year period, the most vulnerable populations (e.g., the aged, previously ill, and lower socioeconomic groups) would respond relatively early to economic trauma, while the least vulnerable would show a longer lag. Thus, a distributed-lag estimate, beginning at year zero and ending at year five, replaced the single optimum discrete lag estimate.

Another significant addition to the explanatory model was developed as a result of stimulation by the rapid development of a research literature on the impact of stressful life changes on morbidity (Holmes and Rahe 1967; Holmes and Masuda 1974). The special importance of this literature was its emphasis on the absolute magnitude of adaptation (Selye 1956; Levi 1972) required to meet a group of relatively ordinary life changes which accumulate over two or more years (Rahe et al. 1964; Thorell and Rahe 1974; Rahe and Romo 1974; Holmes and Masuda 1974). The stress research literature which immediately preceeded the "life change" approach, focusing on the impact of rapid social and cultural changes on the epidemiology of cardiovascular illness, was of equal relevance. These epidemiological studies identified adaptation to urban industrial life, an instance of critical change in the socioeconomic environment, as a particularly important risk factor in cardiovascular disease (Tyroler and Cassel 1964; Levine and Scotch 1970; Scotch 1960; Scotch and Geiger 1963; Syme et al. 1965; Smith 1967; Cassel 1967; Marks 1967). The implication was that for a population which had endured losses of employment and income during recession, and sought to recoup their losses during the following period of rapid economic growth, adaptation to the new work and living environment would be additionally stressful. This view of the harmful effects of urbanization is also strongly supported by evidence from the demographic history of major European cities (Davis 1973).

Since the late nineteenth century, moreover, the expansion stage of the "economic cycle" has come to represent the relatively rapid phases of long-term economic growth. The rapid growth periods are therefore ones of comparatively acute change in the social organization of those industries which are introducing significant innovations or mechanisms toward higher productivity. This stress of organizational growth and development can be problematic not only for the new entrant but for the older worker whose position or job functions may be downgraded with the introduction of more productive technology. While rapid economic growth therefore represents the necessary building block of long-term development, it also carries the threat of obsolescence for the economic positions of specific individuals.

These literatures are also reminiscent of the sociological proposition advanced by Durkheim (1951) that the incidence of societal pathology, e.g., suicide, increases as a result of the anomic conditions accompanying acute change in the social structure; such change is prevalent both in periods of economic decline and expansion. Henry and Short (1954) elaborated Durkheim's thesis and argued that pathology especially prevalent among lower socioeconomic populations, e.g., homicide, increases especially during periods when the majority of the population is gaining economically, thus widening the psychological differential between the lowest and higher socioeconomic strata.

It was possible to infer from these literatures that two different populations were at particularly high risk of morbidity and mortality during periods of rapid economic growth, namely (1) those who had experienced downward mobility through employment and income loss and then sought to be reintegrated into the economy, and (2) persons of low socioeconomic status, highly vulnerable to economic loss during recessions, but vulnerable as well to the relative deprivation of economic expansions in which they are unable to participate fully.

As a result of these theoretical developments, the general model was further expanded to include rapid economic growth as a predictor of mortality. This model was successfully tested with United States data on suicide, homicide, cardiovascular mortality, and age-specific total mortality (Brenner 1978, 1980a, b). With the successful test of the expanded model, it became possible to explain the anomaly discovered by Thomas (1925) that the early phase of business cycle upturns tended to be positively correlated with mortality rates during the late nineteenth and early twentieth centuries in Britain.

Using a graphic analysis, Eyer recently interpreted the Thomas discovery to mean that a comparatively high annual level of *unemployment*, which is moderately inversely correlated with business cycle indices at zero lag, is causative of a *lower* mortality rate at zero lag (Eyer 1977). When, however, this interpretation was tested on United States data by statistical methods, the unemployment rate did not consistently show a negative simple correlation with the mortality rate; usually the relation was positive even at zero lag, and, at lags of two through ten years the relation was consistently positive and significant. In addition, with controls for the effects of long-term economic growth, the lagged relations between unemployment and mortality (for all causes or chronic diseases) became stronger, while the unlagged relations became weaker.

While it was clear that unemployment is occasionally positively related to mortality, the question remained whether another business cycle indicator (Moore 1961) might serve as the explanation for Thomas' early discovery. When, subsequently, business cycle measures which reflected rapid economic growth at zero lag were introduced into the model, these were found significantly positively correlated with mortality rates in the same predictive equation in which unemployment at lags of two to five years was also significantly positively related to mortality rates. These findings supported Thomas' original conclusion, but additionally indicated that *both* unemployment and rapid economic growth are positively associated with mortality even under controls for long-term economic growth, which is inversely related to mortality rates (Brenner 1978, 1980b).

Most recently, attention has been given to the much longer lag of increased chronic disease mortality rates behind recessions as compared with acute pathological reactions such as suicide. It was reasoned that with increasingly larger proportions of total mortality being attributed to chronic disease, the entire distributed lag pattern of heightened mortality behind higher unemployment should become increasingly longer. Tests based on United States data showed that the distributed lag both *began* at a later time (between three and four years) and *extended* over a longer period (ten to fifteen years) as the interval of analysis covered increasingly later time spans, e.g., 1950–1976, as compared with 1940–1976 or 1909–1976.

The findings of elevated mortality rates for chronic diseases beginning with a lag of one year, and running as long as fifteen years subsequent to the initial periods of recession, led to the following conclusions:

(1)   Recession has the effect of causing severe economic loss and downward social mobility, which places many of those affected in a long-term state of vulnerability to subsequent recessions and periods of rapid economic growth.

(2)   Severe economic loss and downward mobility can initiate long-term processes of chronic illness, which may endure for several years, prior to mortality.

(3)   Therefore, in summary, severe economic loss and downward mobility initiate patterns of interaction over several years between chronic disease processes and vulnerability to economic stress.

These findings for chronic diseases are also consistent with the view that the presence of specific illness is only one of several risk factors in mortality (Selye 1960). Thus, the appropriate questions in this research become: (1) Which factors associated with specific illnesses contribute to a higher case fatality rate or to a shorter survival time. (2) Which factors contribute to acceleration of the aging process, rather than only to the course or the severity of a particular chronic disease, and result in death?

ELEMENTS OF THE EXPLANATORY MODEL

The explanatory model which, in this research, enables the development of an equation predicting mortality patterns — probabilistically rather than deterministically — consists of four main components: (1) the smooth exponential trend of long-term economic growth, measured by real per capita income; (2) the rate of unemployment; (3) "rapid economic growth" measured in two ways, (a) deviations from the long-term exponential trend in real per capita income, and (b) annual changes in the rate of growth of real per capita income; and (4) government expenditures for welfare as a per cent of total government expenditures.

The long-term trend in economic growth, with major influences on nutrition, sanitation, and education, tends to dominate the secular history of decline in the mortality rate. The long-term growth in societal wealth probably influenced health levels through stabilization of the availability of nutrition until the time of virtual disappearance of the infectious diseases as important causes of death (approximately 1930–1950) (McKeown 1976; Wrigley 1969). Since that time, the major influence of long-term economic growth on the mortality rate has been in the reduction of the amplitudes of the cycles and fluctuations in national economic behavior that have been intrinsic to the process of economic growth itself. These economic cycles and fluctuations — or "economic instabilities" — remain the sources of substantial life stress, despite greatly improved management at the levels of the national economy and the individual economic enterprise.

Additional important features of technological development accompanying long-term economic growth include sanitary engineering, more effective maternal and child health care, and advances in occupational safety and health. The significance of modern medicine for the extension of the life span in an era of chronic disease and aging populations is currently in controversy. However, it is generally accepted that health care has at least been able to reduce considerably the disability and pain of the chronic disorders, thus improving social functioning. To the extent, then, that disability and pain are substantial contributors to life stress, and cumulative stress is an important component in mortality rates, health care has over the long run contributed significantly to the reduction of chronic disease related mortality.

The unemployment rate is an indirect measure of loss of income, social status, and close personal attachments for individuals and entire families. When used as a national indicator of recession, the unemployment rate becomes an indirect measure of income loss among people who do not necessarily lose employment and a sensitive estimator of work stress based on anxiety over economic insecurity in firms experiencing economic difficulty.

The unemployment variable, indicating economic loss, is theoretically the major source of a long series of subsequent disturbances including pathogenic life habits, breakdown of family and community social structure, and psychophysiologic illnesses and psychological depression. Therefore, we examine the association between the unemployment and mortality rates over a lengthy lag period of zero to ten years.

Rapid economic growth, as compared with long-term growth, is relatively free of major deleterious changes for the majority of the population. For specific minorities, however, it can be a period of anxiety associated with the introduction into industry of technological changes and structural reorganization which seriously threaten employment and income security. For the unemployed and others who earn very low incomes, the rapid growth periods can bring acute feelings of relative deprivation, since the majority of the population is gaining significantly in income.

The indirect deleterious effects of rapid economic growth are most traumatic for minority populations who previously experienced substantial losses in employment and income, and who now have the opportunity to become re-integrated economically. These populations most often suffer a further loss in socioeconomic status in order to secure available employment for which previously acquired skills, experience and seniority are not relevant.

Rapid economic growth is also a period of rapid introduction of new technologies which produces a higher risk of accidents and the threat of job loss or demotion in the process of industrial reorganization.

The government allocation for public welfare is not a necessary explanatory variable in this model, but rather a control variable. The extent to which such allocations are necessary for health maintenance will, of course, depend on the proportion of the population that is impoverished; that proportion, in turn, depends on the level of performance of the national economy for which measures are already found in the explanatory model. However, it can be assumed that in the majority of industrialized nations there is some impoverishment under the most favorable national economic conditions. Therefore, it would at least be important to investigate whether government transfer payments meant to alleviate such distress are found to improve health as well.

FINDINGS

In the present research an attempt was made to test the model by analyzing the relations between trends in economic indices and mortality rates in England and Wales over the years 1936–1976. Table 1 indicates the impact of each of the

TABLE 1

Multiple regression equations on national economic indices of age-specific mortality rates England and Wales, 1936–76 ("t" statistics in parenthesis)[1]

Age	Intercept	Economic growth trend	Growth trend residuals	Annual change in growth rate	Welfare expenditures	Unemployment over 0–10 year period[3]	R^2	Durbin-Watson statistic	F^1 statistic
Total	12.57 (12.05)**	−0.099 (5.20)**	−0.033 (1.33)	0.022 (0.44)	−0.33 (0.30)	20.68 (8.22)**	0.97	2.30	166.66**
Infants	59.76 (10.51)**	−0.05 (5.30)**	−0.004 (0.33)	0.033 (1.55)	−17.79 (2.93)*	156.57 (11.40)**	0.99	1.73	387.98**
1–4	4.31 (2.65)*	−0.002 (3.78)**	−0.033 (1.06)	0.0005 (0.031)	−6.57 (3.78)**	19.59 (4.98)**	0.95	1.69	97.50**
5–9[2]	1.22 (1.68)	−0.001 (1.07)	0.003 (2.30)†	0.007 (0.42)	−0.54 (0.97)	9.97 (6.01)**	0.94	1.92	67.89**
10–14	0.73 (4.03)**	−0.0007 (2.19)†	0.0001 (0.26)	0.002 (2.40)†	−0.14 (0.74)	5.26** (12.12)**	0.98	2.00	232.37**
15–19	0.64 (1.98)†	−0.0003 (0.61)	0.0004 (0.63)	0.004 (3.02)*	−0.075 (0.22)	11.04 (14.20)**	0.98	2.05	197.97**
20–24	1.24 (2.57)*	−0.0009 (1.14)	−0.0005 (0.55)	0.004 (2.49)*	−0.18 (0.35)	13.00 (11.17)**	0.98	1.55	223.17**
25–34	1.86 (4.13)**	−0.001 (1.94)†	−0.001 (1.11)	0.005 (2.72)*	−0.26 (0.55)	10.79 (9.94)**	0.98	1.41	230.35**
35–44	3.91 (7.59)**	−0.003 (3.40)**	0.0001 (0.11)	0.003 (1.76)†	−0.16 (0.29)	12.84 (10.33)**	0.98	1.93	185.32**

(Continued)

Table 1 (Continued)

Age	Intercept	Economic growth trend	Growth trend residuals	Annual change in growth rate	Welfare expenditures	Unemployment over 0–10 year period[3]	R^2	Durbin-Watson statistic	F[1] statistic
45–54	7.59 (8.08)**	−0.003 (1.61)	−0.002 (0.97)	−0.002 (0.48)	−0.70 (0.69)	19.53 (8.61)**	0.95	2.09	95.84**
55–64	21.72 (10.18)**	−0.01 (2.76)	−0.002 (0.42)	−0.002 (0.20)	0.74 (0.32)	27.06 (5.26)**	0.89	2.08	38.16**
65–74	57.63 (11.25)**	−0.030 (0.47)**	−0.006 (0.56)	−0.011 (0.58)	3.82 (0.70)	47.23 (3.82)**	0.85	2.22	26.31**
75–84	145.48 (9.21)**	−0.079 (3.02)*	−0.055 (1.73)†	−0.025 (0.43)	14.09 (0.84)	100.28 (2.63)*	0.82	2.12	21.09**
85+	312.05 (6.94)**	−0.16 (2.19)†	−0.056 (0.62)	−0.12 (0.70)	41.65 (0.87)	300.86 (2.77)*	0.64	2.24	8.48*

1. "t" and F-statistics: † $p < 0.05$, * $p < 0.01$, ** $p < 0.001$.
2. Cochrane-Orcutt transformation used in order to minimize residual autoregression.
3. Second Degree polynomial fit. See Insert 4

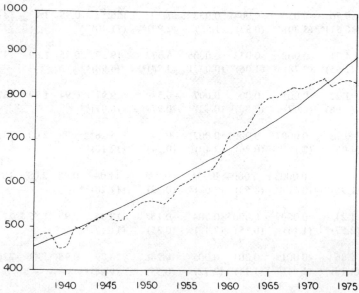

Fig. 1a. Real per caput income and its smoothed exponential trend (in 1970 pounds per person).

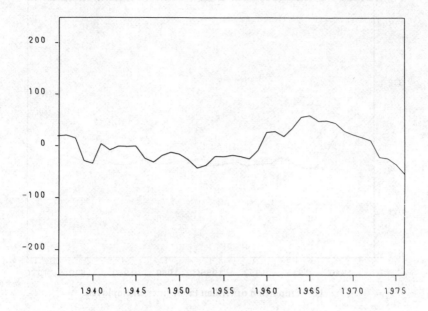

Fig. 1b. Medium-term changes in growth rate, representing departures from smoothed,
exponential trend of real per caput income.

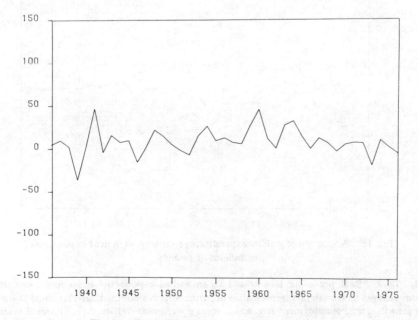

Fig. 1c. Annual changes in real per caput income.

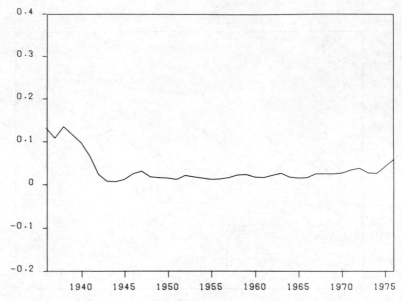

Fig. 1d. Proportion of civilian labor force unemployed.

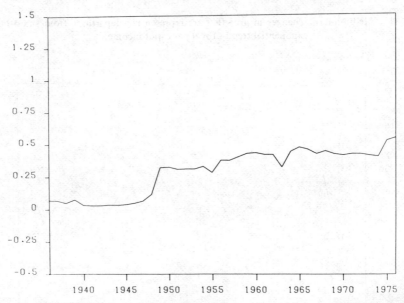

Fig. 1e. Proportion of welfare expenditures to total government expenditures, in millions of pounds

Fig. 1a–e. Real per caput income and its smoothed exponential trend form; medium-term changes in growth rate (representing departures from smoothed curve); annual changes in growth rate; unemployment rate; and percent government welfare expenditures: England and Wales, 1936–76.

independent variables on the mortality rate. The overall hypothesis that long-term economic growth shows an inverse relation, and the unemployment rate — indicating recession — shows a positive relation, to mortality rate trends is sustained for all age groups. The rapid economic growth variables show a relatively weak relation to the mortality rates; the residual from the long-term economic growth rate shows no statistical significance, while the annual growth rate shows significance for the population, aged 10–44. Finally, the relation of government expenditure for welfare is inverse to mortality rates for the infant and 1–4 age groups. The combined effect of all four independent variables yields strong prediction for the total age-adjusted mortality rate (Figure 2) as it

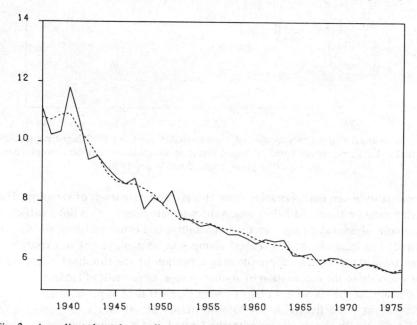

Fig. 2. Age-adjusted total mortality rates per 1000 home population: actual and expected values based on fit of composite economic change model — including long-term and rapid economic growth variables, unemployment rates over 0–10 years, and percent of government welfare expenditures. England and Wales, 1936–76.

does for age-specific mortality rates at nearly all ages (Table 1). The importance of using the entire explanatory model, rather than a single component such as the unemployment rate, is illustrated in Figure 3. Here we concentrate only on annual fluctuations in the total (age-adjusted) mortality rate, in effect, withholding from consideration the long-term trend and all other smooth movements in mortality. In this case, short-term change (i.e., annual change summed over 0–5 years' lag) in the unemployment rate alone is only a moderately good predictor (Table 2).

Figure 3 suggests that short-term changes in unemployment as a measure of economic loss are the most important source of influence on annual fluctuations

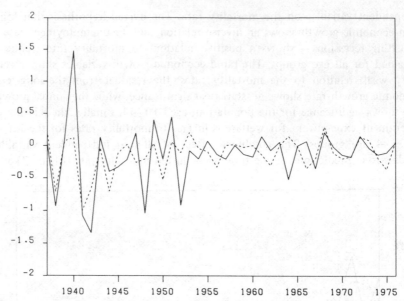

Fig. 3. Annual changes in age-adjusted total mortality rates per 1000 home population: Actual and expected values based on lagged effect of annual changes in the unemployment rate over 0–5 years. England and Wales, 1936–76.

in mortality when both variables show at least moderate levels of variation. This may indicate a threshold below which the unemployment rate is not a sufficient predictor of annual changes in total mortality, and other variables are also required. For example, adding annual changes in unemployment in exponential (i.e., squared) form, thus approximating a portion of the threshold effect, adds considerably to the explanation of annual changes in mortality (Table 2).

Finally, of the six years of lag of unemployment used as predictors, the years of strongest predictive value for total mortality are at lags 1, 2 (particularly) and 5 (Table 2); this coincides with the United States experience for total and especially chronic disease mortality (Russek 1965; Haynes et al. 1977).

The lag structure varies according to the time span and specific causes of death under analysis. Suicide and homicide, for example, show increases within a year following increased unemployment, while cardiovascular mortality begins to increase two to three years following increased unemployment but shows a distributed lag structure which continues for ten to fifteen years. For the period starting in 1950, the lag structure for total and chronic disease mortality following heightened unemployment begins and ends later than when the analysis is started in 1936 or 1940. These findings will be presented in detail in future publications.

Table 3 shows a cross-sectional analysis by county for 1971 indicating the association of unemployment, and relatively high income, to mortality rates, controlling for employment in manual occupations and employment in the

TABLE 2

Coefficients[1] for multiple regression equations of annual changes in
age-adjusted total mortality on annual changes in unemployment
rates, England and Wales, 1936–76

Lagged Effects of unemployment in years	Constant	Sum of regression coefficients – annual changes	Sum of regression coefficients – annual changes squared	Regression coefficients	Rho	R^2	Durbin-Watson statistic	F-statistic
Sum of years 0–5[2]:								
Annual Changes	−0.82E−1	15.68†			−0.34†	0.35	2.25	4.69*
Annual Changes and Annual Changes Squared	−0.17†	70.77†	1572.13†		−0.41*	0.53	2.14	4.30*
Discrete years of lag:								
Annual Changes								
0	−0.13†			4.80	−0.28†	0.09	2.26	3.55
1	−0.11†			8.76†	−0.35†	0.13	2.34	5.86†
2	−0.90E−1			12.69*	−0.24	0.21	2.24	9.99*
3	−0.14†			−1.39	0.24	0.07	2.18	2.69
4	−0.14†			−0.33	−0.25	0.06	2.20	2.62
5	−0.11†			6.80	−0.23	0.11	2.16	4.92†

For t (columns 2–6) and F † $p < 0.05$, * $p < 0.01$, ** $p < 0.001$.
1. Cochrane-Orcutt transformation was used to minimize residual autoregression.
2. Distributed lag: third degree polynomial fit.

chemical industries — a major source of environmental pollution. This analysis
tends to confirm the time series analytic results. Indeed, it can be seen that three
major factors tend to account for over 90 percent of the variance: the unemployment rate (positive relation), high income populations (inverse relation), and
the proportion of the population over age 54 (positive relation). Table 3 also
indicates that, when the cross-section relations are specified further by major
cause of death (adjusted for age, sex and the institutional population) — i.e.,
total cardiovascular disease, ischemic heart disease, cerebrovascular and malig-
nancies — the model is most appropriate for the total cardiovascular and ischemic
heart categories, largely effective in malignancy, and least appropriate for cerebrovascular disease. These cross-sectional findings based on counties are in
general similar to those of Gardner et al. (1969) for county boroughs, but are in
this case tests of a specified model involving unemployment rates and relatively
high incomes.

TABLE 3

Multiple regression equations on county-specific socioeconomic indices of county-specific
mortality rates: England and Wales – 1971
(t-statistic in parentheses)

Mortality rates	Unemployment rate (1)	High income (2)	Manual workers (3)	Self-employed (4)	Farm employment (5)	Chemical industry employment (6)	Population over 54 (7)	R^2 (8)	$\hat{R}^2$ (9)	F-statistic; equation
Crude Total	0.20 (14.64)**	−0.21 (10.42)**	0.04 (0.15)	−0.05 (0.28)	0.02 (0.04)	0.10 (6.87)*	0.79 (168.9)***	0.96	0.95	(103.9)***
Crude Total	0.35 (9.63)**	−0.34 (5.90)*	0.21 (0.98)	0.51 (9.65)**	0.19 (1.34)	0.19 (10.63)**		0.73	0.69	(17.9)***
Infant	0.43 (5.44)	−0.12 (0.005)	0.23 (0.47)	0.09 (0.11)	−0.12 (0.19)	0.01 (0.01)		0.30	0.20	(2.8)
Total minus Infant	0.18 (8.82)**	−0.21 (7.99)**	0.07 (0.31)	−0.03 (0.06)	0.03 (0.12)	0.11 (5.72)**	0.79 (126.3)***	0.94	0.93	(72.6)***
Standardized Total	0.52 (24.30)***	−0.23 (3.08)	0.27 (1.92)	−0.27 (3.08)	0.20 (1.85)	0.28 (10.63)**		0.78	0.74	(22.6)***
Cardiovascular Standardized	0.25 (3.51)	−0.41 (6.19)*	0.34 (1.88)	−0.21 (1.13)	0.27 (1.93)	0.17 (2.49)		0.63	0.57	(10.73)**
Ischaemic Heart Standardized	0.30 (3.93)*	−0.47 (6.41)*	0.11 (0.16)	−0.30 (1.80)	−0.09 (0.16)	0.17 (1.89)		0.53	0.45	(7.07)*
Cerebrovascular Standardized	0.19 (1.74)	−0.16 (0.78)	0.42 (2.42)	−0.13 (0.36)	0.67 (10.39)**	0.17 (1.95)		0.57	0.50	(8.31)**
Malignancies Standardized	0.45 (7.91)**	−0.23 (1.34)	−0.30 (1.01)	−0.26 (1.21)	−0.60 (6.73)*	0.26 (3.98)*		0.47	0.39	(5.63)*

Notes:
1) Unemployment rate = % unemployed of civilian labor force.
2) High income = % of employed with income greater than L 1750.
3) Manual = % of employed with occupation as skilled, semi-skilled, and unskilled labor.
4) Self-employed = % of employed with occupation as self-employed professionals, and own accounts workers.
5) Farm = % of employed with occupation as farm owners, managers, and laborers.
6) Chemical industry = % of employed in chemical industry.
7) Population over age 54.
8) R^2 = estimate of variance explained.
9) $\hat{R}^2$ = adjusted estimate of variance explained.
F-Statistics: * $p < 0.05$, ** $p < 0.01$, *** $p < 0.001$

Sources of Data:

Variable:	Source:
Unemployment for counties and county boroughs	*1971 Census of England and Wales: Economic Activity, County Leaflets*, HMSO. (old county designation)
Occupational groups (SEG categories) employment	"
Chemical Industry employment	"
Income for counties	*Survey of Personal Incomes: 1970–1971*, Board of Inland Revenue, HMSO.
Population for counties and county boroughs	*1971 Census of England and Wales: County Reports*, HMSO. (old county designation; 1966 population data replaced 1971 data for counties where data unavailable.
Mortality for counties	*Registrar General's Statistical Review of England and Wales, 1971*, HMSO.
Mortality for county boroughs	Office of Population Censuses and Surveys, Mortality Division, Direct communication.

DISCUSSION

A theoretical model of the implications of national economic changes for mortality rates has been developed over a period of fifteen years, based on epidemiological, demographic and stress research literatures. The model, which incorporates the long-term trend in economic growth, the unemployment rate, and periods of rapid economic growth, was tested and further refined on the basis of United States data. This model has been applied to the British experience during 1936–76 with results very similar to those based on the United States data for the same time span.

In addition, a cross-sectional analysis of England and Wales county-specific mortality rates for 1971 shows a pattern that is consistent with the over-time predictive equation. These cross-sectional findings, moreover, obtain under controls for, among other factors, age, sex, the institutional population, and the presence of the chemical industry. The importance of this replication of the United States' findings for Britain is that the two populations are distinguished by differences in ethnic groupings, geography and climate, industrial composition, governmental structure, and health and welfare policies. The findings imply that the model is sufficiently general to deal with the experiences of industrialized nations.

The data of this study support the position that three major factors largely explain the trends and fluctuations in British mortality rates during 1936–1976. These are: (1) the long-term trend in economic growth, (2) recessional losses and (3) rapid economic growth. The secular decline in the mortality rate is accounted

for by the first factor, while the majority of fluctuation in the mortality rate
is explained by the latter two factors or, in sum, the incidence of economic
instability. It has been argued that these instabilities in economic growth patterns
partially account for the continuing socioeconomic differential in mortality. The
lower socioeconomic groups are particularly vulnerable to problems of loss and
readjustment resulting from national economic instabilities because of their
comparatively low levels of job skill, lack of seniority and control in industry.

The long-term benefits of economic growth act to moderate the problems
associated with economic instability. The moderating mechanisms include
greater sophistication in the management of the national economy, a higher
quality and greater availability of health care, and more substantial income
supports for displaced workers and other non-participants in the labor force.
In any case, the long-term trend in economic growth or "prosperity" clearly
acts to reduce mortality, and certainly not to increase it as has at times been
suggested. Rapid economic growth, on the other hand, does contribute to
increased mortality within a year, as has been shown in this study.

It is necessary to bear in mind that all three types of major economic change,
additively and interactively, affect mortality trends. It is therefore not correct to
estimate the impact of any one of these factors on mortality in the absence of
statistical controls for the other two in an integrated model. To the extent, then,
that either the unemployment rate or rapid economic growth acts to "increase"
mortality, it actually inhibits or delays the decline in mortality rates which is
associated with long-term economic growth. Thus, for example, the comparatively high unemployment rate in Britain in recent years does not tend to be
expressed in an observable *increase* in the mortality rate trend. Rather, it adds
greatly to the *slowing* of decline in the mortality rate that would ordinarily have
occurred in the course of long-term economic growth.

The mechanism by which unemployment and *rapid* economic growth act to
slow the secular trend of mortality rate decline is through a widening of the
socioeconomic differentials in mortality within the country. To the extent that
one is able to generalize from the United States' and British experience, the
differential mortality rate across countries depends on the interaction of real
per capita income, especially among the lower socioeconomic strata, and stable
rates of economic growth. Countries with the highest real per capita income in
their poorest populations in conjunction with the most stable economic growth
rates should, and typically do, show the lowest mortality rates at all ages.

SOME CONCLUSIONS AND IMPLICATIONS

The state of a population's health can be understood as an adaptation to the
overall environment, including the social and man-made physical environments.
The capacity of a population to adapt successfully to its overall environment is
reflected in the degree to which it is able to produce and utilize material and
organizational resources. This capacity is indicated by the level of economic

development. The health and survival-enhancing potentials of economic development are partially offset by the extent of irregularity, or "cyclic" instability, inherent in the process of economic growth. These instabilities of economic growth, which reflect continuous reorganization of the economic system, represent a primary source of stress in modern society.

In this view, the incidence of illness can be understood to reflect, largely, the failure of social institutions in general – and economic institutions in particular – to interact successfully with the overall environment. Under such conditions of adaptive failure, resources of societal repair are called upon. Among the more sophisticated technologies of societal repair are those associated with scientific medicine. Traditionally, the health professions have played a comparatively minor role in the health status of populations, since they have been called upon only after exposure to physical and social environmental disturbances have already determined the ecological pattern and severity of illness.

However, the increasingly visible research efforts of the epidemiologist in chronic as well as acute disease and disability have made clear the importance of the man-made physical and social environments to the incidence of specific illnesses. Epidemiological research efforts are on the threshold of identifying routinely available information bearing on the prevention or limitation of disease in general populations. As the research findings of this paper indicate, for epidemiological research findings to be utilized to best advantage, they will have to be allowed to influence policies relating to national and regional economic activity as well as to management in a wide variety of industries.

NOTE

* The findings using British data discussed in this chapter were originally summarized in Brenner (1979).

REFERENCES

Antonovsky, Aaron
  1967 Social Class, Life Expectancy, and Overall Mortality. Milbank Memorial Fund Quarterly 47:31–73.
Benjamin, Bernard
  1965 Social and Economic Factors Affecting Mortality. Paris: Mouton and Co.
Benyoussef, A., et al.
  1974 Health Effects of Rural-Urban Migration in Developing Counties – Senegal. Social Science and Medicine 8:243–254.
Brennan, Mary E., and R. Lancashire
  1978 Association of Childhood Mortality with Housing Status and Unemployment. Journal of Epidemiology and Community Health 32:28–33.
Brenner, M. H.
  1971a Economic Changes and Heart Disease Mortality. American Journal of Public Health 61:606–611.
  1971b Time Series Analysis of the Relationships between Selected Economic and Social Indicators. Springfield, Virginia: U.S. National Technical Information Service (March).

1973a Fetal, Infant and Maternal Mortality During Periods of Economic Instability. Int. J. Health Serv. 3(2):145–159.

1973b Mental Illness and the Economy. Cambridge, Mass.: Harvard University Press.

1975 Trends in Alcohol Consumption and Associated Illnesses: Some Effects of Economic Changes. American Journal of Public Health 65:1279–1292.

1979 Mortality and the National Economy: Experience of England and Wales, 1936–1976. The Lancet (September 15):568–573.

1980a Impact of Social and Industrial Changes on Psychopathology: A View of Stress from the Standpoint of Macro Societal Trends. In Society, Stress and Disease: Working Life, Lennart Levi, ed. London: Oxford University Press.

1980b Industrialization and Economic Growth: Estimates of Their Effects on the Health of Populations. In Assessing the Contributions of the Social Sciences to Health. M. Harvey Brenner, Anne Mooney, and Thomas J. Nagy, eds. Boulder, Colorado: Westview Press.

Brenner, M. H., W. Mandell, S. Blackman, and R. M. Silberstein
1968 Economic Conditions and Mental Hospitalization for Functional Psychosis. Journal of Nervous and Mental Disease 145:371–384.

Cassel, J.
1967 Factors Involving Sociocultural Incongruity and Change: Appraisal and Implications for Theoretical Development. Milbank Memorial Fund Quarterly 45:41.

1970 Physical Illness in Response to Stress. In Social Stress. S. Levine and N. A. Scotch, eds. pp. 189–209. Chicago: Aldine.

Cobb, J., S. V. Kasl, G. W. Brooks, and W. E. Connelly
1966 The Health of People Changing Jobs: A Description of a Longitudinal Study. American Journal of Public Health 56:1476–1481.

Davis, K.
1973 Cities and Mortality. International Union for the Scientific Study of Population, Liège, 1973:259–281.

Draper, P., J. Dennis, J. Griffiths. T. Partridge, and J. Popay
1979 Micro-Processors, Macro-Economic Policy, and Public Health. The Lancet (February 17):373–375.

Durkheim, E.
1951 Suicide: A Study in Sociology. Glencoe, Ill.: Free Press. (First published in Paris by F. Alcan, 1897.)

Eyer, J.
1977 Prosperity as a Cause of Death. International Journal of Health Services 7:125–150.

Febvay, M. and L. Aubenque
1957 La Mortalite Par Categorie Socio-Professionelle. Etudes Statistiques. Quarterly Supplement of the Bulletin Mensuel de Statistique (July–September) 1957: 39–44.

Ferman, L.
1964 Sociological Perspectives in Unemployment Research. In Blue Collar World. A. Shostak and W. Gomberg, eds. Englewood Cliffs, New Jersey: Prentice-Hall.

Friedman, M., R. H. Rosenman, and V. Carroll
1958 Changes in the Serum Cholesterol and Blood Clotting Time of Men Subject to Cyclic Variation of Occupational Stress. Circulation 18:852–861.

Friedman, G.
1961 The Anatomy of Work. New York: Free Press, pp. 126–128.

Gardner, M. J., M. D. Crawford, and J. N. Morris
1969 Patterns of Mortality in Middle and Early Old Age in the County Boroughs of England and Wales. British Journal of Preventive and Social Medicine 23:133–140.

Girard, A., L. Henry, and R. Nistri
    1960 Facterus Sociaux Et Culturels De La Mortalite Infantile. Paris: Presses Universitaires De France.
Gove, Walter R.
    1974 Sex, Marital Status, and Mortality. American Journal of Sociology 79(1):45–67.
Gross, Edward
    1970 Work Organization and Stress. In Social Stress. S. Levine and N. A. Scotch, eds. pp. 54–110. Chicago: Aldine Publishing Company.
Haynes, Suzanne G., Anthony J. McMichael, and H. A. Tyroler
    1977 The Relationship of Normal, Involuntary Retirement to Early Mortality Among U.S. Rubber Workers. Social Science and Medicine 11:105–114.
Henry, A. F. and T. F. Short
    1954 Suicide and Homicide. Glencoe, Ill.: Free Press.
Holmes, T. H. and M. N. Masuda
    1974 Life Change and Illness Susceptibility. In Stressful Life Events: Their Nature and Effects. B. S. Dohrenwend and B. P. Dohrenwend, eds. pp. 45–79. New York: John Wiley.
Holmes, T. H. and R. H. Rahe
    1967 The Social Readjustment Rating Scale. J. of Psychosomatic Research 11:213–218.
Kasl, S. V., S. Cobb, and S. Gore
    1972 Changes in Reported Illness and Illness Behavior Related to Termination of Employment: A Preliminary Report. International Journal of Epidemiology 1:111–118.
Kitagawa, Evelyn M.
    1972 Socioeconomic Differences in Mortality in the United States and Some Implications for Population Policy. In U.S. Commission on Population Growth and the American Future, Demographic and Social Aspects of Population Growth, Vol. I, Commission Research Reports, pp. 85–110. Washington: US GPO.
    1977 On Mortality. Demography 14(4):381–389.
Kitagawa, Evelyn M. and Philip M. Hauser
    1973 Differential Mortality in the United States: A Study in Socio-economic Epidemiology. Cambridge, Mass.: Harvard University Press.
The Lancet
    1979 Does Unemployment Kill? Editorial. The Lancet (March 31):708–709.
Levi, L.
    1972 Stress and Distress in Response to Psychosocial Stimuli. Acta Med Scand. 191 Supplement 528. (Simultaneously published in book form by Pergamon Press, Oxford, 1972).
Levine, S. and N. A. Scotch, eds.
    1970 Social Stress. Chicago: Aldine.
Marks, R. V.
    1967 Factors Involving Social and Demographic Characteristics: A Review of Empirical Findings. Milbank Memorial Fund Quarterly 45:51–108.
McKeown, T.
    1976 The Modern Rise of Population. New York: Academic Press.
Mechanic, David
    1978 Medical Sociology, 2nd ed. London: Collier Macmillan Publishers.
Moore, G. H.
    1961 Business Cycle Indicators. Princeton, N.J.: Princeton University Press.
Morris, J. N.
    1979 Social Inequalities Undiminished. The Lancet 1:87–90.

Morris, J. N. and J. A. Heady
  1955 Social and Biological Factors in Infant Mortality. The Lancet 1:343–349.
Morris, J. N. and R. M. Titmuss
  1944 Health and Social Change: I. The Recent History of Rheumatic Heart Disease.
         The Medical Officer (August 26) 1944:69–87.
Palmore, Erdman
  1969 Predicting Longevity: A Follow-up Controlling for Age. Gerontology (Winter).
Paykel, E. S.
  1974 Recent Life Events and Clinical Depression. In Life Stress and Illness. E. K. Gun-
         derson and R. H. Rahe, eds. pp. 134–163. Springfield, Ill.: Charles C. Thomas.
Pepitone, A.
  1967 Self, Social Environment, and Stress. In Psychological Stress M. H. Appley and
         D. Trumbull, eds. New York: Appleton-Century-Crofts.
Rabkin, Judith G. and Elmer L. Struening
  1976 Life Events, Stress, and Illness. Science 194:1013–1020.
Rahe, Richard H.
  1969 Life Crisis and Health Change. In Psychotropic Drug Response: Advances in
         Prediction. P. R. A. May and J. R. Wittenborn, eds. pp. 92–125. Springfield, Ill.:
         Charles C. Thomas.
Rahe, R. H., et al.
  1964 Social Stress and Illness Onset. J. Psychosomatic Res. 8:35–44.
Rahe, R. H., and M. Romo
  1974 Recent Life Changes and the Onset of Myocardial Infarction and Coronary Death
         in Helsinki. In Life Stress and Illness. E. K. Gunderson and R. H. Rahe, eds. pp.
         105–120. Springfield, Ill.: Charles C. Thomas.
Rein, Martin
  1969 Social Class and the Health Service. New Society 14:807–810.
Roemer, Milton I.
  1976 Health Care Systems in World Perspective. Ann Arbor, Michigan: Health Admin-
         istration Press.
Russek, H. I.
  1965 Stress, Tobacco, and Coronary Heart Disease in North American Professional
         Groups. Journal of the American Medical Association 192:89–94.
Sales, S. M. and J. House
  1971 Job Dissatisfaction as a Possible Risk Factor in Coronary Heart Disease. Journal
         of Chronic Diseases 23:867–873.
Scotch, N. A.
  1960 A Preliminary Report on the Relation of Sociocultural Factors to Hypertension
         Among the Zulu. Annals of the New York Academy of Sciences 84:1000–1009.
Scotch, N. A. and H. J. Geiger
  1963 The Epidemiology of Essential Hypertension. A Review with Special Attention
         to Psychologic and Sociocultural Factors. II. Psychologic and Sociocultural
         Factors in Etiology. Journal of Chronic Diseases 16:1183–1213.
Selye, H.
  1956 The Stress of Life. New York: McGraw-Hill.
Selye, H. and P. Prioreschi
  1960 Stress Theory of Aging. In Aging: Some Social and Biological Aspects. N. W.
         Shock, ed. Washington, D.C.: American Association for the Advancement of
         Science.
Smith, T.
  1967 Factors Involving Sociocultural Incongruity and Change: A Review of Empirical
         Findings. In Social Stress and Cardiovascular Disease. S. L. Syme and L. G.
         Reeder, eds. Milbank Memorial Fund Quarterly 45:23–38.

Syme, S. L., N. O. Borhani, and R. W. Buechley
    1965 Cultural Mobility and Coronary Heart Disease in an Urban Area. American
          Journal of Epidemiology 82:334–346.
Thorell, T. and R. H. Rahe
    1974 Psychosocial Characteristics of Subjects with Myocardial Infarction in Stockholm.
          In Life Stress and Illness. E. K. Gunderson and R. H. Rahe, eds. pp. 90–104.
          Springfield, Ill.: Charles C. Thomas.
Thomas, D. S.
    1925 Social Aspects of the Business Cycle. London: Routledge.
Titmuss, Richard M.
    1953 Birth, Poverty and Wealth: A Study of Infant Mortality. London: Hamish Hamil-
          ton Medical Books.
Townsend, Peter
    1974 Inequality and The Health Service. The Lancet (June 15):1179–1184.
Tyroler, H. A. and John Cassel.
    1964 Health Consequences of Culture Change – II: The Effect of Urbanization on
          Coronary Heart Mortality in Rural Residents. Journal of Chronic Diseases 17:
          167–177.
U.S. Congress, Joint Economic Committee
    1976 Estimating the Social Costs of National Economic Policy: Implications for Mental
          and Physical Health and Criminal Aggression by M. Harvey Brenner. Washington,
          D.C.: US GPO. Summarized in: Brenner, M. Harvey, Health Costs and Benefits of
          Economic Policy. International Journal of Health Services 7(4):581–623.
Wolff, H. G.
    1968 Stress and Disease, 2nd ed. Revised and edited by Stewart Wolf and Helen Goodell.
          Springfield, Ill.: Charles C. Thomas.
Wrigley, E. A.
    1969 Population and History. New York: McGraw-Hill.

LIST OF CONTRIBUTORS

Linda Alexander, Unaffiliated, 21225 East Beaver Creek, Cloverdale, Oregon

Arthur J. Barsky, Department of Psychiatry, Harvard Medical School, Massachusetts General Hospital

Marilyn Bergner, Department of Health Services, School of Public Health and Community Medicine, University of Washington

Lisa F. Berkman, Department of Epidemiology and Public Health and Institution for Social and Policy Studies, Yale University

M. Harvey Brenner, Operations Research and Behavioral Sciences, School of Hygiene and Public Health, and Department of Social Relations, The Johns Hopkins University

Leon Eisenberg, Department of Psychiatry, Harvard Medical School, and Department of Psychiatry, Children's Hospital Medical Center, Boston

Alvan R. Feinstein, Departments of Medicine and Epidemiology, Yale Medical School

Betty S. Gilson, Department of Health Services, School of Public Health and Community Medicine, University of Washington

Byron J. Good, Departments of Psychiatry and Family Practice, University of California at Davis

Mary-Jo DelVecchio Good, Departments of Psychiatry and Family Practice, University of California at Davis

Wayne Katon, Department of Psychiatry & Behavioral Sciences, University of Washington

Arthur Kleinman, Department of Psychiatry & Behavioral Sciences and Department of Anthropology, University of Washington

Gilbert Lewis, Department of Social Anthropology, Cambridge University

John B. McKinlay, Department of Sociology, Boston University

Robert G. Petersdorf, Department of Medicine, Harvard Medical School, and Affiliated Hospitals Center, Inc., Boston, Massachusetts

John-Henry Pfifferling, Center for the Well-Being of Health Professionals, Chapel Hill, North Carolina

John D. Stoeckle, Primary Care Program, Medical Service, Harvard Medical School, Massachusetts General Hospital

Andrew C. Twaddle, Department of Sociology and Department of Family and Community Medicine, University of Missouri, Columbia

Howard Waitzkin, La Clinica de la Raza, Fruitvale Health Project, Inc., Oakland, California

Nancy Waxler, Department of Psychiatry, Harvard Medical School

Irving K. Zola, Department of Sociology, Brandeis University

397

NAME INDEX

SUBJECT INDEX